EXPERIENCE WITH ABORTION

EXPERIENCE WITH ABORTION

A Case Study of North-East Scotland

EDITED BY

GORDON HOROBIN

Assistant Director, Medical Research Council
Medical Sociology Unit, Aberdeen

CAMBRIDGE
AT THE UNIVERSITY PRESS · 1973

CAMBRIDGE UNIVERSITY PRESS
Cambridge, New York, Melbourne, Madrid, Cape Town, Singapore, São Paulo, Delhi

Cambridge University Press
The Edinburgh Building, Cambridge CB2 8RU, UK

Published in the United States of America by Cambridge University Press, New York

www.cambridge.org
Information on this title: www.cambridge.org/9780521112772

First published 1973
This digitally printed version 2009

A catalogue record for this publication is available from the British Library

Library of Congress Catalogue Card Number: 73–77171

ISBN 978-0-521-20240-4 hardback
ISBN 978-0-521-11277-2 paperback

CONTENTS

LIST OF CONTRIBUTORS

Jean Aitken-Swan	Research Sociologist, Medical Research Council Medical Sociology Unit, Aberdeen
K. John Dennis	Professor of Human Reproduction and Obstetrics, University of Southampton
Vivien Edward	Psychiatric Registrar, Royal Cornhill Hospital, Aberdeen
Colin Farmer	Assistant Professor of Sociology, St Patrick's College, Carleton University, Ottawa
Gordon Horobin	Assistant Director, Medical Research Council Medical Sociology Unit, Aberdeen
Colin McCance	Clinical Senior Lecturer in Mental Health, University of Aberdeen
Ian MacGillivray	Regius Professor of Obstetrics and Gynaecology, University of Aberdeen
Peter C. Olley	Senior Lecturer in Mental Health, University of Aberdeen

FOREWORD

This study was initiated in 1966 before the advent of the Abortion Act. Recent changes in attitudes and practice had already occurred. A few years earlier, whilst abortions were being performed by some gynaecologists throughout Britain, and whilst a few centres were moving cautiously towards a selective policy of termination, discussion was guarded and information sparse. When any activity is close to illegality or to immorality, the normal scientific processes of research, communication, publication and evaluation are ruled out. Believing, moreover, in the rightness and humanity of their actions, liberal gynaecologists were often more concerned to alleviate the distress of particular patients than to indulge in public debate whose outcome may have led to the restriction of their humanitarian practice. By 1966, however, gynaecologists who had accepted termination as one necessary professional response to the needs of their patients, themselves needed guidance from wider experience about the criteria for decision-making, the appropriateness of available operative procedures, and the specific and general consequences of their decisions.

By 1966, too, the general climate of opinion had changed. The public debate, so long delayed, had begun, forced into the open by changes in sexual behaviour, marital relationships and family formation. The motives which prompted a gynaecologist to terminate a sixth pregnancy and to sterilise a woman worn out physically and emotionally by repeated childbearing and family rearing on a low and uncertain income were not transferable to a newly-emerging demand. What indications, based on strictly medical criteria, were applicable to the young, healthy, middle-class girl who, deliberately or accidentally, had adopted new sexual freedoms without adequate contraceptive knowledge? Psychiatry had already proved, in many spheres, a discipline amenable to the pressure of changing social values and customs, providing justification for the treatment of deviant behaviour rather than its punishment. But could one justify termination on psychiatric grounds for a young woman whose past history showed no signs of behavioural or personality disorder, and whose distress arose from the consequences of thoughtless and hedonistic acts or their stigmatisation by society? Yet the consequences were real enough for the patient whose welfare the physician accepted as part of his professional responsibility.

Contradictions, created by changing mores, were appearing more and more frequently between the traditional professional role of the gynaecologist in regard to abortion (the moral policeman), his professional responsibility to treat the perceived needs of his patients, and his own personal values as a citizen. In the absence of public consensus, did the doctor have the political duty of defending the institutions of marriage and the family, as opposed to the needs of his patients as he perceived them? Did he have the right to impose his personal values about moral issues on patients, or on other doctors who did not share them? Once the line of 'thou-shalt-not' was breached, fresh problems arose, partly ethical, partly scientific. If some women were given terminations by one doctor, or in one city, what were the grounds for refusing others with identical problems in another city? What, across all the range of differing cases, were adequate grounds for termination? And, perhaps more difficult to face as pressure grew, what was the justification for refusal? Did the doctor have any special professional skills in making such decisions, or was he, in this area at least, a technician? Certainly diversity of opinion across the profession and lack of a firm scientific basis for a knowledge of possible consequences threw doubt on the claim that doctors had special knowledge and skills in this area of decision-making – whether it applied to indications, procedures or consequences, its relationship to future reproductive behaviour, or the advisability of concurrent sterilisation in certain situations.

The research reported in this volume constitutes an attempt to provide the kind of information needed, both at the general policy level, and in relation to individual clinical cases. This was certainly my personal intention in initiating the planning meetings which led to the research work reported here. Not all the questions are answered, or could be answered, in this report. Changes in opinion and practice demonstrate that we are dealing with questions of political and social values, not with unchanging natural phenomena. So long as our values about sexual, marital and family behaviour respond to changing conditions, indications for and against termination will change, whether the final decision is made by doctors or by patients themselves. At any stage, and this emerges clearly from the report, individual doctors will vary in their general attitudes and in the weight they attach to particular criteria. The question as to who should make the final decision is likely to remain open so long as such variability continues. And the more emphasis we place on family planning the more likely it is that patients themselves will claim the right to decide. The delicate interchange of hints and clues in the doctor–patient encounter described in this report has already changed and will continue to change towards a more direct exchange of request and opinion.

The authors have made a brave attempt to classify the reasons for granting or refusing a termination. The complexity of the classifications they were forced to employ, using various combinations of medical, psychiatric and social criteria, itself demonstrates the large element of personal judgement involved in a decision. Equally difficult is the task of deciding whether, after the event, the decision was justified. Few patients regretted the operation; reservations related more to the procedures used, particularly in second trimester abortions, than to the decision itself and its consequences. Guilt and fear of stigma remain, but these are consequences of perceived social values and are likely to be lessened as abortion becomes more widely accepted as a necessary and justifiable act. That acceptance is growing. It emerges from the figures showing the great increase in referrals over the period covered by this study. It also emerges, quite dramatically, from the report of a WHO Working Party which in 1972 could recommend that: 'Legislation should allow the woman to decide for herself about the fate of her pregnancy, provided that her choice does not conflict with the interests of her mental and physical health' (WHO Regional Office for Europe 1972). Yet only a few years ago, WHO did not dare to discuss abortion in other than strictly medical terms.

The findings of this report must therefore be regarded as evidence arising at only one stage of a long term trend. It will need to be replicated elsewhere and up-dated as the social context itself changes. Future studies should derive some benefit from the experience recorded here. The technical procedures of termination, and their impact on the woman's feelings clearly deserve continuous attention. The advisability of either concurrent or post-partum sterilisation for some groups of women emerges as a factor of prime importance. More systematic attention should be given to the impact of abortion practice on other obstetric and gynaecological services. Longer-term consequences cannot be fully assessed on the basis of the present limited follow-up.

What happens in later years, and in later pregnancies, to women and their families, when a termination has been refused? Above all, perhaps, the study indicates the need for further and more effective sex education and for the diffusion of family planning services so that birth control becomes an integral part of sexual life, inside and outside marriage.

Director   RAYMOND ILLSLEY
MRC Medical Sociology Unit
Aberdeen

EDITORIAL PREFACE

Gordon Horobin

The role of an editor of a volume such as this is inevitably ill-defined and it is only fair to the contributors and the readers to describe how that role has been defined and taken in this instance. Although I was associated with and involved in the research from the outset, I have not participated in the collection of data. My involvement was at first administrative and to some extent advisory, but latterly became more that of co-ordinator, and, occasionally and reluctantly, arbitrator. When the contributors decided to publish their early findings, in the form of a collection of short papers, I took on the task of subediting the manuscripts and communicating with the editor of the journal.† When, therefore, more extended publication was being considered, a similar task was given to me. Decisions about the form as well as the content of the monograph, however, were made by the group as a whole and are in no sense an editorial imposition. Each chapter, therefore, represents the work of the individual contributor (or in some cases that of two or three contributors), and has only been subjected to fairly minor subediting. Needless to say, I have suggested alternative forms of wording and in some cases more drastic revision, but each author accepts responsibility for the data, analysis and conclusions contained in his or her contribution.

Such a form of presentation has both its advantages and disadvantages. On the positive side it allows each author a greater freedom than would have been possible had every contributor to agree with everything written in the book. By the same token, however, the reader must not expect to find complete consistency across the work as a whole. Occasionally, indeed, there are statements which may appear contradictory but, as I shall try to show in a concluding section, these arise out of the data – the perceptions and accounts offered by the subjects –

† Gordon Horobin (ed.), 'Therapeutic abortion in North-East Scotland', *J. biosoc. Sci.*, **3**, 1971, 87–131.

and from the differing perspectives of the researchers rather than from invalid and unreliable research methods.

Inevitably the work reported in this book is shaped partly by decisions taken several years ago and, with the advantage of hindsight, no doubt many things would have been done differently. Nevertheless I believe that the work as a whole represents a valuable contribution to our inadequate knowledge of this ill-documented field of abortion policy and practice. I further believe that the authors have written about an emotionally explosive subject as objectively and dispassionately as is humanly possible. At the same time, the reader will no doubt be aware that all of the authors, myself included, hold in varying degrees 'liberal' opinions on abortion. If a study with similar research objectives were to be carried out by a group of anti-abortion gynaecologists, psychiatrists and social scientists, its subjects would be different as would the emphasis and hence the findings. Such a comparative study has yet to be carried out.

It seems likely that different sections of the book will appeal to different audiences and this is an additional reason for my not attempting to impose a spurious homogeneity upon it. Nevertheless I am aware, as are the authors, that steering a course between 'talking down' to the non-specialist and providing inadequate information to the specialist is a difficult task and one which may not always have been successfully achieved.

I should conclude by expressing my appreciation of the effort and good humour with which the contributors responded to my 'chivvying'. I owe a special debt of gratitude to Jean Aitken-Swan for the additional help she gave me throughout the study, and especially during the feverish period of editing and re-editing the several manuscripts. The Director of the Medical Sociology Unit, Professor Raymond Illsley, was also, of course, involved with the research from the outset, taking a major role in setting up the study, its design and its realisation. I very much regret that for a variety of reasons, including the very heavy demands upon his time, his influence on the work in general and my own perspective in particular remains implicit rather than receiving overt expression in his own contribution. His help, trust and support are gratefully acknowledged however and I am especially pleased that he has agreed to write a foreword to the book. Finally, my thanks are also due to Miss Anne Forbes who typed many more thousands of words than appear in this volume.

ACKNOWLEDGEMENTS

Research of the kind reported in this book cannot be carried out without the support, co-operation and help of a large number of people and organisations. We have been especially fortunate in this respect and we hope that all those who helped in so many ways will share what is of worth in this book. We ourselves, of course, accept unshared the responsibility for its shortcomings.

Several organisations provided funds and other support for this project and we are grateful to the Scottish Home and Health Department, Nuffield Provincial Hospitals Trust, Nuffield Foundation, Canada Council, University of Aberdeen and the Medical Research Council.

We wish to thank the nursing, social work, administrative, secretarial and clinical staffs of Aberdeen Maternity Hospital, Aberdeen Royal Infirmary, Ross Clinic and Aberdeen University Medical School. Particular thanks are due to the general practitioners and the student health services of the University and College of Education who, as well as facilitating the research in so many ways also agreed to be interviewed about their referral policies and practices. We owe too a special debt of gratitude to those consultant gynaecologists and psychiatrists who so readily allowed their routines to be disrupted and their practices to be examined. The help and advice we received from our colleagues in the University Departments of Obstetrics and Gynaecology, Mental Health, General Practice and Sociology and the Medical Research Council's Medical Sociology Unit are also gratefully acknowledged.

To single out particular people for special mention is in many ways invidious, yet there are some whom we cannot in justice omit. Thus we would like to thank Sir Dugald Baird, Professor Raymond Illsley and Professor Malcolm Millar whose help and encouragement, particularly in the early stages of the work, were invaluable; Staff Nurse Petrie, of the Gynaecological outpatient department, who so conscientiously maintained our notification and 'tracking' system, Mrs Gillian Grant who co-ordinated the long-term psychiatric follow-up study, kept the

ACKNOWLEDGEMENTS

notes and contacted the patients, and Mrs Margaret Johnston, confidential clerk at the Medical Sociology Unit, who also carried out many invaluable tracing and administrative tasks. The data processing and tabulation of the psychiatric sections would not have been possible without the facilities of the Mental Health Research Unit and thanks are due to Professor Millar for making these so freely available. We are grateful too to the technical, clerical and secretarial staffs of that Unit, the Department of Gynaecology and Obstetrics and the Medical Sociology Unit for all their efforts in carrying out the difficult and often tedious tasks we gave them.

Finally and above all we should thank the main subjects of our research – the women who, during what was for many of them a most painful and stressful period of their lives, willingly co-operated in the questioning and testing so essential to the research.

INTRODUCTION

Ian MacGillivray and Gordon Horobin

There are relatively few places in Britain, and perhaps in the world, where the information of the kind given in this book can be adequately documented. There are still fewer where an 'abortion policy' was in existence before the change in the law, making possible an epidemiological study of changes in abortion rates over nearly a decade. It was for these reasons, among others, that the research described here was undertaken in Aberdeen. The decision to make the study was taken before the passing of the 1967 Act at a time when debate about the propriety and efficacy of abortion was in full swing. It was felt that there were many opinions but little systematic evidence about, for example, the effects of terminating pregnancies on the health, both physical and mental, of the women and on their families and social circumstances. At one end of the spectrum of opinion were some of the gynaecologists in Aberdeen (and, of course, elsewhere) who felt that abortion, however undesirable or distasteful it might be, was in certain cases the only solution to the problem of unwanted pregnancy and that, given adequate selection of cases, the results were beneficial. At the other extreme were those like Professor Jeffcoate who argued that the psychological consequences of abortion are such that 'a significant proportion of women – sometimes rated at twenty to thirty per cent in the past – are adversely affected emotionally throughout their life'.[1] Jeffcoate also argued that 'significant illness' follows in up to 15 per cent of cases, that one or two per cent are rendered sterile and that abortion carries a mortality rate of at least 0.3 per 1000.[2, 3]

The fact of the matter is that all estimates of post-abortion morbidity are meaningless unless the characteristics of the at-risk population are known, the methods of assessment stated and the evidence related to the 'abortion policy' of the hospital concerned. Thus, for example, where terminations are carried out only in cases of high physical and/or psychological risk, higher rates (though smaller numbers) of post-abortion morbidity are likely to be reported than where terminations are performed on less stringent grounds. Put more generally, social factors create or at least influence the familial and clinical problem and thus the health and physique of the patients. Therefore the outcome is heavily dependent on the selection of patients, both self-selection (the section of the population requesting abortions) and selection by general practitioners and consultants (the proportion referred and accepted or refused). The subsequent health of a group of aborted women may therefore reflect these processes of social selection much more than the effects of the operation itself. Meaningful research aimed at answering questions about the effects of abortion must then first describe adequately the population at risk, the presenting population, the decision-making procedures and, of course, the mode of assessment. This is what the authors of the present volume have tried to do.

At first sight Aberdeen may not seem the ideal city in which to study the epidemiology of abortion, especially if it is hoped to compare the results with experience elsewhere. Geographically remote, its characteristics and community little known outside Scotland, the city might seem too different from urban centres further south for its experience to have more than a local applicability. However in several ways which will be described later it is particularly suitable for such a study.

Aberdeen, situated at the north-east corner of Scotland, is now the fourth largest city of Scotland and the third largest fishing port in Great Britain. Its population, which reached a maximum of 186,000 in 1963, has been declining, due partly to emigration to England and overseas and partly to movement out to the suburbs. Fishing is Aberdeen's most important industry, employing about 10,000 people in the industry and its ancillary trades. The fishing community lives in certain parts of the city and still maintains some of its traditional way of life. The city also engages in ship-building and engineering, textiles, granite-working, wood-working and the manufacture of paper and paper goods. In addition Aberdeen is a centre for the county, an important predominantly agricultural region containing a fifth of all the arable land in Scotland and renowned for its production of beef cattle. The city provides administrative and commercial services for a wide area of north-east Scotland and is an important educational and medical centre. It is known for its progressive thinking and achievements in the planning of its health services. On most counts Aberdeen is the healthiest of the Scottish cities and it is characteristic of Aberdeen that its teaching hospital is situated on the largest hospital site in Europe.

Besides its fishing and trading activities, Aberdeen is a centre of learning. It has two ancient colleges combined in 1860 into one university with, at the present time, some 6000 students, as well as several other colleges and training schools. Aberdeen is a handsome city with its many buildings of dressed granite, the gateway to a countryside of great natural beauty and a centre for tourists and conferences.

At the same time Scotland as a whole is less prosperous than England and the standard of living, measured in terms of the proportion of families living without the exclusive use of such amenities as water closets, baths and hot and cold water, is lower. Housing is scarce and overcrowding is only very gradually being reduced. A higher proportion of Aberdeen's adult males are unskilled workers than in other Scottish cities or in Scotland as a whole. In common with the rest of Scotland Aberdeen suffers a high rate of unemployment. It remains to be seen what effect the vast oil finds in the North Sea will have on Aberdeen's economy. With 150 oil and oil ancillary companies operating out of the city at the present time it seems unlikely that its economic and social life can remain unaffected, but this development was in the future at the time this study was made.

Studies of abortion have usually been concerned with selected groups of patients often from more cosmopolitan urban areas. This study describes the total abortion experience of a typical Scottish city, predominantly Presbyterian, with a relatively homogeneous and static population where pregnancies have been terminated for many years within the national health service. That doctors were able to do so was a result of differences in the legality of the operation in England and Wales on the one hand and Scotland on the other which must now be mentioned.

LEGAL AND HISTORICAL BACKGROUND

The basic difference lay in the emphasis on statute and case law in England and in contrast to the pre-eminence of common law in Scotland. In England the Attorney General must institute criminal proceedings if there is a prima facie case that a statutory crime has been committed. In Scotland, however, the Lord Advocate (Crown Office) will first have the case investigated by the Procurators Fiscal and only subsequently might or might not take criminal proceedings.

Prior to 1967, then, a doctor who had carried out an abortion on a woman in Scotland could not be charged with any crime, unless a definite complaint was made. Even then the matter would have been investigated by doctors of the Crown Office's choice, and if they were satisfied that the operation had been carried out in good faith and in a proper manner the case would then be closed. Such investigations and decisions would take place in private and the press and public would know nothing of them. In England all such matters were brought before either a magistrate's Court to decide whether there was a prima facie case, or a coroner's court in the case of death from the operation. The famous Bourne case of 1938 in which a well-known London gynaecologist carried out an abortion and then as a test case invited the police to charge him with the crime of procuring an abortion could not have occurred in Scotland. A doctor would either be found guilty of criminal action or nothing whatever would be heard of the matter since all investigations of a 'good faith' case would be held in private. It would have been exceedingly difficult to bring a successful conviction against a doctor in Scotland under the circumstances of the Bourne case for the following reasons: (a) independent proof that the woman had indeed been pregnant would have had to have been obtained – this was not so in England; (b) criminal intent would have to be established; (c) neither the police nor the Procurator Fiscal would initiate any proceedings if the matter came to their notice unless the woman died and an inquiry was instituted into the circumstances; (d) if good faith could be shown then no conviction would be possible. Good faith rests upon such criteria as consultation with other colleagues – a general practitioner, a gynaecologist or a psychiatrist; admission to hospital or a recognised nursing home; observation of the usual ethical procedures such as the consultant being called in by the general practitioner, and reasonable fees being charged where the patient was not being treated under the national health service; and the keeping of proper records.

Until 1967 the law on abortion in England and Wales was based on the Offences against the Person Act of 1861, which made it a felony carrying a maximum sentence of penal servitude for life unlawfully to procure an abortion. Test cases, particularly the Bourne case, caused a gradual change in the law through interpretation by the courts, but the law still remained hostile to the idea of abortion. Justice Macnaghten's judgement in that famous case, however, did a great deal to soften the harshness of the law, and, as Simms and Hindell point out, 'for all lawyers' purposes Macnaghten's opinion was the law of abortion until the Abortion Act, 1967'.[4] That it was not more widely used was probably due more to the traditional attitude that abortion was morally wrong than to fear of prosecution or to any expectation that the statutory penalty might be imposed.

Under the common law of Scotland it had long been possible for a doctor acting in good faith to perform therapeutic abortion where after a careful study of all the circumstances of the case, and after due consultation with colleagues he decided that the disadvantages of allowing the pregnancy to continue were greater than those of termination. There was freedom to practice medicine in this sphere as in all others according to clinical judgement. In some parts of Scotland, particularly in the north-east, gynaecologists had for many years been terminating pregnancies in good faith, and without fear of prosecution. In other areas of Scotland, however, the legal right to terminate pregnancies was not used by gynaecologists nor were the differences between English and Scottish law in this regard made clear to medical students. As a result graduates, with few exceptions, believed that procuring an abortion was always a crime unless the woman's life was in imminent danger.

While the Abortion Act 1967 which changed the law from case law to statute law transformed the situation in England and Wales, it made little difference to the freedom already existing in Scotland apart from the requirement to notify all terminations of pregnancy to the Chief Medical Officer of the Scottish Home and Health Department and to register nursing homes carrying out such operations. Abortion is now legal in England, Wales and in Scotland in the circumstances described in the following extract from the Abortion Act 1967:

1 (1) Subject to the provisions of this section, a person shall not be guilty of an offence under the law relating to abortion when a pregnancy is terminated by a registered medical practitioner if two registered medical practitioners are of the opinion, formed in good faith –
- (a) that the continuance of the pregnancy would involve risk to the life of the pregnant woman, or of injury to the physical or mental health of the pregnant woman or any existing children of her family, greater than if the pregnancy was terminated; or
- (b) that there is a substantial risk that if the child were born it would suffer from such physical or mental abnormalities as to be seriously handicapped.

(2) In determining whether the continuance of a pregnancy would involve such risk of injury to health as is mentioned in paragraph (*a*) of subsection (1) of this section account may be taken of the pregnant woman's actual or reasonably foreseeable environment.

The effect of the Act on abortion 'policy' in the north-east region of Scotland has been rather limited. The grounds for termination allowed in the Act are substantially similar to those indications previously considered acceptable by the gynaecologists in this area. Prior to and at the time of the Act, Aberdeen and the north-east were considered to have a very 'liberal' attitude towards abortion and to have a high abortion rate. While it is true that doctors' attitudes to abortion were in general more liberal than in many other parts of the country this applied almost exclusively to termination of pregnancies in married women. In Sir Dugald Baird's 'A Fifth Freedom?' the emphasis was on the liberation of women from the burden of frequent childbearing and his policy was to terminate the unwanted pregnancies of women of high parity and to offer them sterilisation.[5] Termination of illegitimate pregnancies, particularly in unmarried women, was rare prior to 1965. The pregnancies being terminated were therefore mostly in lower social class women and were virtually all done in the public wards of the hospitals under the National Health Service.†

Sir Dugald Baird was also a strong protagonist of abortion law reform and this helped to create the impression that large numbers of abortions were carried out in Aberdeen; indeed there were many who thought the situation was one of 'abortion on demand'. This was and still is far from the truth; abortion on demand was much more likely to have been practised in 'Harley Street type' practices before the Act than in Aberdeen.

THE RESEARCH AND ITS SETTING

In the winter of 1966–7 discussions were held between members of the university departments of Mental Health, Obstetrics and Gynaecology, and the Medical Sociology Unit of the Medical Research Council with the object of setting up a collaborative study of abortion in Aberdeen. Each department had its own special interests in the topic, its own

---

† It is noteworthy that in Scotland only 1.4 per cent of abortions are performed in 'approved places', although some abortion patients are admitted to private beds in national health service hospitals.

perspectives and, of course, its own methodology. The study, then, became an inter-departmental one rather than a combined one, or, perhaps more accurately, a series of separate, but related, studies. These different emphases and interests are reflected in the form and content of this book, each researcher reporting on his or her topic, method and results. It is therefore appropriate to deal with them only briefly in this introduction.

The study as a whole had both a retrospective and a prospective component. Because of the completeness of the record system in Aberdeen hospitals, information in considerable detail was available on all women considered by consultants for termination of pregnancy under the National Health Service. Thus it was possible retrospectively to examine the characteristics of the women considered for abortions, compare them with the total at-risk population, and further to compare those who had abortions with those who were refused. Detailed information was available from 1963 onwards, although some data could have been obtained for the decade before that. This part of the study was undertaken by Jean Aitken-Swan, a member of the MRC Medical Sociology Unit.

Valuable as such retrospective data are, however, most of the questions which interested all the investigators could only be answered by prospective study. Among such questions were: what were the circumstances surrounding the unwanted pregnancy? what influenced the woman's decision to seek abortion as a solution to her problem? what factors in the patient and her circumstances as well as in the organisation of medical practice influenced the decision to terminate the pregnancy or to allow it to continue? what were the woman's social, psychological and physical characteristics before and after the decision was taken?

To gather data relevant to these questions, it was decided to set up an administrative procedure to ensure that each woman referred to a specialist for consideration of termination would be interviewed by one of two sociologists and by a psychologist before she saw the consultant, and hence before the decision was made. This was important because if the decision had been given the patient would be unlikely to present her story again in the same way, and if not recommended for abortion might understandably feel less inclined to co-operate in the research. In the majority of cases, referral was directly from a general practitioner to the gynaecology outpatient department of Aberdeen Royal Infirmary and in these cases there was little or no administrative problem. A minority, however, were referred to a psychiatrist in another hospital, or occasionally from a medical or surgical department of the hospital to the gynaecologist or psychiatrist. It was, therefore, extremely important to ensure that every woman so referred was 'picked up', even though occasionally this meant that she had to be seen by both sociologist and psychologist after the decision had been made.

At these interviews, the client was asked about events leading up to the pregnancy, her social and economic circumstances, her reasons for requesting termination, her sources of advice and knowledge and so on. The psychologist administered a battery of standardised psychological tests in order to evaluate her mental state at referral and her more enduring personality traits.

Two sociologists shared the interviewing, one of them (Farmer) using the interview partly to gain knowledge of the patient so as to be able subsequently to discuss the decision with both consultant and general practitioner. His part of the study then was to elucidate the professional decision-making process while the research role of the other sociologist (Aitken-Swan) was more directly concerned with what might be called the 'client's perspective'.

Pilot work on the construction and testing of interview schedules, smoothing out administrative problems and gaining knowledge of the clinicians and their procedures began in the late summer of 1967 and continued until August 1968.

To the sociologists but not to the psychiatrists this group comprised a pilot study. When the time came for follow-up it would have been undesirable from the woman's point of view for her to be seen by both the sociologist and psychiatrist and it was arranged that the psychiatrists alone should follow up this group. The sociological study proper began in September 1968 and comprised all the women referred over a nine-month period, none of whom was psychologically tested. These women underwent a sociological and gynaecological follow-up only, usually at the same attendance. A comparison of the social characteristics of the two series showed no significant variations so that each can be considered a representative sample of the total series referred about abortion between September 1967 and June 1969. More detailed methodological and technical issues are discussed in the separate sections so that it is only necessary here to mention a few further points of general concern.

Ideally any study aimed at measuring the effects of clinical intervention, in this case termination of pregnancy, should attempt to randomise cases in the 'operation done' and 'operation not done' categories. The ethical problems involved in the clinical trial method, however, are always difficult and in this instance were deemed quite overwhelming. Where a new drug is in question the problems are relatively slight, but in this case not only was the clinical procedure well established, but there was inevitably strong pressure from patients, their families and often general practitioners for the operation to be performed. In any case it was felt that the clinical trial method would be inappropriate even if it could be justified ethically, since there is no single clinical entity for which drug A might or might not show better results than drug B, or no drug at all. Each 'abortion case' is a unique combination of physical, psychological and social forces rendering simple comparisons impossible.

Thus it was decided to try, where possible, to maintain the preexisting selection procedures throughout the research, with one exception. At the outset of the research one or two of the gynaecologists were seeing a disproportionately large number of cases. Some more equitable distribution of abortion requests would in any case have to be made at some stage so it was decided, with the agreement of general practitioners, to suspend the normal system of referring to specific consultants and instead to have all referrals to the outpatient department allocated randomly to consultants. This procedure was maintained throughout the research although a few direct referrals of a 'semiprivate' nature did occur and, of course, private patients were treated on a personal basis as before.

A major concern of a study of abortion in a comparatively small city such as Aberdeen is the confidential nature of the material collected and the need to safeguard the identity of the subjects. Considerable thought was given to this in the initial planning and a method of notification of referrals was devised making use of one individual at the receiving end (the staff nurse in charge of the gynaecological clinic who routinely received the general practitioners' referral letters), and one confidential clerk at the interviewer's end. Every patient was given a survey number and only the number appeared on the research cards for the whole of the epidemiological study, so that they could be dealt with by clerical workers without fear of identification. The same numbers were used on the interviewing schedules and for linking the sociological and psychiatric sections of the study.

There are, of course, other ethical considerations in a research project of this type, concerned as it is with the intricate and intimate relationships between general practitioners, consultants and patients. Once again the research procedures adopted represented a compromise between the need to obtain data from both doctors and patients and the wish to protect the woman from unnecessary stress and invasion of her privacy. For women referred in the period 1967–8, the demands were quite heavy – an hour-long interview immediately followed by a further hour of psychological tests a day or two before their appointment to see the consultant.

The necessity to interview the clients before they were seen by the gynaecologist raised another problem. Inevitably many women interpreted the interview as part of the decision-making procedure despite being told that it was 'for research purposes'. Indeed in one respect these clients were correct in their assumption for, in order to reduce demands on patients as well as their own work load, consultants were given a brief statement of the 'factual' situation (e.g. age, marital status, occupation, housing, economic circumstances, etc.) by the research interviewer. Thus, not only might the woman's account of her problem and reasons for requesting abortion have been coloured by her perception of the interviewer's role, but the interviewer too had to be extremely careful in wording the report not to influence, however inadvertently, the gynaecologist's decision. This point is referred to in Chapter 3, p. 96.

We may conclude this brief introduction by mentioning some of the more essential characteristics of the setting of this research. As mentioned earlier there are few places in Britain where a research project of this kind could have been carried out. By the same token, of course, Aberdeen is in some respects unique and generalisation of the research findings to other situations would be dangerous. Among these unique features are the high degree of integration of obstetric, gynaecological and family planning services. Although the Aberdeen Family Planning Clinic is run by the local health authority and not by the hospital board, close liaison is maintained partly through referrals, and partly through the personal contacts of the hospital and clinic staffs. The study refers entirely to women applying through the 'public sector'. All national health service patients, as well as the few private patients, are seen by the small number of gynaecologists, and sometimes psychiatrists, all of whom co-operated in the study. As a consequence of the small numbers of consultants the research was made immeasurably easier to accomplish but at the same time variations in acceptance and refusal rates occur within narrower limits than would be the case in large metropolitan areas. It is perhaps somewhat surprising therefore that there is nevertheless a good deal of variation and there is certainly no agreed policy or set of agreed criteria. This point is documented more fully in a later section, so that here it is important only to note that consultant services are sufficiently integrated to allow total co-operation in the research, but not so fully integrated as to remove individuality of ideology and practice.

Much the same can be said of the general practitioner services. With over a hundred GPs referring patients, there is clearly more variability in practice than among consultants, but all were sufficiently a part of a 'medical community' as to co-operate fully in the research enterprise. Without their agreement to allow their normal referral procedures to be interrupted by the research routines, for example, the research would have been extremely difficult if not impossible to carry out.

To what extent does this uniqueness limit the usefulness and interest of the study? In one sense, of course, all case studies are specific to their own place and time, and extension of findings to other situations becomes hazardous. At the same time, we would argue, what is happening in regard to, for example, trends in abortion requests, in acceptance or refusal rates or the decision criteria used by consultants, can only be explained when seen against the interplay of institutional and demographic forces in a specific context. Uniqueness, then, is one side of the coin; concreteness is the other. The authors of this book hope that their reports will be interpreted and judged in this light.

REFERENCES

1 T. N. A. Jeffcoate, 'Abortion', in *Morals and Medicine*, BBC, London, 1970, p. 32.
2 Ibid.
3 A full and interesting discussion of the debate leading up to the Act of 1967 is contained in: Sally MacIntyre, 'The medical profession and the 1967 Abortion Act in Britain', *Social Science and Medicine*, 1973, **7**, 121–34.
4 M. Simms and K. Hindell, *Abortion Law Reformed*, Peter Owen, London, 1971, p. 14.
5 Sir Dugald Baird, 'A Fifth Freedom?', *Brit. med. J.*, 1965, **2**, 1141–8.

1 EPIDEMIOLOGICAL BACKGROUND

Jean Aitken-Swan

In several ways Aberdeen is particularly suitable for an epidemiological study of abortion. To begin with, legal abortions have been performed there for a longer time and in proportionately greater numbers than was possible in England and Wales before the Abortion Act of 1967. The differences in Scottish and English law prior to 1967 have already been mentioned. At a time when most doctors, although they were often faced with illness and debility in women of high parity, did not see it as part of their responsibility to help them to limit the size of their families, Sir Dugald Baird was prepared to perform post-partum sterilisation 'frequently', as he says, and therapeutic abortion 'in certain cases'.[1] As long ago as 1938–47, 233 women in north-east Scotland had their pregnancies terminated in Aberdeen and were sterilised, mostly on the grounds of multiparity and debility. Aberdeen has therefore an impressive experience of therapeutic abortion over a period of more than thirty years.

In the second place, probably more is known in Aberdeen than in any other British centre about the totality of women resident in its area applying for abortion. Certain aspects of the population and of the organisation of medical services facilitate epidemiological studies in Aberdeen; a comparatively stable and homogeneous population, patients mostly known to their family doctors, a medical professional world small enough for its members to interact on a personal level, a centralised system of medical care and a comprehensive maternity records system built up over a period of more than twenty years. All gynaecologists in Aberdeen are on the staff of the hospitals.

The count of patients seeking abortion in Aberdeen through the national health service is remarkably complete. There is no 'advisory service' to which women can go if they are not recommended abortion by the hospital consultant, unless they go outside the area. During the period of the study there were no private nursing homes for abortion patients,† although women could be admitted to the hospital's private wards. Before 1968 private abortions formed a negligible proportion of the whole but this is no longer true since the Act. Numbers of private abortions have been increasing and in 1970 probably between 12 and 15 per cent of abortions in Aberdeen were done privately. It is true that the number of women normally resident in Scotland who go south to have their pregnancy terminated has increased since the Act. Of all abortions notified in England and Wales, the numbers of women said to have a home address in Scotland are reported to be 65 in 1968, 173 in 1969 and 309 in 1970.‡ However, most probably the majority of these came from parts of Scotland where the policy regarding abortion is less liberal than in Aberdeen. General practitioners in Aberdeen know that their patients will have a sympathetic hearing at the hospitals so that they would be unlikely to refer them elsewhere, at any rate in the first instance. Some Aberdonians may go to London or elsewhere for reasons of anonymity but this is likely to be a small minority. Others may go because they know (or think) that their doctors would be unwilling to refer them about an abortion, and it is known that a very small proportion obtained an abortion elsewhere when they were unsuccessful in having it done in Aberdeen. These last, however, are included in the number of referrals, and the total omissions are unlikely to amount to more than a small fraction of the whole.

The range of data available is unique to Aberdeen. Abortions can be related to nearly all the pregnancies of Aberdeen women in the same age, parity and socio-economic groups as well as to the population of all women of reproductive age over three periods of time. The first two years (1963–4) cover a period before abortion became a major public issue. During the next three years, which culminated in the Abortion Act (1965–7), the subject was being widely debated and reported. The third phase of nearly four years (April 1968–71) deals with the situation obtaining under the new legislation. At the time of writing rates of abortion in other areas can be shown for the period 1968–70 only.

Although Aberdeen hospitals admit patients from the whole of the north-east region, the study is confined to women resident in the city, including students and temporary workers but excluding visitors.

† One nursing home has been approved for abortions under the Act since the study ended.
‡ Figures kindly supplied by the Chief Medical Officer, Department of Health and Social Security.

The first part of this chapter presents rates of abortion in Aberdeen between 1963 and 1971 and the second part describes some socio-demographic characteristics of the women referred.

ANNUAL RATES OF ABORTION

Between 1963 and 1971 the total number of known pregnancies to Aberdeen women, married or single, fell by 8 per cent. There were fewer legitimate live-births and spontaneous abortions, and stillbirths also showed a slight fall. A small but increasing proportion of legitimate pregnancies was terminated but by 1971 these still only represented 6 per cent of the total. Illegitimate pregnancies showed a different pattern. Their numbers for 1963 had increased nearly 2½ times by 1971. In 1963 illegitimate pregnancies comprised 6 per cent and in 1971 16 per cent of all known pregnancies. Numbers both of illegitimate live-births and therapeutic abortions increased together until 1968 but in 1969–70 it seemed as if the sharp rise in therapeutic abortions might have halted the upward trend of illegitimate births (Table 1:1). In 1971, however, the number of illegitimate pregnancies terminated was only 11 more than in 1970 while illegitimate live-births increased by 40, a larger increase than in any of the previous years. This is likely to be related to another unusual finding for 1971 – a fall for the first time in the proportion of women with illegitimate pregnancies referred for consideration of abortion (Table 1:6). Whether this is due to a change in attitude of the general practitioners or to a greater willingness on the part of the women themselves to continue an illegitimate pregnancy we cannot say, nor do we know yet if this is the beginning of a new trend. Which age and occupational groups have been affected is shown later. At any rate there is no sign of any slowing down in the steadily increasing number of illegitimate pregnancies although their outcome shows different trends over the nine years. Table 1:1 shows the extent to which abortion in Aberdeen has become associated with the problem of illegitimate pregnancy.

Of every 1000 women, married or single, in the age group at risk the numbers who had a therapeutic abortion rose from fewer than 2 in 1963 to 10 in 1971 (Table 1:2), but the increase is seen most clearly in the relationship of abortions to live-births. In 1963 in Aberdeen 21 pregnancies were terminated for every 1000 live-births compared with 146 in 1971.

It is not known how these rates would compare with those in a city of similar size and type because data are not available for other cities. Differences are to be expected if numbers of abortions in a relatively small homogeneous population are compared with numbers in a larger more diversified population. In England and Wales rates in urban areas are invariably higher than in rural areas; for one thing abortion is more readily accessible to women living in cities than it is to country women. Social and demographic differences between populations affect rates; one population may contain a higher proportion of the especially 'at risk' groups than another. Differences in medical attitudes and practice account for part for the variation in different regions and the smaller the region studied the more effect such differences are likely to have on rates. However, to put Aberdeen experience into some kind of perspective rates for 1969 and 1970 are shown for several areas, the hospital regions of Scotland, Scotland as a whole and England and Wales, in Table 1:3.

The comparatively low rates for Scotland as a whole reflect the fact that a considerable part of the population lives in the urban west where the Catholic proportion of the population is high and medical practice in regard to abortion conservative. Although in the western region the ratio of abortions to live-births has risen from 27 per 1000 in 1969 to 44 in 1970 it is still lower than in any other Scottish (or, for that matter, English) region. It will be noted that the north-east with Aberdeen as its centre, which had the highest ratio in 1969 with 66 abortions per 1000 live-births, has fallen to fourth place in 1970, ratios being higher in the north, the east and south-east regions. The ratio for Aberdeen city appears high but might not be so in comparison with some other cities, for practice in Aberdeen is less liberal than its reputation would suggest, as will be seen later.

The effect on abortion rates of the increasing number of illegitimate pregnancies is seen in Table 1:4. The small number of widowed and divorced women produce the highest rates each year, followed by single women. Rates for married women are the lowest and increase the most slowly over the years.

When multiparous married women ceased to be the main candidates for abortion the age of women having abortions began to fall. Since 1965 the highest rates are in the age group 20–24, about half this population being unmarried. The number of girls under age 20 having an abortion, fewer than 1 in 1000 in 1963–4, has increased to 18 in

1000 in 1971, still a very small proportion of the teenage population (Table 1:5).

So far abortions in Aberdeen have been shown in relation to all births and population. The increasing rate is seen to be associated with the growing number of illegitimate pregnancies, although at the same time there has been a small increase in rates for married women. Overall, rates were rising before the Abortion Act became law, but the rise was more rapid from 1967 on. This does not necessarily reflect a more liberal policy on the part of Aberdeen gynaecologists towards the termination of pregnancy, but rather an increase in referrals made to them by family doctors and student health services. In the section that follows the number of abortions performed is related to the number of referrals and some socio-demographic characteristics of the women seeking abortion are described.

REFERRALS AND ABORTIONS

How many women unintentionally pregnant want to have their pregnancy terminated is not known as some may get no further than discussing the possibility with their family or with the family doctor. All who took the next step and who were referred for either gynaecological or psychiatric consultation through national health service channels are included in the study, whatever the outcome. It has already been said that it is unlikely that many Aberdeen women seeking abortion go to consultants outside this area and the number of private patients is still relatively small.

Those who are not referred and who do not come into the study may have a weaker case for abortion or may be less persuasive in presenting it than those who reach the gynaecological or psychiatric clinic, or they may change their minds on talking it over with their doctor. Prior to the publicity surrounding the Abortion Act and the pressures from patients that this may have produced, general practitioners appear to have been more selective about whom they referred and a high proportion were accepted for abortion. It has become increasingly usual to allow a patient a second opinion so that selection now takes place at the gynaecological clinic and the number of abortions in relation to the numbers referred has fallen. Table 1:6 shows the percentage of all known legitimately and illegitimately pregnant women who were referred to a gynaecologist or psychiatrist for consideration of termination of pregnancy during the years 1963–71.

The proportion of married women referred remained at under 3 per cent until 1967 when there was a slight and continuing rise, flattening out in 1971. Referrals of women with an illegitimate pregnancy rose steadily from 1963 to a peak in 1970 when two-thirds of all women illegitimately pregnant were being referred about abortion. In 1971 the proportion fell for the first time.

In the analyses that follow single women are kept as a separate category. Married, widowed and divorced women are combined under the heading 'ever-married'.

REFERRALS AND ABORTIONS: EVER-MARRIED WOMEN

The numbers of ever-married women who had a pregnancy between 1963 and 1971 are shown by age group, parity (live-births and still-births) and husband's socio-economic group in Table 1:7 (a), (b) and (c). Spontaneous abortions are omitted as the details are not available but even with this omission rates are based on some 90 per cent of all known pregnancies.

Over the years referrals have increased in all three age groups, under 25, 25–34 and 35 and over, the proportion referred increasing with age. The only marked change in the upward trend is the fall in the high proportion of referrals in those aged 35 and over from 44 per cent in 1970 to 38 per cent in 1971. Women who had had 2 births or fewer had the least chance of being considered for abortion although their referrals increased from 1.5 to 7 per cent over the years. Women with 3 or 4, or 5 or more, previous births were the most often referred, the proportion reaching a peak in 1970 when 42 per cent and 51 per cent respectively were referred. The ever-married women most likely to be considered for abortion therefore are still older women of high parity, the group for whom abortions have been performed in Aberdeen for many years.

The 'total' line shows little change in referral rates of ever-married women to 1966 and until then there was little difference between rates in the various socio-economic groups. The increase in referrals that took place after 1966 affected each of the groups favouring, if any one, the wives of semi-skilled and unskilled workers. (The reverse is true of unmarried women as will be seen later; in their case women in semi-skilled and unskilled occupations were least likely to be referred.)

Even if private patients are included in Table 1:7(c) the advantage in number of referrals of this group is not lost. (It is assumed that private patients come into the professional and managerial category although of course this is not always the case.) In 1970, the last year for which the calculation was made, and the year in which up to then the small proportion of private patients was at its highest, their inclusion would only increase the referral rate of women in the professional and managerial group from 9.0 to 11.8 per cent compared with 13 per cent of women in the semi-skilled group and 19 per cent in the unskilled group referred.

These results indicate the selective bias of general practitioners as well as the self-selection of patients while Table 1:8, showing abortions performed as a percentage of referrals, indicates the selective bias of consultants. Abortions as well as referrals vary according to age and parity, the proportion accepted for abortion being highest in older rather than younger women and in those who had had 5 or more previous births. If social class is cross-tabulated with parity the non-manual group has a slight advantage where previous births number 2 or less but with 3 or more births the proportion of abortions in each broad socio-economic category is almost the same.

The relation between numbers of referrals and terminations is illustrated in Fig. 1:1(a).

The most striking of the tables showing abortion rates in ever-married women is Table 1:9 in which abortions are shown as a percentage of all pregnancies to women in the various age, parity and socio-economic groups over the nine-year period. The proportion of terminations has risen slowly from 2 per cent in 1963–4 to 8 per cent in 1971, a rise which has affected each group. Since 1967 the trend has been for a higher proportion of wives of semi-skilled and unskilled men to have their pregnancies terminated than wives of skilled men or non-manual workers. This may reflect not only the generally higher parity of the former but the considerable socio-economic pressures which underlie so many of the requests for abortion from these women and which doctors may have been readier to take into consideration since the Act.

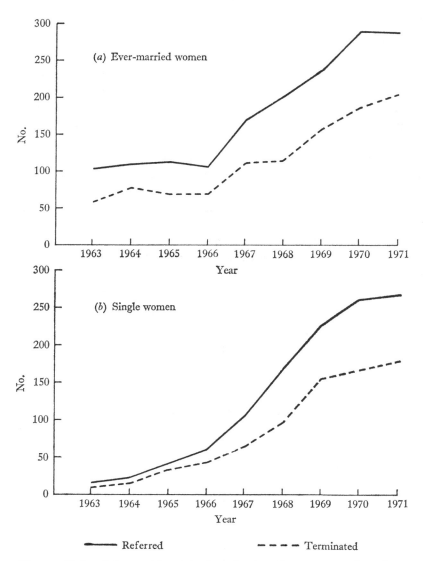

Fig. 1:1. Referred for consideration of termination of pregnancy and numbers terminated: 1963–71

JEAN AITKEN-SWAN

ILLEGITIMATE PREGNANCIES TO EVER-MARRIED WOMEN

Between 1963 and 1971 illegitimate pregnancies to Aberdeen married, widowed or divorced women accounted for between 18 and 35 per cent of all illegitimate pregnancies each year. Their actual numbers showed an upward trend over the nine years but the proportion they formed of all illegitimate pregnancies fell because of the increasing number of pregnancies to single women. In 1963 there were 75 illegitimate pregnancies to ever-married women (or 33 per cent of all illegitimate pregnancies) compared with 97 in 1971 (or 18 per cent). Changing attitudes in the 1960s are seen in the considerable increase in the proportion referred for consideration of abortion, from 17 per cent in 1963 to 58 per cent in 1971, and in the increasing proportion being accepted for termination.

Nearly half (48 per cent) of the 293 ever-married women who applied for termination of an illegitimate pregnancy between 1963 and 1971 were separated from their husbands and another 29 per cent were divorced. A small number of both groups were recorded as cohabiting.

Married, separated (12 cohabiting)	142
Divorced (8 cohabiting)	84
Married, living with husband	42
Widowed	25
	293

Dr Olley suggests that psychological factors may play an important though probably not an exclusive part in the occurrence of many illegitimate conceptions. The amount of social pathology in this group of broken and unhappy marriages is high. Psychiatric histories are commonly mentioned, instability, cruelty, previous abortions, previous illegitimate pregnancies, psychopathic husbands, suicidal attempts and so on. Although the couples in the group 'married, living with husband' are technically together, the husband was often absent from home through working in another part of the country, at sea for long periods or sometimes in prison; or the wife might be alone because her young husband spent his time with his parents and was said to take no interest in his own family. It is not unusual for pregnancies to occur after parties and following excessive drinking. 'I was drunk at a wedding and anything could have happened', as one woman explained.

Among the ever-married women referred, those aged under 30 were twice as likely as those aged 30 or more to be seeking abortion of an illegitimate pregnancy. The group is weighted with wives of semi-skilled and unskilled workers. About half the separated and divorced women were in social classes IV and V. Forty-three per cent of the whole group were already supporting 3 or more children.

Almost two-thirds (64 per cent) of the women had their pregnancy terminated, the same proportion as in the case of married women with legitimate pregnancies.

REFERRALS AND ABORTIONS: SINGLE WOMEN (Fig. 1:1(*b*))

Single women have been responsible for an increasing proportion of all illegitimate pregnancies occurring in Aberdeen between 1963 and 1971, the number of their illegitimate pregnancies having tripled over the nine years. In 1963 67 per cent of all illegitimate pregnancies were to single women, in 1971 82 per cent. Older teenagers contributed most to this increase.

Illsley and Gill,[2] studying the changes which have been occurring in Britain in regard to illegitimacy, have drawn attention to the reversal which has taken place in past patterns. Illegitimacy has ceased to be primarily a problem of the rural areas, with rates in Scotland higher than in England and Wales. Evidence links illegitimacy ratios to population density so that the highest ratios are now found in urban areas, and England's ratios have at last overtaken those for Scotland. Changing attitudes and freer sex relations have affected all social classes so that illegitimate pregnancy, for long predominantly a problem of the lower socio-economic groups, now appears to be becoming more frequent among girls at the other end of the social scale. They seek to explain these trends in terms of changes taking place in society and in the whole conception of marriage, and suggest the emergence of a new pattern in the incidence of illegitimate birth, associated with youth, urban living and sophistication.

It is not surprising in this context that referrals for abortion in Aberdeen should have increased most rapidly among single women and that the age of those referred has been falling. Up to the early 1960s it was not usual for a single girl who became pregnant to be referred for consideration of abortion – in those days it is unlikely that either the family or the family doctor thought of it as a practical possibility, apart from the exceptional case. Abortion in Aberdeen mainly concerned married, multiparous women. By 1963, however, one pregnant unmarried girl in ten was being referred, and by 1971 this proportion had increased to six in ten.

Barbara Thompson[3] in a social study of illegitimate maternities in Aberdeen in 1949–52 found that at that time illegitimacy in unmarried women tended to be associated with unskilled, unattractive or menial occupations (this being the woman's own pre-pregnancy occupation). In the present study, *ever-married* women having an illegitimate pregnancy still come predominantly from the lower socio-economic groups but since 1965 this is no longer true of *single* women. By 1971 professional women, students, nurses and clerical workers as a group accounted for 43 per cent of all pregnancies to single women compared with 25 per cent to women in semi-skilled and unskilled work, including fish-workers. (Fish-workers in Aberdeen form a distinct group and are usually shown separately in the tabulations.)

The steady rise in the number of pregnancies to single women, matched by a rise up to 1970 in the proportion referred for consideration of abortion, is shown in the various age and occupational groups in Table 1:10(a) and (b). A disturbing feature not confined to Aberdeen is the increase in the number of very young girls becoming pregnant; this is discussed later. A high proportion of them is referred, particularly since 1968. The greater willingness of doctors to refer single women is seen in all age groups, and by 1970 abortion was being considered for two-thirds of all pregnant single women in Aberdeen. Such a high referral rate makes the other third of great interest and one wonders by what process they are missed out from consideration of abortion. If the trend continues, the only single women not considered for abortion could be those who wish to continue their pregnancy. However it may not continue, for 1971 shows for the first time a fall in the proportion referred.

The change in the occupational distribution of referrals is strikingly shown in Table 1:10(b). Omitting the miscellaneous group bracketed together, less than 10 per cent of any group other than professional women, students and nurses were referred in 1963–4, whereas by 1970 referrals were not only more common but were becoming more evenly distributed over the occupational groups, with the exception of women in semi-skilled and unskilled work. In 1971 these women and fish-workers were still the least often referred.

For some reason, perhaps to do with which consultants are practising at a particular time, a higher proportion of the single women referred were accepted for abortion in 1965–6 than in any of the other years under consideration (Table 1:11). Each occupational group 'benefited', except the 32 pregnant fish-workers, but none of them was referred in those two years. Small numbers could account in part for the fluctuating percentages. On average about two-thirds of the single women referred succeeded in having an abortion. Not all the rest were 'refused'; each year between 10 and 15 per cent of applications fell through because of changes of mind, spontaneous abortion or other happenings (see footnote to table on p. 31 below).

The percentage of women referred who had their pregnancy terminated shows no clear trend if age alone is considered, nor is there a consistent pattern if abortions are related to total pregnancies in a particular age group (Table 1:12(a)). In 1971 59 per cent of all pregnancies to girls of 16 or under were terminated, a higher proportion than in any previous year. There is however a clear occupational class gradient in single women's abortions (Table 1:12(b)). The proportion of women in semi-skilled and unskilled work and fish-workers who obtained an abortion has risen more slowly than the proportion in any other occupational group and by 1970 was still only about 16 per cent of the total compared with a third in skilled and distributive workers, well over half in clerical workers and nearly two-thirds in professional women, students and nurses. 1971 shows no change in the fish-workers' rate but some increase in the rate for semi-skilled and unskilled workers although this still remains well behind the others. In 1971 for the first time the percentage of pregnancies aborted in the clerical worker group showed a marked fall.

Besides the single women whose pregnancies ended in birth or abortion ('spontaneous' or therapeutic) are several hundreds each year who though appearing in the statistics for married women were single at conception and who, if anything had stood in the way of marriage, would have added to the numbers of single pregnant women. Data for all primiparous single pregnant women in Aberdeen show that in 1963 nearly three-quarters had married before the birth of the baby while by 1971 this proportion had fallen to just over half. After 1964 the drop in pre-nuptial conceptions was most marked in professional women, students and nurses, coincident with the considerable rise in the number of therapeutic abortions in this group.

One can only speculate on why so comparatively few women in the lower occupational categories have their illegitimate pregnancies aborted. Traditionally this is the group in which pre-marital pregnancies occurred most frequently and which is most tolerant of them. Among fish-workers, for instance, it is more common for conception to take place before marriage than after marriage. Customarily the young woman keeps the baby and it is accepted into her family. Abortion may be less acceptable to them than it is to women higher in the social scale for whom the repercussions of an illegitimate pregnancy on their reputation and career may be more severe. But Dr Olley's evidence does not support this view (Chapter 5). In his group of Aberdeen single women he found a gradient of 'distress' increasing down the occupational scale from students to manual workers, with the manual workers the most hostile, guilt-prone and depressed. If, as his evidence suggests, it is the more intropunitive and neurotic section of unmarried pregnant women who are referred for abortion, one would expect referral rates to be higher in these lower occupational groups. This suggests a differential access to abortion. Women in semi-skilled and unskilled work may know less about the opportunity for abortion than the better educated (this is indicated by the interviewing study reported further on), or may feel more diffident about raising the question with their doctor. If they do they may not present their case so strongly or may be more easily discouraged from pursuing the matter with him. There is evidence too that some general practitioners can be subject to class bias. They may be less able to sympathise with the problems of the lower social class girl who is illegitimately pregnant than they can when dealing with a student or nurse. Whatever the reason, the comparatively low proportion of abortions to women in the lower occupational groups is due more to the differential in referrals than to what happens after they reach hospital, except perhaps in the case of young women who have been pregnant before.

SINGLE WOMEN PREGNANT MORE THAN ONCE

Illsley and Gill mention the tendency, reinforced by methods of compilation of British statistics, to treat illegitimacy as a unitary phenomenon – first births to unmarried girls. It has already been noted that separated, divorced and widowed women account for a considerable though declining proportion of all illegitimate pregnancies between 1963 and 1971. In addition, one in five of the single women is having a second or later pregnancy (Table 1:13). This proportion has not changed very much over the eight years.

There would appear to be a social class gradient in illegitimate pregnancy-repeating. The proportion of single women who had no pregnancy before referral and, as far as is known, none after (up to 1970) declines from 88 per cent in the professional–student group to 57 per cent in semi-skilled, unskilled workers and fish-workers combined. The proportion who had had one pregnancy, or two or more, prior to first referral, rises as occupational class falls (Table 1:14). It is true that mobility follows the same gradient and any later illegitimate pregnancies of professional women and students are less likely to appear in Aberdeen's statistics than those of clerical or manual workers. Even so, the difference between the percentages in more static groups, the skilled and semi-skilled and unskilled workers, suggests that illegitimate pregnancy-repeating is associated with low occupational status. Thus the traditional pattern for all illegitimate pregnancy, which was reversed in Aberdeen in 1965, is now perhaps only applicable to pregnancy-repeating.

In addition to the 131 women who had had one or more pregnancies *before* they were first referred, another 60 who had had no previous pregnancy became illegitimately pregnant again *after* referral. These are shown in a separate column of Table 1:14. It is striking that in their case there is no class gradient; indeed the proportion is the same – 6 per cent – in four groups, professional–students, nurses, distributive–skilled workers and the unskilled group.

However one must be careful about drawing conclusions about pregnancy-repeating in the population of single women from single women referred for consideration of abortion. If it is true that fewer upper class single women have a second illegitimate pregnancy than lower class single women and that in general a much higher proportion of upper class women are referred for consideration of abortion when they become pregnant then a lower rate of previous pregnancies in referred upper class women is to be expected. Conversely pregnancy-repeating is thought to be more common in manual workers, but manual workers as a group are less likely to be referred for consideration of abortion than upper class women. The fact that they have been pregnant before, and may already have a child to support, may be a factor in the referral of the lower class women. This group is therefore weighted with pregnancy-repeaters. It is striking that when pregnancy-repeating is considered in young women who all start at the same point – that is, previously nulliparous and referred for consideration of abortion of their first pregnancy, the rate of pregnancy-repeating is practically the same in all the occupational groups, which suggests that selective factors are operative. The slightly higher proportion (10 per cent) in the category 'at home, school or not stated' is probably due to the number of single women in this category who were cohabiting.

STUDENTS

Table 1:10 has shown that known pregnancies to professional women and students total 370 over the nine years 1963–71. Students account for all but 50 of these. The numbers of pregnancies to students have been increasing each year but at the same time the student population of Aberdeen has also been increasing. Although precise figures are not available an attempt has been made to ascertain the number of unmarried women attending the university and other colleges in Aberdeen during the period of the study. When related to this total population, the increase in the number of student pregnancies is seen in perspective. In 1970–1, all known pregnancies amounted to 13 per 1000 unmarried women students and 8 per 1000 had had an abortion (Table 1:15).

It seems likely that this is an underestimate of the number of pregnancies. Even in 1966 when illegitimate pregnancy was less common than it is now, the Honorary Secretary of the British Student Health Association, reporting at a conference on abortion in Britain,[4] stated that between 2 and 3 per cent of unmarried women students in British universities became pregnant each year. In Aberdeen the rate of known pregnancies had only reached 1.3 per cent of *all* students by 1970–1. It seems unlikely that there are significantly fewer pregnancies to non-university students and that their inclusion has lowered the rates. The difference may be a measure of the numbers who marry or go outside the area on finding themselves pregnant without approaching either their own student health service, general practitioner or the gynaecological or ante-natal services in Aberdeen. One medical officer dealing with Aberdeen students gave the following figures from his own experience of four consecutive academic years.† Of these, the students referred

† Figures kindly provided by Dr Campbell Murray.

about abortion, whether accepted or not, and others who continued the pregnancy in Aberdeen are included in the survey.

	1967–8	1968–9	1969–70	1970–1
Students who thought they might be pregnant	66	79	90	101
Number who were pregnant	35	37	39	48
Outcome:				
Therapeutic abortion	12	17	24	26
Got married	16	11	9	17
Continued pregnancy unmarried	5	7	4	5
Left area, lost touch with	2	2	2	—

A recent study by McCance and Hall[5] provides figures about pregnancies in unmarried female undergraduates at Aberdeen University in 1971 with which the figure of 13 pregnancies per 1000 Aberdeen students can be compared. At the time of that survey 6 of their 1552 respondents said they were pregnant and another 49 thought they might be pregnant. The tabulation above suggests that approximately half the students who thought they were pregnant actually were, so it could be hypothesised that some 30 of McCance and Hall's respondents were in fact pregnant at that moment in time, or 2 per cent. This again indicates that the pregnancy rate for 1970–1 in Table 1:15 of 1.3 per cent or less for all students is too low.

Abortion statistics in a university city are likely to be inflated by the inclusion of students who, though resident in the city, do not necessarily belong to it. A check made in 1969 of the home-town of university students referred for consideration for abortion showed that just under two-thirds of them (63 per cent) came from areas outside Aberdeenshire, Kincardineshire and the north-east of Scotland. Most came from other parts of Scotland with a few from south of the border and abroad. The proportion of all full-time women university students whose home was outside the north-east was estimated to be 47 per cent so that they would appear to be over-represented in the abortion referral group. If these non-Aberdonians are omitted from the figures for 1969, the rate of abortions in Aberdeen single women (Table 1:4) would be reduced from 11.2 to 8.5 per 1000 population.

JEAN AITKEN-SWAN

PREGNANCY IN VERY YOUNG TEENAGERS

A high proportion of Aberdeen girls who get pregnant at a very early age do so in socially pathological circumstances. Over the nine years of the study 60 girls under age 16 have been pregnant, one of them twice. Numbers have increased slightly each year from 2 in 1963 to 15 in 1971 (Table 1:10). Forty-seven were referred for consideration of abortion so that some information is available on the great majority.

In 6 cases the girl herself or her family had a psychiatric history, 2 girls having been under the care of the child psychiatric unit at an earlier age because of behaviour disorders. One mother was a schizophrenic and the father of another girl had committed suicide – this girl was on probation as being out of her mother's control. In all 8 girls came from broken homes, the mother having deserted to cohabit with another man or the parents separated or divorced; one of these girls had suffered serious childhood deprivation. Two girls were the victims of alleged rape, in one case by several youths. Four other girls had been made pregnant by members of their own family. This was the type of background or situation underlying 21 of the 47 pregnancies to girls of 13 to 15 years of age. Nearly all these pregnancies were terminated. Whatever the deficiencies in parental care in the other 26 cases, the adverse factors were not quite so obvious. Some of the girls were serious about their boyfriend with whom they had been friendly for months or even years. Others were experimenting when the opportunity presented, such as when left alone baby-sitting with a boy. It is sometimes said that pregnancy may have a symbolic significance to some girls and that in getting pregnant they are meeting an emotional need in themselves, but our data are not adequate to assess this possibility. In some there may have been an element of sexual precocity. Certainly 11 of the 47 were pregnant again quite soon.

Five of 15 with a disturbed background became pregnant again within a year or so but by then they were old enough to marry, and 3 did so. Six of the other girls became pregnant again but only one married the father.

A remark often made by unmarried girls pregnant for a second time is: 'I never thought it could happen again.' Unfortunately parents and doctors share this misapprehension and feel that it would be bad for such young girls to have the protection of contraception. If the girls were of stable temperament and learnt by experience and if they were fortunate enough to come from a secure and happy home this would be so, but then they might not have got pregnant in the first place. It is precisely because of the circumstances in which many of them get pregnant at that age, their disturbed home circumstances and perhaps in some cases lack of parental care, that this attitude is unrealistic. The measure of the inadequacy of their aftercare is the fact that in this small series nearly a quarter of the 14- and 15-year-olds were pregnant again so soon.

MORE THAN ONE REFERRAL FOR ABORTION: EVER-MARRIED AND SINGLE WOMEN

It is sometimes feared that if people think that abortion is freely available they will become careless about the use of contraception and abortion will be increasingly relied upon as a method of birth control. In the present series there is no indication so far that the number of *ever-married women* seeking abortion more than once is increasing but cases would have to be followed up for another three years before experience in 1969 is comparable with that in 1963. Combining the seven years, 87 ever-married women (or 8 per cent of the total referred) had had more than one referral or a previous therapeutic abortion elsewhere. Eight of these were referred on 3 occasions and 3 on 4 occasions.

Among *single women* the porportion was about the same (7 per cent of all referrals), or 45 women in all between 1963 and 1969. One of the 45 was referred more than twice. This is not a large number considering that one in five of all pregnancies to single women in Aberdeen are second or later pregnancies (Table 1:13).

Table 1:16 shows the outcome of the second referral in relation to what happened the first time in those cases where there were 2 referrals only. It would appear that the second unwanted pregnancy of the ever-married women occurred in much the same circumstances which had made the first termination necessary, for 27 of the 34 obtained a second abortion. (Fifteen of the 27 were sterilised at the same time.) Twenty-two of the 24 who had been refused abortion the first time succeeded in getting it done the second time they applied (17 of these were concurrently sterilised). Nine of the 18 whose first application had ended in spontaneous abortion, changes of mind, etc. ('not done for other reasons') had their pregnancy terminated when they applied again

(8 of the 9 being sterilised). In all over two-thirds of the 58 ever-married women whose second referral resulted in therapeutic abortion were sterilised at the same time.

Compared with married women, the single women's second applications were less successful. Only half those whose pregnancy had been terminated the first time had it done the second time. A second request for abortion by a single woman sometimes seems to put the doctor in a difficult position and may raise problems for him of where to draw the moral line. He is understandably irritated with someone who appears to be taking the availability of abortion for granted and he may feel that to agree to a second abortion would only encourage immorality, or at least carelessness. Yet it seems no more desirable the second time than it was the first time for a baby to be born in order to teach its mother to be more careful in future; in fact from the potential child's point of view it might be less desirable in view of the personality problems common in the group of unmarried pregnancy-repeaters. Expressions such as giving her 'the benefit of the doubt' or 'whether she is deserving of abortion' suggest that doctors sometimes see their role as judgemental. Ingham and Simms[6] give an example in their description of patients applying for abortion to a London hospital: 'Two girls were refused because they had already had previous unwanted pregnancies *and had still not used birth control on this occasion*' (my italics). Yet 'deservingness' has always been difficult to define and is not a legal requirement for obtaining abortion; indeed this appealing quality may not be offered by the very women most in need of abortion on psychiatric grounds. A second illegitimate pregnancy may be as much a measure of bad home conditions, defective family relationships and the poor quality of aftercare after the first pregnancy as of irresponsible sex. It would be unreasonable to expect a doctor to make his decision in a moral vacuum even if his legitimate concern is less with deservingness and more with the risks of repeated abortion to a woman's future maternal health and fertility. Partialities are apparent in the fact that 50 per cent of the professional women, students and nurses as a group pregnant a second time had both pregnancies terminated compared with only 8 per cent of women in all other occupations.

OUTCOME WHEN THE PREGNANCY IS NOT TERMINATED: EVER-MARRIED AND SINGLE

During the nine years of the study, 970 (35 per cent of all those referred for consideration of abortion) did not have their pregnancy terminated for the reasons tabulated below. Omitting the 92 who aborted spontaneously about the time of their application and the 31 found not to be pregnant leaves 847 pregnancies to be accounted for. Their outcome is known in all but 10 per cent (Table 1:17), these mostly being the most recent cases, as at the time of writing the follow-up for 1971 is incomplete.

	Total	Ever-married	Single
(a) Not accepted for abortion by consultant	683	366	317
(b) Patient changed her mind	137	92	45
(c) Being considered when had spontaneous abortion	92	64	28
(d) Found not to be pregnant	31	24	7
(e) Not done for other reasons†	27	22	5
	970	568	402

† E.g. abortion not necessary on medical grounds and not wanted, decision delayed and then pregnancy too far advanced, etc.

The majority of the women who were unsuccessful in obtaining an abortion went on with their pregnancy and arranged for their confinement in Aberdeen. A few, mostly single women, went elsewhere to have the baby. In the nine years only 17 who were refused abortion by the Aberdeen consultants were known to have obtained a legal abortion elsewhere, 10 of them between 1968 and 1970 and 7 in 1971. These pregnancies were all illegitimate. Up to 1970 the abortions had been obtained in London (3) or Scotland (7) but in 1971 only 2 of the 7 were obtained in Scotland and the other 5 women (all students) went to Birmingham or Brighton where clinics run by the Pregnancy Advisory Service had been opened.

Patients who change their minds or who come into the category 'not done for other reasons' are unlikely to have sought abortion elsewhere (although one withdrew her application and then decided to have the abortion as a private patient). This leaves the 66 in Table 1:17 not accepted by the consultants for whom the outcome is not known. Some of these may have obtained an abortion elsewhere; two stated this to be their intention. A quarter of them attended before the Abortion Act came into operation and it is unlikely that women referred before the Act went elsewhere, at least for a legal abortion. More probably the single women anyway went to a relative or out of town for their confinement and others will have married and attended the ante-natal clinic under a new name.

To sum up the abortion situation between 1963 and 1971, Aberdeen practice, for long comparatively liberal, has been overtaken by the wave of illegitimacy which reached Scotland from the urban centres of the south during the sixties. This affected better educated girls, teachers, nurses, students and clerical workers, many of whom were reluctant to solve the problem by precipitous marriage or by placing the baby for adoption. Requests for abortion were multiplying before the Abortion Act became an issue and the increase in abortions preceded, and was not a consequence of, the new law. The rate of abortion of legitimate pregnancies on the other hand did not change until the Act was passed in 1967 when there was an increase in the numbers referred and a proportionate increase in abortions performed.

More illegitimate pregnancies and abortions and fewer live-births have occurred in the context of a declining number of total pregnancies – from 3640 in 1963 to 3370 in 1971. Post-partum sterilisation, the introduction of oral contraception to Aberdeen in 1964, and the extension of the work of the family planning clinics that followed, all contributed to the decrease. In view of the reliability of oral contraception and its availability in Aberdeen (without charge to the patient since 1966 in local authority clinics), it might be expected that the need for abortion, in married women at least, would lessen rather than increase, but this is not yet the case. Thompson et al.[7] report that of a series of married women resident in Aberdeen and attending an ante-natal clinic in 1968, who were asked if they had ever taken oral contraception, about a quarter gave an affirmative reply. (This proportion will almost certainly have doubled by now.) Just under two-thirds of those attending with their fourth or later pregnancy had never taken 'the pill', and an earlier Aberdeen study[8] has shown that a high proportion of fourth and later pregnancies are unintentional and unwanted. Abortion, and also sterilisation, are obviously still needed to help people to have the size of family they want and feel able to afford.

The non-use and failure of contraception plays a major part in the circumstances leading to referral for abortion and is considered in more detail in Chapters 3 and 4. But what decides each patient to seek this solution and what are the circumstances that make it necessary in her opinion? What of her family relationships and how are they affected by the abortion or the decision not to terminate the pregnancy? In her opinion later on, was the decision the right one? To answer these questions an interviewing study was made of a consecutive series of women applying for abortion between September 1968 and June 1969, a total of 342. This gives the patient's own description of the circumstances surrounding the application for abortion and her views on the outcome, whether successful or not (Chapters 3 and 4).

REFERENCES

1 Baird, D. (1967). 'Sterilisation and therapeutic abortion in Aberdeen', *Brit. J. Psychiat.*, **113**, 701–9.
2 Illsley, R., Gill, D. G. (1968). 'Changing trends in illegitimacy', *Soc. Sci. and Med.*, **2**, 415–33.
3 Thompson, B. (1956). 'Social study of illegitimate maternities', *Brit. J. prev. soc. Med.*, **10**, 75–87.
4 Finlay, S. E. (1966). 'Abortion in British universities', in *Abortion in Britain*, proceedings of a conference held by the Family Planning Association, Pitman Medical Publishing Co. Ltd., London, p. 46.
5 McCance, C., Hall, D. J. (1972). 'Sexual behaviour and contraceptive practice of unmarried female undergraduates at Aberdeen University', *Brit. med. J.*, **2**, 694–700.
6 Ingham, C., Simms, M. (1972). 'Study of applicants for abortion at the Royal Northern Hospital, London', *J. biosoc. Sci.*, **4**, 351–69.
7 Thompson, B., Durno, D., MacGregor, J. E., McGregor, M. S. M. (1969). 'Some aspects of oral contraception and married women', *Med. Officer*, **cxxi**, 8, 93–6.
8 Scott, E. M., Thomson, A. M. (1956). 'A psychological investigation of primigravidae, Part 1', *J. Obstet. Gynaec. Brit. Emp.*, **63**, 311.

TABLE 1:1. *All known pregnancies, Aberdeen city: 1963–71*

All known pregnancies	Legitimate									Illegitimate								
	1963	1964	1965	1966	1967	1968	1969	1970	1971	1963	1964	1965	1966	1967	1968	1969	1970	1971
Live-births	3034	2889	2938	2640	2553	2557	2282	2380	2373	164	157	185	195	201	221	210	200	240
Stillbirths	39	39	29	22	20	25	26	29	30	7	6	2	2	1	—	3	1	3
Spontaneous abortions	288	279	281	269	243	201	219	232	243	36	33	40	39	39	44	53	45	43
Therapeutic abortions	52	70	58	53	91	94	131	141	163	16	20	42	59	84	118	181	211	222
Other and not known†	1	2	—	3	3	3	2	3	10	3	3	7	6	12	28	25	30	43
Total	3414	3279	3306	2987	2910	2880	2660	2785	2819	226	219	276	301	337	411	472	487	551

† In the detailed analysis of pregnancies that follows account cannot be taken of 'transferred-in' cases, that is, deliveries of Aberdeen residents occurring elsewhere and transferred by the Registrar General to Aberdeen's birth statistics. There are, however, pregnancies to Aberdeen women (known to us because the woman applied for an abortion) which ended elsewhere or where the outcome is not known, and these are included above. They are of numerical importance only in the case of illegitimate pregnancies.

TABLE I: 2. *Annual rates of abortion: 1963–71*

Annual rate	1963	1964	1965	1966	1967	1968	1969	1970	1971
Annual rates of abortion per 1000 women aged 15–44†	1.8	2.3	2.6	2.9	4.5	5.5	8.1	9.1	9.9
Annual ratios of abortion per 1000 live-births	21.3	29.5	32.0	39.5	63.5	76.3	125.2	136.4	146.5

† As it makes no difference to the rates if the base population is taken from the 1961 census or from the 10 per cent sample of 1966, the 1961 census population has been used for all the years.

TABLE I:3. *Annual rates of abortion† per 1000 female population aged 15–44 and per 1000 live-births, by area: 1969–70*

Area	Per 1000 women		Per 1000 live-births	
	1969	1970	1969	1970
Aberdeen	8.1	9.1	125.2	136.4
Scotland	3.5	5.3	39.2	59.8
North	5.8	7.8	62.0	88.0
North-east	5.3	6.3	65.6	78.5
East	5.0	7.6	58.6	90.7
South-east	4.4	6.6	52.8	81.0
West	2.5	4.0	26.9	43.8
England and Wales‡	5.3	8.1	62.5	96.8

† Abortions in the regions taken from Annual Report of the Registrar General for Scotland, Part II, 1970.
‡ Figures for England and Wales taken from the Registrar General's Supplements on Abortions, 1969, 1970, and from the Registrar General's Statistical Review for these years. Non-residents are excluded from the abortion totals.

TABLE I:4. *Rate of abortions by marital state: 1963–71*

Marital state	1961 census population women aged 15–44	Rate per 1000 population						
		1963–4	1965–6	1967	1968	1969	1970	1971
Single	13,844	0.8	2.8	4.5	6.9	11.2	12.0	12.6
Married (incl. separated)	24,045	2.7	2.5	4.2	4.4	5.9	7.1	7.8
Widowed and divorced	741	3.4	9.4	16.2	12.1	18.9	21.6	16.2

TABLE I:5. *Rate of abortions by age group:†* *1963–71*

Age group	Population		Rate per 1000 population						
	1961 census	1966 sample	1963–4	1965–6	1967	1968	1969	1970	1971
15–19	6989	8366	0.6	2.0	2.3	5.4	8.6	9.7	17.6
20–24	6704	6220	1.6	4.8	8.8	9.2	16.4	16.7	21.7
25–29	6257	5340	2.7	2.6	5.6	6.7	9.4	9.2	15.7
30–34	6170	6040	4.2	4.2	6.1	5.5	7.6	7.3	6.5
35–39	6542	5940	2.2	1.9	3.7	5.4	4.9	9.6	6.9
40–44	5968	6570	1.1	1.0	1.8	1.4	2.0	2.3	3.5

† 1963–5 based on 1961 census population; 1966–71 on the 10 per cent sample.

TABLE I:6. *Women referred: legitimate and illegitimate pregnancies,* *1963–71*

Year	Legitimate		Illegitimate	
	All known pregnancies	Per cent referred	All known pregnancies	Per cent referred
1963	3414	2.6	226	12.4
1964	3279	2.9	219	16.4
1965	3306	2.9	276	21.4
1966	2987	2.8	301	25.9
1967	2910	4.9	337	38.9
1968	2880	5.5	411	51.0
1969	2660	7.3	472	57.0
1970	2785	8.3	487	65.3
1971	2819	8.2	551	58.6

TABLE 1:7. *Referrals by age group, parity† and socio-economic group: ever-married women*

Age, parity,† socio-economic group	Per cent referred									Pregnancies†								
	1963	1964	1965	1966	1967	1968	1969	1970	1971	1963	1964	1965	1966	1967	1968	1969	1970	1971
(a) By age group																		
<25	0.9	1.2	1.7	1.5	2.2	3.1	5.3	5.8	5.2	1329	1324	1390	1277	1278	1338	1273	1418	1453
25–34	3.9	4.6	3.6	4.6	8.1	8.4	11.1	12.2	13.7	1545	1445	1428	1250	1181	1159	1036	1027	1008
35+	9.2	9.1	13.9	11.1	16.6	25.3	26.1	43.9	38.3	316	296	281	252	271	249	211	189	193
(b) By parity†																		
0–2	1.5	1.6	1.6	1.7	2.7	4.0	5.3	6.4	7.3	2504	2415	2464	2256	2213	2250	2082	2302	2232
3, 4	10.1	9.0	11.8	12.9	22.9	22.6	30.6	41.7	29.5	543	512	506	419	414	402	350	295	366
5+	5.6	16.5	10.8	11.5	13.7	20.2	21.6	51.3	24.5	143	139	129	104	102	94	88	37	53
NS	—	—	—	—	—	—	—	—	—	—	—	—	—	—	—	—	—	3
(c) By socio-economic group																		
Professional and managerial	3.2	2.5	2.5	3.2	5.2	5.5	6.7	9.0	6.5	524	472	515	436	481	471	432	445	542
Other non-manual	2.5	1.6	3.8	2.0	3.6	3.1	4.9	4.6	7.1	362	306	343	296	276	380	263	237	255
Skilled manual	3.6	3.5	2.8	3.9	6.0	7.1	9.1	9.3	9.3	1277	1276	1242	1106	1102	1015	1007	1137	1044
Semi-skilled and armed forces	2.4	5.4	5.5	4.3	7.8	8.8	12.2	12.6	12.3	654	615	596	576	561	545	482	500	488
Unskilled	3.3	3.6	4.5	4.2	7.8	12.4	11.7	18.8	15.8	362	389	396	359	295	323	317	303	297
NS	—	—	—	—	—	—	—	—	—	11	8	7	6	15	12	19	12	28
Total	3.2	3.5	3.7	3.8	6.2	7.3	9.4	11.0	10.9	3190	3066	3099	2779	2730	2746	2520	2634	2654

† Excluding spontaneous abortions.

TABLE 1:8. *Abortions by age group, parity† and socio-economic group: ever-married women*

Age, parity,† socio-economic group	Per cent aborted							Referrals								
	1963–4	1965–6	1967	1968	1969	1970	1971	1963	1964	1965	1966	1967	1968	1969	1970	1971
(a) By age group																
<25	46.4	55.8	57.1	51.2	48.5	47.6	64.5	12	16	24	19	28	41	68	82	76
25–34	63.8	68.8	66.7	58.8	72.2	62.6	73.2	61	66	51	58	96	97	115	123	138
35+	75.0	53.7	71.1	60.3	74.5	81.9	75.7	29	27	39	28	45	63	55	83	74
NS	—	—	—	—	—	—	—	—	—	—	—	—	—	—	2	—
(b) By parity†																
0–2	53.8	54.4	66.1	45.5	54.9	55.8	60.4	38	40	40	39	59	90	111	147	164
3, 4	68.3	62.3	65.3	65.9	72.0	69.9	78.7	55	46	60	54	95	91	107	123	108
5+	80.6	80.8	71.4	73.7	94.7	89.5	69.2	8	23	14	12	14	19	19	19	13
NS	—	—	—	—	—	—	—	1	—	—	—	1	1	1	1	3
(c) By socio-economic group																
All non-manual	67.4	63.0	71.4	57.9	73.8	64.7	75.5	26	17	26	20	35	38	42	51	53
Skilled manual	72.5	60.3	65.1	59.7	65.2	67.0	71.1	46	45	35	43	66	72	92	106	97
Semi-skilled and armed forces	61.2	65.5	65.9	50.0	67.8	68.2	68.3	16	33	33	25	44	48	59	63	60
Unskilled	42.3	63.6	65.2	65.0	56.7	57.9	76.6	12	14	18	15	23	40	37	57	47
NS	—	—	—	—	—	—	—	2	—	2	2	1	3	8	13	31
Total	64.4	61.6	66.3	57.7	66.0	64.1	71.5	102	109	114	105	169	201	238	290	288

† Excluding spontaneous abortions.

TABLE I:9. *Abortions as percentage of total pregnancies to ever-married women, by age group, parity† and socio-economic group*

Age, parity,† socio-economic group	Abortions as percentage of all pregnancies in group							Abortions								
	1963–4	1965–6	1967	1968	1969	1970	1971	1963	1964	1965	1966	1967	1968	1969	1970	1971
(a) By age group																
<25	0.5	0.9	1.2	1.6	2.6	2.7	3.4	3	10	12	12	16	21	33	39	49
25–34	2.7	2.8	5.4	4.9	8.0	7.5	10.0	36	45	35	40	64	57	83	77	101
35+	6.9	6.7	11.8	15.3	19.4	36.0	29.0	20	22	20	16	32	38	41	68	56
NS	—	—	—	—	—	—	—	—	—	—	—	—	—	—	2	—
(b) By parity†																
0–2	0.8	0.9	1.8	1.8	2.9	3.6	4.9	20	22	19	24	39	41	61	82	109
3, 4	6.5	7.7	15.0	15.0	22.0	29.1	23.2	33	36	38	33	62	60	77	86	85
5+	8.9	9.0	9.8	14.9	20.4	45.9	17.0	6	19	10	11	10	14	18	17	9
NS	—	—	—	—	—	—	—	—	—	—	—	1	1	1	1	3
(c) By socio-economic group																
All non-manual	1.7	1.8	3.3	2.6	4.5	4.8	5.0	15	14	16	13	25	22	31	33	40
Skilled manual	2.6	2.0	3.9	4.2	5.9	6.2	6.7	32	34	19	28	43	43	60	71	69
Semi-skilled and armed forces	2.4	3.2	5.2	4.4	8.3	8.6	8.4	8	22	23	15	29	24	40	43	41
Unskilled	1.5	2.8	5.1	8.0	6.6	10.9	12.1	4	7	9	12	15	26	21	33	36
NS	—	—	—	—	—	—	—	—	—	—	—	—	1	5	6	20
Total	2.2	2.3	4.1	4.2	6.2	7.1	7.8	59	77	67	68	112	116	157	186	206

† Excluding spontaneous abortions.

TABLE 1:10. *Referrals, by age group and occupation: single women*

Age and occupation	Per cent referred							Pregnancies†								
	1963–4	1965–6	1967	1968	1969	1970	1971	1963	1964	1965	1966	1967	1968	1969	1970	1971
(a) By age group																
13 or 14	—	—	—	—	—	—	—	—	—	—	1	1	2	2	2	2
15	—	—	—	—	—	—	—	1	2	3	2	4	6	7	11	13
16	—	—	—	—	—	—	—	7	9	13	8	6	16	16	27	34
16 and under	30.0	29.6	45.4	79.2	72.0	80.0	81.6	9	11	16	11	11	24	25	40	49
17–19	6.2	19.0	31.8	52.8	60.2	73.2	58.9	38	42	62	101	107	123	156	138	175
20–24	14.9	31.4	48.6	52.3	66.4	59.2	51.7	65	56	76	80	107	128	140	174	176
25+	11.9	16.1	40.6	41.5	44.7	60.0	61.5	36	31	34	28	32	41	47	40	52
NS	—	—	—	—	—	—	—	3	2	5	10	3	14	3	—	1
(b) By occupation																
Professional, students	54.5	74.5	78.4	92.6	94.0	94.1	80.5	7	4	21	30	37	54	67	68	82
Nurses	50.0	58.8	85.7	81.2	77.1	100.0	75.9	9	11	9	8	21	16	35	26	29
Clerical workers	9.4	17.2	34.4	52.9	70.0	80.0	56.6	31	33	36	51	61	87	90	80	83
Distributive	5.1	16.7	28.6	39.3	35.1	52.3	52.3	23	16	20	28	28	28	37	44	44
Skilled manual	7.0	11.7	31.4	47.5	56.7	76.2	53.1	17	26	36	41	35	40	30	42	64
Semi-skilled, unskilled	4.7	14.9	15.8	26.4	38.5	22.2	43.5	35	29	46	41	38	53	65	54	62
Fish-workers	5.1	0.0	20.7	17.2	17.2	33.3	25.5	17	22	14	18	29	29	29	45	51
Schoolgirls }								4	—	3	4	5	9	12	20	18
At home }	38.5	20.8	45.4	43.5	72.2	72.7	92.1	3	1	2	1	3	2	1	4	2
NS								5	—	6	8	3	12	5	9	18
Total	12.6	23.2	40.0	50.9	60.9	66.3	58.9	151	142	193	230	260	330	371	392	453

† Including spontaneous abortions.

TABLE I:II. *Abortions, by age group and occupation: single women*

| | Per cent aborted | | | | | | | Referrals | | | | | | | | |
Age and occupation	1963–4	1965–6	1967	1968	1969	1970	1971	1963	1964	1965	1966	1967	1968	1969	1970	1971
(a) By age group																
13 or 14	—	—	—	—	—	—	—	1	—	—	1	1	—	3	2	2
15	—	—	—	—	—	—	—	—	1	2	3	2	6	5	8	11
16	—	—	—	—	—	—	—	—	1	3	1	2	13	10	22	27
16 and under	(3)	(6)	(1)	—	(9)	—	—	3	2	10	5	5	19	18	32	40
17–19	(4)	77.4	52.9	52.6	65.9	62.5	72.5	4	5	21	21	34	65	94	101	103
20–24	55.5	79.6	75.0	50.8	75.3	55.4	55.3	8	10	21	28	52	67	93	103	91
25+	(5)	(8)	(5)	88.2	66.6	83.3	81.2	3	5	6	4	13	17	21	24	32
NS	—	—	—	—	—	—	—	—	—	—	—	—	—	—	—	1
(b) By occupation																
Professional, students }	75.0	85.4	72.3	55.5	78.9	64.4	71.6	3	3	14	24	29	50	63	64	66
Nurses								5	5	5	5	18	13	27	26	22
Clerical workers	(3)	66.6	52.4	50.0	69.8	70.3	59.6	1	5	8	7	21	46	63	64	47
Distributive }	(2)	76.5	(7)	63.3	63.3	56.4	71.9	1	1	4	4	8	11	13	23	23
Skilled manual								—	2	1	8	11	19	17	32	34
Semi-skilled, unskilled }	(2)	76.9	(8)	63.1	50.0	59.2	57.5	—	3	6	7	6	14	25	12	27
Fish-workers								—	2	—	—	6	5	5	15	13
Schoolgirls }	(3)	—	—	—	—	—	—	—	—	—	—	—	6	11	18	18
At home								2	—	1	3	4	3	1	2	1
NS								2	1	1	—	1	1	1	4	16
Total	59.4	78.6	60.6	57.1	68.6	63.8	67.0	15	22	40	58	104	168	226	260	267

NOTE. Figures in parentheses = *N* < 10.

TABLE I:12. *Abortions as percentage of total pregnancies† to single women, by age group and occupation*

Age and occupation	Abortions as percentage of all pregnancies in group							Abortions								
	1963–4	1965–6	1967	1968	1969	1970	1971	1963	1964	1965	1966	1967	1968	1969	1970	1971
(a) By age group																
13 or 14	—	—	—	—	—	—	—	—	—	—	1	—	—	2	1	2
15	—	—	—	—	—	—	—	—	—	—	2	—	—	4	6	10
16	—	—	—	—	—	—	—	1	1	1	1	1	4	3	13	17
16 and under	15.0	22.0	9.1	41.7	36.0	50.0	59.2	2	1	2	4	1	10	9	20	29
17–19	5.0	14.7	16.8	26.8	39.7	40.6	32.6	—	4	8	16	18	33	62	56	57
20–24	8.3	25.0	36.4	29.7	50.0	40.2	37.5	6	4	18	21	39	38	70	70	66
25+	7.5	12.9	15.6	36.6	29.8	50.0	50.0	1	4	5	3	5	15	14	20	26
NS	—	—	—	—	—	—	—	—	—	—	—	—	—	—	—	1
(b) By occupation																
Professional, students	36.4	64.7	64.9	55.5	71.6	61.8	54.8	2	2	13	20	24	30	48	42	45
Nurses	40.0	47.0	47.6	31.2	65.7	61.5	62.1	4	4	5	3	10	5	23	16	18
Clerical workers	4.7	11.5	18.0	26.4	48.9	56.2	33.7	—	3	5	5	11	23	44	45	28
Skilled, distributive	2.4	10.4	11.1	27.9	28.3	36.0	38.0	—	2	4	9	7	19	19	31	41
Semi-skilled, unskilled	1.6	11.5	13.1	15.1	16.9	16.7	24.2	—	1	5	5	5	8	11	9	15
Fish-workers	2.6	0.0	10.3	13.8	13.8	15.5	15.7	—	1	—	—	3	4	4	7	8
Schoolgirls, at home and NS	23.1	12.5	27.3	30.4	33.3	48.5	63.1	3	—	1	2	3	7	6	16	24
Total	7.5	18.2	24.2	29.1	41.8	42.3	39.5	9	13	33	44	63	96	155	166	179

† Including spontaneous abortions.

TABLE 1:13. *First and subsequent pregnancies to single women*

Pregnancy order	Percentage of total							Pregnancies								
	1963–4	1965–6	1967	1968	1969	1970	1971	1963	1964	1965	1966	1967	1968	1969	1970	1971
First	75.4	76.8	80.4	78.4	78.4	79.8	78.3	108	113	151	174	209	259	291	313	355
Second	14.3	14.2	13.1	13.4	17.3	15.1	13.7	24	18	25	35	34	44	64	59	62
Third	3.8	3.3	3.8	2.7	1.3	3.3	4.2	5	6	6	8	10	9	5	13	19
Fourth or more	4.4	1.9	1.2	1.5	1.1	1.5	1.8	10	3	6	2	3	5	4	6	8
NS	2.1	3.8	1.5	4.0	1.9	0.3	2.0	4	2	5	11	4	13	7	1	9
	100.0	100.0	100.0	100.0	100.0	100.0	100.0	151	142	193	230	260	330	371	392	453

TABLE I:14. *Previous pregnancies of single women and subsequent illegitimate pregnancies, by occupational group: 1963–70 combined*

Occupational group	Total referred between 1963 and 1970		Previous pregnancies before first referral			One or more pregnancies after but none before referral (% of all referrals)
	No.	%	None %	One %	Two+ %	
Professional, students	250	100	94.4	5.2	0.4	6.0
Nurses	104	100	88.5	11.5	0.0	5.8
Clerical workers	215	100	86.5	12.6	0.9	7.9
Distributive, skilled manual	156	100	82.7	15.4	1.9	6.4
Semi-skilled, unskilled and fish-workers	106	100	62.3	29.2	8.5	5.7
Home, school and NS	62	100	85.5	6.4	8.1	9.7
	893	100	85.4	12.4	2.2	6.7
			(N = 762)	(N = 111)	(N = 20)	(N = 60)

NOTE. In addition 9 women had pregnancies both before and after the index referral, 5 in the distributive–skilled manual category, 3 semi-skilled, unskilled or fish-workers and one in the miscellaneous group.

TABLE 1:15. *Pregnancy and abortion rates in unmarried Aberdeen women students: 1963–70*

Year	Unmarried women students (approx.)	All known pregnancies	Pregnancies per 1000 students	Referred about abortion	Aborted	Abortions per 1000 students
1963–4	2350	5	2.1	2	1	0.4
1964–5	2600	2	0.8	2	2	0.8
1965–6	3000	18	6.0	13	12	4.0
1966–7	3500	27	7.7	22	18	5.1
1967–8	3850	35	9.0	28	23	6.0
1968–9	4000	46	11.5	42	25	6.2
1969–70	4300	58	13.5	57	44	10.2
1970–1	4400	59	13.4	58	36	8.2
	28,000	250	8.9	224	161	5.7

TABLE 1:16. *Outcome of first and second referrals: 1963–9 combined*

	Outcome of second referral							
	Ever-married				Single			
Outcome of first referral	Total	Ter-minated	Refused	Not done for other reasons	Total	Ter-minated	Refused	Not done for other reasons
Terminated	34	27	3	4	31	16	13	2
Refused by doctor	24	22	1	1	10	6	3	1
Not done for other reasons	18	9	3	6	3	3	—	—
	76	58	7	11	44	25	16	3

TABLE 1:17. *Outcome of pregnancy when abortion not done: ever-married and single women*

	Not accepted for abortion by consultants (*a*)			Changed mind, not done for other reasons (*b*) and (*c*)		
	Total	Ever-married	Single	Total	Ever-married	Single
Had baby in Aberdeen	510	310	200	126	93	33
Had baby elsewhere	61	9	52	8	2	6
Had spontaneous abortion	29	21	8	9	9	0
Obtained abortion elsewhere	17	2	15	1	0	1
Died before operation	—	—	—	1	1	0
NK	66	24	42	19	9	10
	683	366	317	164	114	50

2 GYNAECOLOGICAL ASPECTS

Ian MacGillivray and K. John Dennis

INTRODUCTION

Doctors have traditionally been concerned with the preservation of life, and abortion like euthanasia was generally regarded as something which a good doctor would not do; besides it was part of the training of the doctor in forensic medicine that to procure an abortion was a criminal act unless it was to save the woman from imminent death. Apart from such an emergency it was supposed that abortions were only performed by 'back-street abortionists' using dirty instruments, or by doctors who were charlatans and doing the operation for financial gain. Against this sort of background very few gynaecologists were willing to perform termination of pregnancy for conditions other than gross medical indications.

There were a few pioneers and they influenced the thinking of others, in particular their junior staff. Not only did they have to satisfy their own consciences that it was desirable to terminate pregnancies for conditions other than gross medical illness, but they had to overcome the prejudices and opposition of other members of medical staff, the nursing staff and the administration. The report of the inquiry into 'The Attitude of Consultant Gynaecologists to Termination of Pregnancy' organised by the Royal College of Obstetricians and Gynaecologists in England and Wales indicates that the great majority of gynaecologists would prefer not to have to do abortions.[1] Being a profession which is traditionally conservative and in which the opinions and attitudes of colleagues can influence greatly the career prospects of junior staff and indeed senior staff, in terms of both financial rewards and status in the profession, it is not surprising that conservative attitudes are maintained. Although doctors have long recognised the influence of 'social factors' on disease, the social factors operating in pregnancy have tended to be ignored. This may be to some extent because pregnancy is considered to be a physiological condition, and if social factors were operating adversely on pregnancy, then it was the social factor which should be changed rather than the pregnancy terminated. Even those gynaecologists who recognised the major influence played by social factors in determining the outcome of pregnancy tended to react adversely toward the attitudes of those who appeared to be advocating that gynaecologists should 'cure' the conditions produced by social ills by performing abortions. Some gynaecologists resented being put in a position of dealing with social problems which they felt were the patients' own fault, or, if not, should be dealt with by social welfare or government agencies.

In most parts of the country at the time of the Abortion Act controversy there was a shortage of gynaecological beds and an insufficient number of maternity beds to hospitalise all the women deemed to require hospital confinements. Many gynaecologists feared that women with other gynaecological conditions would be kept out of hospital or be kept waiting an unduly long time because abortion cases had to be admitted urgently. This is of course true but the difficulty is in deciding on the priorities of dealing with an unwanted pregnancy or some other gynaecological problem which might not have such an adverse effect on the woman's well-being, at least in the short term.

Against this background of professional conservatism and relative lack of facilities it was not surprising that the majority of gynaecologists were unwilling to adopt any active policy to try to produce a more liberal attitude to abortion. Only those with a strong social conscience, and who were aware of and wished to be concerned with the miseries of women who are forced to produce unwanted babies or to risk the immediate or long-term effects of an illegally procured abortion, were likely to play an active part in the fight to produce a more liberal attitude to abortion. Even those gynaecologists who actively supported the Abortion Act were divided over the question of which women and under what circumstances abortion should be performed. The latter problem was possibly even more acute for those gynaecologists who, while not wishing to take an active part in promoting the Abortion Act, did not feel strongly against it and were willing to accept the Act and to try to make it work. This conflict arises because of the vagueness of the Act and the difficulty of interpreting what is 'good health' and what is 'ill health', and even more so of determining what the ultimate outcome will be whether pregnancy is terminated or not. It is only after fairly long experience of dealing with abortion cases that a gynaecologist can assess whether his decision has been the correct one or not. Gynaecologists who had not previously been involved in the decision-making in abortion cases were at a comparative disadvantage here, and the reaction of many was to feel that they were not competent to decide and that they were unwilling to become involved. It seems, however, that with the passage of time and the gaining of some experience gynaecologists mostly arrive at some personal standards which they adopt and employ, since there now appears to be relative uniformity of practice throughout the country apart from a few specific areas where some senior gynaecologists have adopted an anti-abortion stance.

This uncertainty about the standard to adopt and the dearth of specific information on the sequelae of abortion in this country were among the reasons for undertaking the present study. Experience in other countries was not felt to provide sufficiently comparable information because of their obvious differences in populations, laws and contraceptive practices. Swedish experience was probably nearest to our own but again there are differences which make direct comparison invalid. A study of a British population was needed, in part epidemiological covering the years before and after the Abortion Act of 1967, and in part an intensive prospective study of the women themselves taking into account all the aspects of abortion, gynaecological, psychiatric and sociological. This inter-departmental study was thus set up with the co-operation of the three university departments concerned and began in 1967, ten months before the Act came into operation. Consultants and general practitioners alike were eager to participate in it.

The consultant gynaecologists, all of whom took part in the study, had all trained under or worked with Sir Dugald Baird for some considerable time and had been fairly equally exposed to his influence. It is of interest to note therefore that there is no uniformity of opinion among them regarding termination of pregnancy, although none could be considered 'anti-abortion'. Most of the general practitioners in the city had been taught by him when they were medical students but again there is a wide spectrum of opinion among them regarding termination of pregnancy.

'LIBERALS' AND 'CONSERVATIVES'

In deciding whether to recommend termination of a pregnancy or not a consultant takes into account many factors such as stage of gestation, medical and psychiatric conditions, social influences such as illegitimacy and living conditions, and the number and health of other children in the family, and any significant genetic history. His assessment of these factors is inevitably coloured by his thinking on the moral aspects of abortion. Assuming that overall there is no great variation in the type of patient being seen by each consultant, his 'refusal' rate over a period of time such as two years must reflect his personal philosophy and will categorise his attitude as liberal or conservative. (The proportion of the consultant's abortion applicants who are 'refused' is a better indication of 'liberality' than abortions done because of a third category in the denominator, 'not done for other reasons', i.e. changes of mind, spontaneous abortion, etc., which accounts for between 7 and 14 per cent of each consultant's patients.)

The 'refusal' rates for city cases for the eight years 1963–70 combined divide the eight consultants into three distinct categories: three conservatives with refusal rates of between 37 and 40 per cent, four liberals with a rate of 16–21 per cent and one ultra-liberal who refused only 4 per cent (see Table 2:1). In the eight years the conservatives had refused more than twice the proportion of patients refused by the liberals. This was so for both married and single women. There was a tendency among the conservatives and one liberal to refuse more single than married women. The rest made no difference by marital state.

Looking at 1963–70 in four two-year intervals (see Table 2:2), while there is no consistent trend, by 1969–70 the conservatives had become rather more conservative, refusing 37 per cent compared with 27 per cent in 1963–4, while the liberals' refusal rates had remained the same (18 per cent). The greatest discrepancy between the two groups was in 1965–6 when the liberals refused 9 per cent to the conservatives' 41 per cent. By 1969–70, 18 per cent were refused by the liberals and 37 per cent by the conservatives.

It is worth noting that attempts have been made to see if it would be possible to arrive at a common policy for abortion and to arrive at defined criteria for determining which cases should be terminated and which not. All attempts failed because the doctors concerned differed in their evaluation of the risks of continuing as against terminating the pregnancy. This is in large measure due to inability to assess accurately the outcome in terms of mental health, one reason why the gynaecologists were anxious that psychological testing and follow-up should be carried out.

The refusal rate could very well have been influenced by the general practitioner who was referring the woman in the first place for a consultant opinion. Knowing the attitudes of the consultants, a general practitioner could send the patient to a liberal consultant if he wished the termination done, or conversely to a conservative consultant if he (the general practitioner) was not in favour of termination in that case. In the event, it was the liberal gynaecologists who were seeing most of the women seeking abortion, so much so that it became necessary to distribute the load more evenly in order to reduce the pressure on this group and also to avoid delay and adverse effects on teaching. This had the effect of randomising the allocation of abortion patients to consultants and the method (agreed with the general practitioners) was maintained for the duration of the sociological study. When the study had ended it was decided that patients would go to the consultant of the general practitioner's choice except when the numbers being referred to any individual consultant became too large and an undue delay would have occurred before he could see all the patients referred to him. In such circumstances the excess patients were transferred to another consultant. In this way that was still a fairly even distribution of cases amongst the consultants, but there is now more of a chance of the woman being seen by the consultant requested by the general practitioner than was likely to happen while the study was in progress.

It was also decided by the consultants that if a woman was refused termination she would not be seen by a second consultant unless under exceptional circumstances or after he had conferred with the first consultant. This has tended to ensure that the liberal consultants are not having to see an undue proportion of the women. As shown in the epidemiological section only a very small proportion obtained an abortion elsewhere when they were unsuccessful in having it done in Aberdeen.

GENERAL PRACTITIONERS

It is possible that the narrowing of the difference in the two groups in 1967–8 was due to the redistribution of the referrals. The general practitioner is in a particularly strong position to determine whether a termination is carried out or not, because he can tell the woman that he does not consider there are grounds for termination and that he will not refer her to a consultant. Unless the woman is persistent and determined this may be the end of the matter, but even though she insists on being referred to a consultant the general practitioner can choose a consultant who he knows would be likely to refuse termination. The general practitioner is, therefore, in a stronger position in this respect than the consultant to decide whether a woman should have a termination or not, and in this way they have a considerable influence on the abortion rates of an area. It is difficult to assess how much variation there is between them because their referrals cannot be expressed as rates when the number of women who ask their doctor for a termination is not known. It is unlikely that the requests are evenly distributed among general practitioners – indeed which doctor in a practice an applicant sees may be determined by her idea of which would be the most sympathetic to her request. Some idea of the variation can be gained by comparing referrals from different practices rather than from individual doctors and relating them to the numbers of women at risk, that is, women of reproductive age in the practice. We must then assume that about the same proportion of these women in each practice ask for termination and that overall there is no bias between practices in regard to applicants' length of gestation or severity of presenting indications for termination. Differences in referral rates might then reflect 'liberal' and 'conservative' attitudes in the practices. These are rather large assumptions to make, but in default of more precise data we have looked at referral rates in 34 practices in Aberdeen (as they were in 1971) run by 79 doctors (Table p. 53). All referrals between 1968 and 1970 are related to the population of women aged between 16 and 44 in the practice.†

In most of the practices (27) between 30 and 40 per cent of their female patients were aged 16–44. Referral rates in this group ranged from 1.3 (the lowest proportion referred in all practices) to 5.5 per cent. There was only one higher rate – 6.1 per cent in a practice in which 43 per cent of its women patients were in the at-risk age group.

If the woman happens to be on the practice list of a conservative practitioner, her only alternative really is to change her general practitioner or to seek an abortion elsewhere. Either of these solutions pre-

† Based on data made available by the local Health Executive Council for the research purposes of the University of Aberdeen departments of General Practice, Mental Health and Social Medicine and the MRC Medical Sociology Unit.

Percentage of women aged 16–44 referred	No. of practices
1.0–1.9	2
2.0–2.9	10
3.0–3.9	5
4.0–4.9	12
5.0–5.9	4
⩾ 6.0	1
	34

supposes that the woman is both determined and knowledgeable about the attitudes of general practitioners in the area or of alternative facilities. Such a strategy of 'shopping around' is further complicated by the urgency of the matter since a factor which influences the gynaecologist considerably more than the general practitioner or even psychiatrist in his decision-making is the duration of pregnancy. Some gynaecologists are quite willing to adopt a liberal attitude to a very early abortion but a conservative attitude to a later abortion, some indeed refusing to terminate an advanced pregnancy except under very extreme conditions. The length of gestation which is considered to be too long for termination varies, some considering the upper limit to be 20 weeks, others being willing to extend it to 24 weeks in exceptional cases. The method of termination varies, particularly in later gestations. Saline terminations, prostaglandins and hysterotomy all have their protagonists and antagonists. All the common methods of termination of pregnancy were used in this study but some were used only by a proportion of the gynaecologists. The methods are described on pp. 67–76 below.

DECISION-MAKING

The time spent by gynaecologists on decision-making varied considerably. Some were able to come to a fairly rapid decision in most instances. Although no two cases are quite comparable it is possible to sift them in broad categories, and for most gynaecologists it was a matter of collecting the basic facts to determine the group into which the patient fitted and then making the decision. Others spent considerable time not only interviewing the patient but in contacting the patient's doctor, usually by telephone, and having long discussions with him. Even then

53

they may have had difficulty in arriving at a decision and could only do so after consultation with their gynaecological colleagues and sometimes with a psychiatrist. Undoubtedly most of them found decision-making in abortion cases much more difficult than in straightforward gynaecological cases. Most were conscious of the fact that their decision-making could be influenced by many factors and that it was not always consistent. For example, the number of patients being seen for consideration of abortion at one session, the number of other urgent gynaecological cases known to be waiting for admission, the attitude of the nursing staff, junior medical staff and even medical students who might be present at the interviews, could all consciously or subconsciously play a part in influencing the gynaecologist's decision.

Once the decision was made the termination itself did not usually present problems to the gynaecologist although most would admit that they preferred ordinary gynaecological surgery even though the operation itself might be technically more difficult. It is difficult to determine the reason for this but possibly it was associated with the fear that something might go wrong and there was the feeling that a maternal death or a serious morbidity was particularly undesirable in these patients. All the gynaecologists at one time or another had had a case of termination which had caused them serious worry because of complications at the time of operation or soon afterwards, and although of course complications sometimes occur with other gynaecological conditions the degree of worry seems to be greater in cases of abortion.

This tends to strengthen the view that gynaecologists perform abortions either because they feel they have to or in a few cases because they are strongly motivated to do so mainly for socio-medical reasons.

ILLEGAL ABORTION

One of the greatest hopes of the abortion law reformers was that the number of illegal septic abortions would be greatly reduced when abortion was legalised. It is very difficult, however, to get any precise figures on illegal or septic abortion rates, although it is usually said that most septic abortions are illegally procured. This is by no means certain, and conversely by no means all illegal abortions are septic. Again the so-called spontaneous abortions which form the major part of abortion admissions are probably not all spontaneous. The number of unwanted illegitimate pregnancies has probably risen, as judged by the numbers being terminated. Some idea of the number of illegal abortions can be obtained by studying the figures for spontaneous abortions admitted to hospital. In the married women, however, this picture is confused by the fact that many more are now using contraceptives, and possibly they have a smaller number of unwanted pregnancies. Certainly there would seem to be a lesser number for which women would wish to risk having an illegal abortion. It is not surprising then that in Aberdeen the proportion of legitimate pregnancies ending in spontaneous abortion has remained the same. Possibly more informative are the figures for illegitimate pregnancies. Table 1:1 (p. 34 above) shows that the proportion of illegitimate pregnancies ending in so-called spontaneous abortions has fallen, and this may be due to a decrease in illegal abortions as legal abortions have increased.

Rhodes in 1966 stated that among 5000 abortions of all kinds he had dealt with in recent years, unequivocal evidence of the use of instruments was almost non-existent and objective evidence of the use of douches was rare.[2] We have no information of this sort from Aberdeen, but MacGillivray, also in London, showed that in a high proportion of admissions with incomplete abortions the abortion had been procured.[3]

The septic abortion rate has fallen, but whether this is due to the use of antibiotics by illegal abortionists or to better handling and care of patients with spontaneous incomplete abortions is uncertain. Septic abortions in Aberdeen numbered in 1962–4, 25 or 8.3 per annum; 1965–7, 15 or 5.0 per annum, and 1968–70, 7 or 2.3 per annum. The more reasonable explanation would seem to be that fewer illegal abortions are now being done. Diggory et al. suggest that between 20 and 25 per cent of all criminally induced abortions later require hospital admission, their estimate being based on questioning the women and on experience in general practice with patients who admitted interference and did not require hospital admission.[4] If the same applied in Aberdeen the number of illegal abortions in Aberdeen would be around 100 in 1962–4, 60 in 1965–7 and 28 in 1968–70.

Table 1:17 on p. 46 has shown that of the 617 women who were refused termination during the study and the outcome of whose pregnancy is known, 4.2 per cent had 'spontaneous' abortions. Even if some of the 66 pregnancies where the outcome was not known had ended in spontaneous abortion the total would not exceed the 10 per cent which, it is generally accepted, terminate in spontaneous abortion. It would seem therefore that very few of the women who were refused abortion resorted to illegal methods although, as Table 1:17 shows, a few (2.7 per cent of those known) obtained a legal abortion elsewhere.

INDICATIONS FOR REFERRAL AND TERMINATION

The Abortion Act sets out in general form the conditions under which termination of pregnancy is legal. In the nature of the case it does not, and cannot, set out the indications for abortion since these are myriad and occur in a virtually infinite number of combinations and permutations. Each case has its unique features and the consultant is, in effect, forced to make some overall judgement about the possible effects of intervening or not intervening on a variety of aspects of a family's life. Thus each patient, each referring doctor and each consultant has to have some idea, however vague and general, of what are acceptable grounds for having a pregnancy terminated. In some instances the woman's medical history or her present physical state is a predominating factor in her request and in the decision. In others the social circumstances may appear more relevant while in yet other cases the emotional stability of the woman assumes greater importance, though seldom does a single factor dominate to the exclusion of all others.

It follows from the above that any attempt to categorise patients according to the indications for termination is fraught with difficulty, since the referring doctor and the consultant are quite likely to place their emphasis on different elements in the total situation, and the client's own view of her situation may be quite different from either (see Chapters 3 and 4, 'The Woman's Story'). Despite these problems it was felt that some sort of retrospective classification would be worthwhile in order to uncover any systematic variations in referrals and terminations over time and as between consultants. Two of the gynaecologists (IMacG and KJD) examined the case notes on a hundred patients and on that empirical basis decided upon five main categories: medical, social, eugenic, socio-psychiatric and medico-psychiatric. There were, however, 'social factors' present in a large proportion of cases other than those where the main indication seemed to be the social circumstances of the woman and her family, so that three further 'mixed' categories seemed appropriate. The next hundred cases were classified independently by the two consultants and considerable agreement was achieved. Agreement became virtually complete after the third hundred and the rest were then shared by the two, a total of 1671 case records being examined. It must be emphasised that the classification was devised retrospectively by the two consultants taking into account all the available information on each case (including, for example, psychiatric and social reports, where they existed). As such it remains a *post hoc* classification and it does not therefore follow that every single case in the category 'socio-psychiatric', for instance, was referred on 'socio-psychiatric grounds' by the general practitioner, nor the decision made on those grounds by the consultant, nor does it follow, one might add, that the psychiatrists would have classified patients referred to them in the same way, although, as is noted in Chapter 5, the findings of the psychological study in regard to character disorder are broadly consistent with the gynaecologists' operational definitions.

Before going on to consider each category in more detail, it might be helpful to examine the distribution of all referrals over the several categories and the proportions in each which were terminated. These data are set out in Table 2:3. It will be observed that about three-quarters of the referrals for the years 1963–9 fell into either the category 'social' or one of the three combined categories in which there was a strong social component. The proportion in these categories increased from 57 per cent in the earlier to 79 per cent in the last year of the series. At the same time the proportion classified as primarily medical declined although absolute numbers remained fairly stable.

Medical indications

When a patient suffers from a recognised medical condition which is likely to deteriorate during pregnancy and/or to be aggravated by the care of a child. Examples are heart disease, emphysema, nephritis, serious varicose veins with previous thrombosis or embolism and also, although this is declining in incidence, debility through frequent and complicated child-bearing.

A decreasing proportion of women each year present with solely medical indications for termination of pregnancy, 4 per cent in 1969 compared with 11 per cent in 1963–4. However in the parity group 0–2 medical indications comprised the most frequent reason for referral. The great majority of the pregnancies were legitimate. Just over two-thirds of the women (68 per cent) had their pregnancy terminated.

EXAMPLES

(1) A nulliparous unmarried woman aged 20 was referred at the 14th week of pregnancy. The uterus was equivalent in size to 12 weeks gestation. She had had sexual intercourse with more than one steady boyfriend and the only contraception (used irregularly) was by condom. She suffered from severe asthma from the age of 4 and had had numerous admissions to hospital in status asthmaticus; in addition, at the age of 12 she developed juvenile diabetes and her co-operation in its control since then had been imperfect. There was no problem so far as insulin dosage was concerned, but she did not stick to her diet and in consequence was overweight.

The pregnancy was terminated on medical grounds by suction curettage and at follow-up examination the question of contraception was thoroughly discussed. The patient felt that she had 'learnt her lesson' and was most unwilling to contemplate contraception. Subsequently she approached her general practitioner having changed her mind and was referred to the contraceptive clinic. Because of her diabetic state she was fitted with a diaphragm but did not attend for follow-up examination. Two years later she was referred once again with an illegitimate pregnancy at 8 weeks gestation. This was again terminated by suction curettage on the same indication. After this, however, she readily accepted contraceptive advice and was fitted with an intrauterine device.

(2) This married woman of 24 had had two babies without complications. Two months prior to referral she had noticed a swelling in her neck and this was being investigated and treated at the thyroid clinic. Her general practitioner had referred her for consideration of abortion as he had gained the impression from the thyroid clinic that the pregnancy was likely to make the thyroid swelling worse. The patient was quite unsure about her menstrual data but the uterus corresponded in size to approximately 16 weeks gestation.

Full consultation then took place between the gynaecologist involved and the physician and the surgeon at the thyroid clinic. It was found that the patient had a degenerative colloid goitre and that, although surgical treatment appeared to be indicated, this should be postponed until the end of the current pregnancy. This recommendation was passed on to the family doctor and the patient duly had her baby without any complications. At follow-up examination she was well but requested sterilisation, which was subsequently performed.

Social indications

Where the external environment, both economic and cultural, is considered to be seriously prejudicial to continuation of the pregnancy. The woman's reaction to the pregnancy is thought to be in proportion to the effects of the unfavourable environment and there is no evidence of abnormality in the patient's previous personality. Social indications cover a wide range of environmental factors.

A quarter of the women referred had no grounds other than their social difficulties for requesting abortion. By 1969 their numbers had doubled. In 1963–4 few of these pregnancies were illegitimate but by 1969 women with illegitimate pregnancies applying for abortion for social reasons outnumbered women with legitimate pregnancies by two to one. Social reasons are presented more often by women who had had 4, or 5 or more, previous pregnancies than by women of lower parity. Acceptances for abortion were lower in this category than in any other group (38 per cent terminated), with no significant difference between legitimate and illegitimate.

EXAMPLES

(3) A first-year student, aged 18, pregnant to a student in the second year of a four-year course. The couple had discussed contraception with the doctor and had asked to be referred to the family planning clinic, but she had already fallen pregnant. The doctor was impressed by them and thought they were a sensible, responsible pair who had a stable relationship. He felt that termination would be the most satisfactory solution to their immediate problem and probably the least damaging to their relationship in the long term. The gynaecologist thought she was an immature person and that the putative father was not prepared to support her if she had the baby. Accordingly she had a suction termination of an 8 weeks pregnancy. When seen for follow-up eight months later she was very well and was on an oral contraceptive.

(4) A woman of 34, married for eleven years to a man who had recently set up his own business but had found that the business was encumbered with debts. He was trying to pay these off and she had to

manage on £6 per week. They had three children aged between 10 and 20 months and lived in a three-roomed flat up three flights of stairs, at a rent of £9 per month. She was worried and tired and did not feel able to cope with another baby. A hysterotomy and sterilisation was performed on a 16 weeks pregnancy and when seen for follow-up eight months later she was very well.

Eugenic indications

Where there is serious risk of abnormality in the baby. This is best exemplified by rubella which in this group was the commonest reason for referral. Other examples are muscular dystrophy, some forms of hydrocephaly and mongolism. It is now possible in certain cases to determine whether an abnormality is present by examining the liquor amnii, which is obtained by passing a needle through the abdominal wall.

The number of patients referred because of the possibility of serious risk of abnormality in the baby fluctuated in any one year from 2 to 20 and comprised only 3.5 per cent of all referrals.

EXAMPLES

(5) A single woman, aged 21, when 8 weeks pregnant had an attack of rubella during a rubella epidemic. The pregnancy was terminated at 10 weeks by dilatation and curettage. At follow-up five months later she was symptom-free and there was no pelvic abnormality.

(6) A married woman, aged 26, requested abortion because one of her two children had rubella and she was afraid she might have developed the disease. She had no clinical evidence of the disease and this was confirmed serologically. She was therefore allowed to continue with the pregnancy.

Socio-psychiatric indications

Where the woman's personality structure is not judged to be markedly deviant but where the stress of the pregnancy and of the total external environment produce a disproportionate emotional reaction. Thus most of the referrals of unmarried women with a first illegitimate pregnancy would be classified 'social', but if the stress was producing an 'excessive' response, e.g. an inability to sleep, deterioration in examination results, a socio-psychiatric indication might be considered to be present.

Ten per cent of all women referred were considered to have a disproportionate emotional reaction to the stress of the pregnancy and the total external environment. This proportion has remained much the same over the seven years. In this category the ratio of legitimate to illegitimate pregnancies was over two to one, and about 70 per cent of the patients were given terminations.

EXAMPLES

(7) A student aged 20, engaged to be married, was referred for termination of pregnancy when approximately 8 weeks pregnant. Contraception had not been used on all occasions, and when she found herself pregnant she assumed that the wedding would simply be put forward. Her fiancé, however, refused and this caused a great deal of emotional upset. At the time of referral she had just failed all her professional examinations. The gynaecologist to whom she was referred got the impression that she would become more depressed and perhaps morbid if the pregnancy were permitted to continue and abortion was performed by suction curettage from which she made an uneventful recovery.

(8) A woman aged 28 was referred by her family doctor for consideration of abortion after he had been treating her for some months for depression due principally to marital disharmony. She had been married for ten years and had three children, two girls and a boy. She had been on oral contraception but had not taken it regularly as she had felt it did not agree with her. At the time of referral she had had 10 weeks' amenorrhoea.

The gynaecologist's report stated that he thought she was fond of children and, provided that she had adequate support during her pregnancy, she would not be unwilling to have the baby. He also discussed contraception with her but found that she was unhappy about tubal ligation. He felt that abortion was not the answer and that perhaps marriage guidance counselling should be considered. A few months later she reported to the ante-natal clinic. She had now changed her mind and requested post-partum sterilisation. This was duly performed.

Medico-psychiatric indications

Where there was evidence taken from the previous psychiatric history or as a result of psychiatric examination during the pregnancy, that

61

the patient's personality structure before pregnancy was markedly deficient. This also includes some cases where the reaction to pregnancy was psychotic in degree.

Numbers in this category have fallen throughout the seven years. In all they account for 6 per cent of the total referred. Most (72) of the 103 pregnancies were legitimate. Medico-psychiatric indications became less common as family size increased, comprising 13 per cent of all indications among married women with 0–2 previous pregnancies, 7 per cent in those with 3 and 4 per cent in those with 4 or more. This group was second highest in regard to percentage terminated (78 per cent).

EXAMPLE

(9) This patient, aged 25, was a diabetic who had suffered from endogenous depression and had a previous history of attempted suicide. She had two children and was separated from her husband. There was no prospect of marriage to the putative father. In view of her long-standing mental history and previous admissions to a mental hospital termination was carried out by the injection of hypertonic saline when the pregnancy was of 17 weeks size. She was seen for follow-up three months later when an intrauterine contraceptive device was inserted. She was then quite well.

Medical/social indications

Nine per cent of women were referred with a combination of medical and social indications (as defined above) for requesting abortion. Nearly all were married (117 of the 143). Among these the proportion referred on 'medical/social' grounds increases with parity, only 6 per cent of women with 0–2 previous pregnancies being referred on these grounds, 12 per cent of those with 3 and 24 per cent of those with 4 or more. Seventy per cent of the women with both medical and social indications for abortion had this done, the medical component having the greatest weight.

EXAMPLE

(10) This patient, aged 32, was pregnant when she married at age 17 and was divorced four years later. Of her 7 previous pregnancies only the first 2 were to her husband. Four ended in the birth of live babies although 3 of these were pre-term and of low birth weight. Three pregnancies ended in abortion. She had custody of her four children.

Following the abortion which occurred two years prior to this referral, she had a prolonged spell in hospital with infective myocarditis. From this she had made a slow but steady recovery. She was a heavy smoker with marked chronic bronchitis. She had previously requested sterilisation but this had not been recommended due to her unstable marital state. In his referral letter, the family doctor stated that she was in poor physical health and fully extended, but she looked after her children as well as her hard-pressed financial circumstances would allow. He recommended that her pregnancy be terminated and that she be sterilised. This was done by curettage and laparoscopic sterilisation.

Socio-psychiatric/social indications

These combined indications are put forward by the largest proportion of the women seeking abortion in Aberdeen, one-third of the total, and this is the fastest growing category. Numbers have increased from 51 in 1963–4 to 209 in 1969. The rise is clearly associated with the great increase in illegitimate pregnancies over the seven years. Among married women with legitimate pregnancies socio-psychiatric/social grounds are associated with increasing parity, women with 4 or more previous pregnancies applying for abortion on these grounds more often than on any other. From 1965 onwards this was the largest category for single women applying for abortion. A high proportion of women referred on socio-psychiatric/social grounds had their pregnancy terminated (74 per cent) although not as high a proportion as in the medical/psychiatric categories.

Four examples are given from this numerous category.

EXAMPLES

(11) This woman, aged 29, had been married for ten years. Her first baby was born two months after marriage and was a difficult forceps delivery. The second pregnancy was complicated by a post-partum haemorrhage and varicose veins were troublesome throughout the pregnancy and also throughout her third pregnancy. In this, her fourth pregnancy, she was referred with the following letter:
'This woman requests termination of pregnancy threatening suicide if this is not done. As she is an anxious individual whose family are all neurotic, I believe she would attempt to carry out her threat. The situation between herself and her husband is not too happy,

and I should be very pleased to discuss this more fully by telephone. She has obviously been hoping for a miracle as her fundus suggests twelve to thirteen weeks gestation. Her menstrual cycle is very irregular. Physically, she is not very robust, although she has had no serious illness. She had severe varicosities, and was admitted because of them, before her last confinement. After much thought, I think that termination is the correct course. Failure to do so could have diastrous effects on the present family through her.'

The question of sterilisation had not been discussed with the patient by her doctor, but she readily grasped at the opportunity when it was mentioned to her. Termination was done by suction curettage, this was combined with a Pomeroy type sterilisation through a small incision. At follow-up four months later the patient's menstrual pattern had not changed although her periods were heavier than before. Pelvic examination was negative.

(12) A patient aged 27 had been married at age 16 and was divorced on the grounds of cruelty seven years later. While married she had been pregnant three times, resulting in the birth of two girls aged 7 and 4 and a stillborn boy. She lived with her two girls and her widowed mother of 60, who looked after the children while the patient was at work. The patient was the sole breadwinner for this household.

In his letter of referral the doctor stated that he did not consider the patient to be promiscuous and he believed she had had intercourse on one occasion only. He felt that in view of the social circumstances and the disastrous effect another pregnancy would have on the patient's mental well-being the pregnancy should be terminated. At operation suction curettage was performed and a cystic mass was felt behind the uterus. At laparotomy this was found to be a benign para-ovarian cyst which was removed. The patient failed to attend for a follow-up examination.

(13) A married woman of 25 requested termination of her pregnancy because of her fear of another pregnancy and fear that the child might not survive. Her first pregnancy had ended with a neo-natal death following a difficult forceps delivery. Her second baby was delivered by Caesarean section because of cephalo-pelvic disproportion. Her third child was also delivered by Caesarean section. Her husband was a motor mechanic and she also felt that there would be

financial difficulties if she had another baby. It was felt that there were not sufficient grounds to terminate this pregnancy and she was persuaded to continue with the pregnancy and have a post-partum sterilisation.

(14) A nulliparous first-year student of 20, presenting with 10 weeks' amenorrhoea, said she had had intercourse on one occasion only with the young man to whom she was engaged to be married. Her relationship with him was excellent and their plans for marriage unaffected by the pregnancy. She had, however, hoped to complete her training before marrying and starting a family.

The gynaecologist who saw her felt that a termination of pregnancy was not in the patient's best interest, but as she showed a very emotional reaction throughout the interview, she was referred for a psychiatric opinion. The consultant psychiatrist agreed with the gynaecologist's recommendation and stressed to the patient that it was important that her parents be informed of the situation. It was recommended to the family doctor that, should the patient's emotional state give rise to anxiety after the family had been informed, he would be very willing to reconsider the matter. Following this decision the couple were married and the pregnancy progressed uneventfully.

Medico-psychiatric/social indications

This small group of 92 comprises only 5.5 per cent of all referrals but where indications fall into this category the women concerned are more likely to have the pregnancy terminated than in any other category (85 per cent terminated). Illegitimate pregnancies predominate in this group.

EXAMPLES

(15) A young woman of 20 was referred when she had approximately 8 weeks' amenorrhoea. She had married at age 16 after she had known her husband for six months, and her first child was born, 10 weeks before term, a month after her marriage. The child had a congenital heart defect. The patient's mother helped a great deal with the care of the child. Nine months after the confinement the patient was admitted to a psychiatric hospital for three months, but while on leave of absence she became pregnant again to her husband. This pregnancy was terminated elsewhere on the advice of the psychiatrist and of her

family doctor, as her other baby was not yet a year old at the time. The patient then started oral contraception. Five months after the abortion she left her husband and took up residence with the putative father of the present pregnancy.

The decision about the second termination was not made in Aberdeen. After she was seen by the gynaecologist she was asked to go home to England and have the whole matter investigated there. It transpired that eventually she had a spontaneous abortion about a week later. The following year she was admitted to another psychiatric hospital as a Tuinal addict.

(16) A patient of 30 was referred when 6 weeks pregnant because of anxiety about the possible effect another child might have on her husband's ambitions and on their plans for the future of their only child, then at school. Some years earlier she had been seen by a psychiatrist for consideration of termination of a second pregnancy. She was then considered to be neurotic and hysterical. While a decision was being awaited she was admitted to hospital with an incomplete abortion. She was emphatic that this third pregnancy should not continue but the gynaecologist who saw her thought that the pregnancy should be allowed to continue and that she should have psychiatric supportive therapy throughout the pregnancy. She was, however, admitted when she was 10 weeks pregnant having attempted a self-induced abortion with soapy water douching.

On admission she was pyrexial and had lower abdominal tenderness. An antibiotic was commenced and the symptoms settled. A pregnancy test was positive and sonar examination showed a continuing pregnancy. She was warned that it would be dangerous to terminate the pregnancy in view of the pelvic sepsis. She continued through the pregnancy and was delivered of a baby weighing 2 lb. 14 oz. and it survived after being delivered at 29 weeks. A sterilisation was carried out three months after the birth of the baby and it was noted at operation that the left ovary was bound down by multiple adhesions. She had the right ovary and tube removed two years previously because of the presence of an ovarian cyst.

(17) This young married woman of 23, living apart from her husband, had two children aged 3 and 2. She said that the putative father of the present pregnancy had assaulted her. She had taken an overdose of Valium and was admitted to hospital because of that. She had had a

previous admission to a mental hospital for depression. Both a gynaecologist and a psychiatrist considered that there were sufficient grounds for terminating the 10 weeks pregnancy and this was done by suction.

Given that there are variations between consultants in the proportion of cases they accept for termination, one might expect that there would be greater differences between the conservatives and the liberals in the so-called 'social' indications than in those where a medical factor predominated. In fact, as Table 2:4 shows, the conservatives are more conservative over all the indication categories with the possible exception of 'eugenic', where, however, numbers are very small.

METHODS OF TERMINATION

It is only in fairly recent years that much attention has been given to developing new effective methods of termination of pregnancy, because in Britain gynaecologists formerly performed only small numbers of abortions and these were usually done by curettage or by hysterotomy. With the greatly increased numbers of abortions being done in hospitals, doctors wish to see the present rather unsatisfactory methods replaced by methods that are efficient, rapid and safe. Some of the methods most commonly used by women were developed by criminal abortionists, and so-called abortifacients were and still are sold in chemists or rubber goods shops. Many substances were advocated which could be taken by mouth, the most common being apiol, pennyroyal, aloes, lead, quinine and ergot. These substances are not likely to be effective except in dosages which would endanger the life of the woman. Other methods developed by criminal abortionists involve the introduction of foreign bodies such as the crochet hook or similar implements, into the uterus. Rubber catheters, sounds, needles, slippery elm bark and even slivers of wood have been used in the past. In a survey of procured abortions carried out in London[5] the syringe or douche using soap and Dettol was found to be the method most commonly used. The resulting complications which may occur are haemorrhage, infection, renal failure, soap intoxication and trauma of the vagina, cervix, uterus or bladder.

Gynaecologists in the past also used substances which were introduced into the uterus, in particular Utus paste (medicated soft soaps). This is fairly effective but there is a risk of infection, embolism or haemorrhage occurring. Laminaria tents (seatangle tents) were also used. These were introduced into the cervix and as they absorbed the water they became swollen and caused the cervix to dilate. Again sepsis was the problem and the abortion was often incomplete. In more advanced pregnancies gum elastic bougies, catheters or balloons were introduced through the cervix into the uterus. These caused irritation of the uterus and were liable to produce sepsis.

It is now recognised that there is no effective means of procuring abortion by any oral drug, and that any drug that is going to be effective must be given parenterally or into the uterus. Intramuscular or intravenous ergometrine or pitocin or syntocinon have been tried but are not effective in causing an abortion, although continuous syntocinon infusion intravenously can aid in the emptying of the uterus if another method, e.g. the intra-amniotic injection of a substance, has been employed. The recently introduced prostaglandins are proving fairly effective.

It has been known for a long time that substances introduced into the amniotic cavity will cause the uterus to contract and expel the contents. This was found to be one of the disadvantages of using radio-opaque substances injected into the amniotic sac for the identification of placenta praevia. Various substances (dextrose, saline, inulin and formalin) have been used. These are quite effective in causing abortion, but there is a considerable risk of intrauterine sepsis particularly if dextrose is used, and fatalities have been reported with the use of saline due to intravascular injection causing cerebral infarction. These methods must be employed with considerable care and obviously can only be employed if the uterus is enlarged to a sufficient size to allow the amniotic sac to be entered with assurance. Although the technique is usually employed after the uterus is enlarged to 16 weeks size or more through the trans-abdominal route the method has also been employed in earlier pregnancies through the trans-cervical route.

In pregnancies before about 12 weeks the usual method employed is to dilate the cervix and remove the contents of the uterus with forceps and curette, or more recently the method has been introduced of evacuating with a suction aspirator. This is generally done under anaesthesia but can be done under a local anaesthetic. It is possible to evacuate a uterus by suction up to 14 or 15 weeks gestation, but generally at this stage or later a vaginal or abdominal hysterotomy is performed under a general anaesthetic if an operative procedure is decided on.

The vaginal operation is technically more difficult but leaves no abdominal scar. For the abdominal operation a vertical incision can be made or a low transverse incision which will be less visible. The latter might be of advantage psychologically because a woman might react badly to being constantly reminded by an abdominal scar of a termination of pregnancy.

There have been claims recently for a new method which promises to be hopeful. This is the use of prostaglandin. There are several different prostaglandins, but the ones most commonly used are E and F. The results so far reported are encouraging but there are too few cases and from too small a number of centres to allow a true assessment of their value.

The methods most commonly in use will now be considered in more detail and an assessment made of their advantages and disadvantages and the specific indications and contra-indications for each method.

1   Dilatation and curettage (D & C)

A general anaesthetic is usually given and the cervix is dilated with a graduated dilator sufficiently to allow an ovum forceps or sponge-holding forceps to be passed through the cervical canal into the uterus. The conceptus is then grasped and removed piecemeal with the forceps. The small pieces remaining are then scraped out with a curette. It is usually recommended that a blunt curette is used. It is considered essential that an oxytocic preparation, either syntocinon or ergometrine or a combination of the two, is given before the uterus is evacuated, otherwise haemorrhage can be considerable. There is a danger too that the uterus might be perforated either with the forceps or with the curette. Care must be taken to try to avoid tearing of the internal cervical os, as this might lead to incompetence of the cervix and spontaneous abortion of a subsequent pregnancy. Dilatation of the cervix can often be facilitated by an injection of a local anaesthetic into the para-cervical tissue. Sepsis can usually be avoided by attention to technique. This method is indicated in early pregnancy, but is contra-indicated after the 12th week of pregnancy. It was the method of choice in early pregnancy until the advent of the next method.

2   Vacuum aspiration

This method was used in China and then in Russia and Czechoslovakia before it was introduced to Britain. It has become increasingly popular here over the past five or six years. The cervix is dilated in the same way as for curettage after an oxytocic substance has been given. The metal or plastic aspirator is then introduced through the cervix. The size of the aspirator depends on the duration of pregnancy. A negative pressure of 0.4–0.6 kg./sq. cm. is then applied and the uterine contents aspirated. This can be usually done almost bloodlessly, but if the uterus is relaxed then very considerable haemorrhage will occur. Sepsis should not be a problem if the technique is employed properly, but again there is danger of causing damage to the cervix in dilating it. This is particularly true the further on the pregnancy is and the more the cervix has to be dilated. This method can be used up to 14 or 15 weeks pregnancy size, but the dangers and complications increase as gestation advances In pregnancies before 10 weeks local analgesia induced by paracervical block is sufficient for the operation. A plastic aspirator (Karman) is gaining in popularity for use in early pregnancy.

3 Intra-amniotic injections

Of the various substances used, hypertonic saline is now the most commonly employed. A wide-bore needle is introduced into the abdomen about two or three finger-breadths above the symphysis pubis, after injecting a local anaesthetic into the abdominal wall. It is important that in this technique the patient is not anaesthetised as her reaction to the intra-amniotic injection must be observed while she is conscious. The amniotic fluid is then aspirated. Usually about 200 ml. are removed, and 200 ml. of 20% saline are injected either through the needle or through a fine plastic catheter. Abortion usually occurs within twenty-four hours but may be delayed in some cases and have to be assisted by an oxytocin infusion. The method is effective and safe if great care is employed. The dangers are the introduction of infection, intravascular injections or the injection of too large a volume of saline causing cerebral infarction. In some cases the placenta is retained and has to be removed after dilatation of the cervix under general anaesthesia. The method is contra-indicated in cases with severe medical conditions such as renal disease, cardiac disease or hypertension. It is most suitable for the physically healthy woman for whom termination has been recommended on psychiatric or social grounds.

4 Utus paste

After cleansing the vulva and vagina with an antiseptic solution the cervix is grasped and the cannula is introduced into the uterus through the cervical canal. The Utus paste is injected slowly at a rate of 2 ml. per minute in an amount of 1–2 ml. per week of gestation. Pre-medication is given but it is usually not necessary to give a general anaesthetic. This method has the advantage that the procedure is easy and it is possible to cause abortion of advanced pregnancies. It is, however, not an infallible method and further stimulation with a syntocinon drip or a further injection of Utus paste is sometimes necessary, and occasionally complete evacuation of the uterus can only be achieved by dilatation and curettage. Other disadvantages of the methods are the risks of infection and trauma. The method is not popular in Britain.

5 Hysterotomy

This is done either by the abdominal or the vaginal route. In the abdominal operation a vertical or low transverse incision is made. In the vaginal operation an incision is made high in the cervix and the isthmus of the uterus is opened after the bladder has been displaced upwards out of the way. The advantages of hysterotomy are that sepsis and haemorrhage are usually avoided and sterilisation can be carried out while the abdomen is opened. The disadvantages, however, are a longer stay in hospital and scarring of the uterus. The operation is carried out in women where sterilisation is also going to be performed and in other girls or women with pregnancies enlarged beyond 14 weeks.

6 Prostaglandins

From the reports which are available it appears that the continuous infusion of prostaglandins intravenously is a fairly effective method of emptying the pregnant uterus. Distressing side effects, such as diarrhoea and vomiting, are unfortunately common. Both extra-amniotic and intra-amniotic injections and infusions of prostaglandins are being evaluated and the early results suggest that the extra-amniotic infusion is the more effective method. Early results of the use of vaginal prostaglandins appear to be encouraging. If this method is indeed successful then it will rapidly take the place of all others when prostaglandins become freely available.

All these methods have been used in Aberdeen and their frequency of use is shown in Table 2:5. Prostaglandins were not available for use in Aberdeen until after 1969 and have not yet been used extensively because of limitation in supplies. There has been a change in the type of abortion performed since 1963 partly because of the different type of patients having termination, in particular the rising number of primigravidae, and partly because of the new methods which have become available, in particular suction. Another change has been brought about by the new methods employed for sterilisation when termination is also being performed. It was the usual practice to do a hysterotomy and tubal ligation through a fairly large abdominal incision. This has been replaced particularly in early pregnancies by vaginal termination followed by either laparoscopic sterilisation or sterilisation through a very small supra-pubic incision. The technique for laparoscopic sterilisation is to make a small stab wound below the umbilicus and to introduce the laparoscope. The Fallopian tubes are identified and can either be coagulated with an electric cautery or divided and cauterised. The alternative method of sterilisation through a small supra-pubic incision has taken advantage of part of the laparoscopic sterilisation technique in that an assistant anteverts the uterus and pushes the Fallopian tubes upwards towards the small incision so that the tubes can be reached easily. The tubes are then crushed, ligated and a portion excised.

The number of hysterotomies without sterilisation has never been large, indeed the highest number reached was in 1968 when 21 were done. The fall in the number of hysterotomies in 1969 occurred mainly because unmarried women attended earlier in pregnancy and also because cases formerly done by hysterotomy could now be done by suction termination up to 14 weeks pregnancy size. The percentage of cases having a hysterotomy and sterilisation was high in 1963–4 when many of the terminations were for multiparity. When all sterilisations in association with termination of pregnancy are considered together, that is, hysterotomy and sterilisation, and sterilisation with either D & C, suction or saline, the total number had risen from 72 in 1963–4 to 87 in 1969, including pregnant hysterectomies.

Dilatation and curettage was the common method of terminating early pregnancies until 1968 when suction termination became popular. The suction method had been introduced to Aberdeen in 1967 when 14 suction terminations were performed on city patients. By 1969 the number of terminations by suction had risen to 116 compared with 50 by dilatation and curettage. Hysterectomy was a common method of terminating pregnancy between 1963 and 1966 but thereafter only a few cases were done by this method, possibly due to the introduction of the vaginal termination combined with the simpler sterilisation techniques. Saline terminations were fairly common between 1963 and 1966 but the percentage of cases fell thereafter. This coincided with the introduction of the suction method of termination and cases that would have been considered too far advanced for dilatation and curettage were then done by suction rather than saline.

The introduction of the suction method considerably reduced the duration of the patient's stay in hospital. This was achieved in several ways. First, in patients having a sterilisation as well as termination a major abdominal operation is avoided which before had necessitated a stay of up to two weeks in hospital. Secondly, the pregnancy considered too far advanced for D & C is terminated by saline instead of hysterotomy, necessitating a stay of usually only three or four days in hospital. Patients presenting early enough, that is before the 8th week of pregnancy, are now aborted as outpatients, but unfortunately the number of such patients is still relatively small.

Suction termination seems at the moment to be the most satisfactory method provided that the length of gestation is less than 14 weeks. The earlier the pregnancy the easier and safer the method, not only in terms of immediate risk of haemorrhage but also in avoiding damage to the cervix which would interfere with future child-bearing. The cervix should only be dilated sufficiently to allow the appropriate size of suction tube to be inserted. If the pregnancy is early enough a plastic catheter of the Karman type can be used. General anaesthesia is not required in such cases, but infiltration of the cervix with local anaesthesia makes dilatation of the cervix easier and painless for the patient. Sterilisation can be carried out immediately following the suction termination, but a general anaesthetic is usually required and again the sterilisation is usually easier if the pregnancy is of short duration because a bulky uterus makes the tubes difficult to identify through the laparoscope or through a small supra-pubic incision.

The real problem is in dealing with the pregnancy which is over 12 weeks in duration. Up to 14 weeks termination can be done by suction but the chances of haemorrhage or damage to the uterus and cervix are increased. Abdominal or vaginal hysterotomy are not desirable because of the greater magnitude of the operation, the greater likelihood of

73

complications and the longer hospital stay. Intrauterine injection of substances such as saline, dextrose and urea have their disadvantages and their dangers, but if sepsis is avoided and great care is taken to ensure that the injection is made into the amniotic sac the methods are still acceptable. However, the patient may have to spend several days in hospital awaiting the start of uterine contractions and it is then not uncommon for the abortion to be incomplete and for it to be completed with a suction or a curettage, usually under general anaesthetic.

The introduction of prostaglandins appeared at first to go a long way towards resolving the problem but it was fairly soon appreciated that intravenous use was associated with a high incidence of side effects, for example diarrhoea and vomiting, and also that in some cases the infusion was not effective and had to be augmented with an infusion of syntocinon. The intra-amniotic injection appeared to be an improvement but was also associated with some failure and at present the extra-amniotic intrauterine infusion seems to provide the best answer for cases with gestation lengths of 14 weeks or more.

Clearly the method of termination employed is to a considerable extent dictated by the duration of pregnancy, and one of the problems facing Aberdeen gynaecologists has been the late stage of pregnancy of many of the women accepted for abortion, particularly when the pregnancy is illegitimate. As can be seen in Table 2.6, up to 1967 the duration of pregnancy of nearly two-thirds of the women aborted was 13 weeks or later at the time of operation, with a third of the illegitimate and a quarter of the legitimate pregnancies at 18 weeks or later. More recently, however, there has been a trend towards earlier attendance, and in 1969 half the women accepted for abortion had the operation before the 13th week, with only 9 per cent at 18 weeks or later. Unfortunately the number being aborted at an early stage (i.e. before 8 weeks) is still very small.

Efforts are being made in Aberdeen and in most other centres to encourage women with unwanted pregnancies to apply for abortion as early as possible. General practitioners are being advised to refer such women to a gynaecologist before waiting to see if the next period comes and then sending a urine specimen for pregnancy test or, even worse, giving a hormone pill to see if this would bring on the period, before they get the pregnancy test done. Patients who are referred early enough are having their pregnancies terminated as outpatients whenever possible. This necessitates some reorganisation of theatres and working timetables, but no centre should find any particular difficulty in organising an outpatient termination of pregnancy service. Even when it is considered that the patient might be nervous and a general anaesthetic required this can still be done on an outpatient basis. It does mean that patients have to be checked at the outpatient department to see if they are fit enough for a general anaesthetic. As the majority of such cases are physically healthy young women this does not usually present any great problem. It is also necessary, of course, to take blood for blood grouping, not only in case a blood transfusion should be required but also so that anti-D immunoglobulin can be given to rhesus negative women, thus preventing haemolytic disease in a baby of a subsequent pregnancy.

There are many reports now of outpatient abortion units and the 'lunch-time abortion' is now quite common. Most of the reports are from enthusiasts and not unnaturally suggest that troubles are few and easily dealt with. Some who are less enthusiastic are more critical and have reported an unusually high incidence of complications.[6,7] It is argued that the doctors doing outpatient abortions are not able to report on complications because they do not keep the patients in hospital long enough to observe immediate complications and do not usually carry out any follow-up. While it is possible to determine immediate complications with considerable accuracy subsequent follow-up and determination of complications is much more difficult. It is not sufficient, however, to report on the immediate or even the late complications of termination without reference to what might have happened if the pregnancy had gone to a viable stage, or if a spontaneous abortion had occurred. So far no such study has been carried out, but it is hoped that one might be undertaken in Aberdeen. The intention would be to compare the subsequent reproductive performance in nulliparous single women who have had a spontaneous abortion, a therapeutic abortion or an illegitimate pregnancy to try to determine whether there are differences in the subsequent pregnancies of the three groups, particularly in terms of mid-trimester abortions and premature labours.

One difficulty which arises in dealing with outpatient terminations is that a recovery area is necessary. If there is no recovery area, of if this is being occupied by patients having other operations, beds in the ward have to be used for this purpose which could otherwise be used for patients with other gynaecological conditions. The recovery time after an outpatient abortion is usually quite short so that beds are not usually occupied for very long. It might be necessary to use other facilities such as delivery beds in a maternity hospital for this purpose and this has been done to a limited extent in Aberdeen for the past two years. Problems of bed utilisation are examined further in the next section of this chapter.

UTILISATION OF BEDS FOR TERMINATION OF PREGNANCY

For several years there has been a growing demand for gynaecological treatment. This has occurred in Aberdeen as in other parts of the country and has resulted in long waiting lists for gynaecological beds. Several factors operate in increasing the demand for gynaecological treatment. The increasing safety of operations and of anaesthesia encourages women to seek treatment and also allows the gynaecologist to operate on patients who would otherwise have been considered too great a risk. With increasing sophistication women are less likely to put up with annoying symptoms such as heavy periods or urinary incontinence even though these are not going to cause risk to her life. As the life expectancy of women has been increasing not only is there more time to develop gynaecological conditions, but also there are more chances of her developing atrophic conditions the further she is past the menopause. This increase in demand has been only partly compensated for by a shorter duration of stay in hospital after operation and by outpatient treatment, which are now much more common.

The increasing use of hospital beds for abortions has aggravated the problem even though some abortions are done early and on an outpatient basis; this still means theatre time and occupation of beds which could be used for other minor operations suitable for outpatient treatment. In general abortions are considered as urgent cases because the longer the pregnancy lasts the greater the risk of complications with termination of pregnancy. This means that they cannot go on to a waiting list and there is, therefore, bound to be a hold-up on the admission of other cases. It is, therefore, inevitable that the pressure on beds has been increased and efforts have had to be made to accommodate these cases without jeopardising too much the chances of the other cases of being admitted.

In Aberdeen the situation has been eased by the fall in the birth rate. Unlike many other areas where it was only recently that a high proportion of women had been confined in hospital (85 per cent in England and Wales in 1970), hospital confinement has been the practice in Aberdeen for many years. The NHS hospital confinement rate for all parities in Aberdeen has now reached 95 per cent. The annual number of births to city women alone has fallen by about 600 between 1963 and 1970, which has obviously reduced the demand for obstetric beds. Before the introduction of the Abortion Act very few terminations were performed in the Maternity Hospital. These were mainly for hyperemesis gravidarum or some serious medical condition, and the majority were performed by hysterotomy. Now many vaginal terminations and intra-amniotic saline and prostaglandin terminations are carried out in the Maternity Hospital. However, over this period of time there has been an increasing number of higher risk cases admitted from the country districts to the main Maternity Hospital, so that the total number of deliveries in the Maternity Hospital has not been reduced. Otherwise it might have been possible to do many more terminations in the Maternity Hospital, but as mentioned elsewhere, there tends to be more resistance on the part of midwives to therapeutic abortion than amongst gynaecological nurses. During 1963–70, 1421 therapeutic abortions further decreased the demand for obstetric beds for deliveries, but some of these beds were used for the abortions. Over these years there has been no change in the number of obstetric beds in Aberdeen, but there has been a slight increase in the gynaecological bed complement from 96 in 1965–7 to 114 in 1969–70.

The numbers on the waiting list vary throughout the year so that the mean of the number at the end of each quarter of the year has been taken. A more accurate picture is also given by dividing the cases into major abdominal, major vaginal and minor operations (Table 2:7). There was an increase in the numbers of both majors and minors from 1965 to 1967, but the total number fell in 1968 because of a fall in major abdominal operations and again in 1969 because of a reduction in the numbers of major vaginal cases awaiting operation. This in turn was due both to a conscious attempt to reduce the numbers of major cases and to an unexplained fall in the actual numbers being put on the waiting list. The numbers in 1970, however, had risen again, but the position was not as bad as it was in 1967, because although there were more minor cases on the waiting list there had been a reduction in the major cases. The number of major cases on the waiting list fell from 667 in 1967 to 574 in 1968, and was about the same in 1970. The total numbers rose again in 1971 but this rise was almost entirely due to major abdominals and more particularly to the greatly increased numbers of sterilisations. In 1971 there were 222 cases for sterilisation among the 446 for major abdominal operation.

Although the cases for termination must undoubtedly have caused some of the increase in the waiting time for gynaecological beds the figures in Table 2:8 show that this is not the whole reason. This table shows the number of obstetric and gynaecological beds required for termination of pregnancy in North-east Scotland, which has a population of about half a million, and also the number of bed days for these cases. It also shows how the beds in the Maternity Hospital are now being used for doing terminations. There were only 30 cases terminated in the Maternity Hospital obstetric beds in 1967, but this number went up to 181 in 1970. This amounted to a saving of 677 bed days for the gynaecological wards. The number of gynaecological bed days used for termination was 2549 for 254 patients in 1967 and 3336 for 552 patients in 1971. The average bed days were almost halved (from 10.0 to 5.3). Thus in spite of the increased number of patients the bed occupancy has not increased correspondingly. This is due to a higher proportion of minor termination operations.

The change in the type of operations and number of operations done in the obstetric beds and in the gynaecological beds is shown in Table 2:9, for Aberdeen city cases in 1968–71. The number of cases for suction or curettage in obstetric beds has increased from 3 in 1968 to 80 in 1969 and 88 in 1970, with a fall in the number of abdominal operations from 9 in 1968 to nil in 1971. Admissions to obstetric beds for saline terminations also increased from 5 in 1968 to 33 in 1969 and 39 in 1970, and fell in the gynaecological wards from 37 in 1968 to nil in 1971. Although there was an increase in the number of suction terminations and curettages from 1968 to 1971 in the gynaecological beds from 78 to 186, the relative increase was not nearly so great as in the obstetric beds. A slight fall in the number of such terminations in obstetric beds is apparent in 1971. The number of abdominal operations in the gynaecological beds did not alter significantly and the number of saline termination cases fell markedly from 37 in 1968 to 4 in 1970 and to zero in 1971. It was a result of deliberate policy that saline terminations should be performed only in the Maternity Hospital where the facilities were better, in that there were more single rooms, whereas in the gynaecological ward there was no privacy for the supervision of abortion. Although there has been some help in easing of pressure on the gynaecological beds by utilising obstetric beds it was felt that there was a limit to the number of terminations which should be put into obstetric beds. This was mainly because it was felt that if large numbers of terminations of pregnancy were put into the obstetric wards there might be resistance from the midwives.

The total gynaecological bed days (used for abortion in the gynaecological wards) were 1490 in 1968, 1233 in 1969, 1522 in 1970 and 1630 in 1971, whereas obstetrical bed days rose from 181 in 1968 to 439 in 1969. There was no further increase in 1970 in the usage of obstetric beds, and there was a significant decrease to 291 in 1971. If the number of cases of terminations increases further it may become necessary to use more obstetric beds in the Maternity Hospital for abortions, but it is felt that it would be preferable if more gynaecological beds could be provided.

Table 2:10 compares the length of stay in hospital for abortion of Aberdeen ever-married and single women from 1968 to 1971. For single women the average number of bed days fell from 6.0 in 1968 to 3.6 in 1971, and for the ever-married it was 9.4 in 1968 and 6.3 in 1971. The reason for the longer average stay of the ever-married women is that many were also sterilised and required an abdominal operation (Table 2:11). Those ever-married women who were also sterilised as well as having a termination were in hospital for an average of 11.9 bed days in 1968, compared with those aborted without sterilisation who were in for an average of 4.8 bed days. In 1971 the comparable figures were 8.2 for the sterilised as against 3.6 for those who were not sterilised. The bed days for the married women who were not sterilised are comparable to those for the single women. The length of stay for women being terminated and sterilised has been reduced because in most cases in which the pregnancy is of sufficiently short duration a suction termination is carried out followed by sterilisation through a laparoscope or a small supra-pubic incision. Previously a hysterotomy and sterilisation was carried out through a fairly large abdominal incision and this necessitated a longer stay in hospital.

There is no doubt that too much time is being spent by the women in hospital for termination. This is due in part to their not consulting the general practitioner early enough and partly because they are not referred early enough by the doctors to the clinic. An appeal has been made to all the doctors in the region to send the women as early as possible if they are likely to be seeking termination of pregnancy. As a result of earlier referral it has now become possible to operate on some women as outpatients. Apart from the necessity of restricting this to early pregnancies there is an additional limitation on outpatient abortions, however, because many of our patients come from a considerable distance outside the city, and have in any case to stay overnight.

Outpatient time, theatre time and beds must be used for termination of pregnancy cases. Even if special abortion clinics were to be set up, this requires clinic time and even though many of the cases can be done as outpatients this requires the provision of theatre space and recovery beds. The population served by the consultants in Aberdeen is small enough to allow them to deal with termination cases at the gynaecological clinics and in gynaecological and obstetrical beds without the necessity to set up special clinics or have a special abortion unit. This means that all the consultants take part in dealing with abortion cases and the load is spread fairly evenly, and in addition the consultants do not require to see a concentration of termination cases at one time. They all prefer to do this rather than deal with a large number on one occasion. They feel that this would place more strain on them than seeing a small number interspersed with gynaecological cases even although they are seeing abortion cases more frequently than if they were to take turns at running an abortion clinic. In larger centres the consultant gynaecologists might find it preferable to set up separate abortion clinics and abortion units.

GYNAECOLOGICAL FOLLOW-UP

Because of the difficulties of getting good follow-up data in pregnancy termination cases, much uncertainty still exists concerning the physical effects of the operation. The operation is, in any case, often performed where a woman has pre-existing symptoms, especially dysmenorrhoea in the nullipara, and menorrhagia and vaginal discharge in the parous woman.

An attempt was therefore made to evaluate the woman's physical well-being, and the incidence of certain gynaecological symptoms. For those whose pregnancy was terminated this was done at a point in time when, had the pregnancy been allowed to continue, the stage of gestation would have been 34 weeks; whereas the assessment was carried out at the time of the post-natal examination, 6 to 8 weeks after delivery, in those whose termination was not carried out.

At this time the patient was submitted to a structured interview, and, at the same time, an abdominal, pelvic and vaginal examination was carried out, and a cervical smear was taken for cytological examination. The 'symptoms' emerging from this interview, and the findings on examination were compared with the gynaecological history and findings obtained at the original 'referral' examination. For the purpose of the subsequent tabulations each symptom in each case was assessed as being 'unchanged', 'better' or 'worse'. It must be emphasised that these categories are mostly dependent on the patient's own assessment of her symptoms and well-being rather than on any objective tests.

Menstruation

Table 2:12 shows that menstrual flow and associated symptoms were thought to be unchanged in approximately one-half of those whose pregnancy was terminated. In nulliparae, whether the pregnancy was terminated or not, an improvement was more commonly experienced than a deterioration, whereas in multiparae this position was reversed. The table shows that menstruation, where it has been changed at all, appears to have been affected more by the fact that the patient had been pregnant rather than by any termination operation. The only exception to this general statement (see Table 2:17) appears to be in cases where a hysterotomy and sterilisation operation had been performed in an elderly multiparous patient. These women appeared to experience menstrual problems very frequently.

Abdominal and pelvic pain

In Table 2:13 most of those classified as 'same' had no pain either before or after their pregnancy. It must also be stressed that all positive responses to the question 'Have you any pain in your abdomen, down below, or with intercourse?' were taken into account. This explains the relatively high proportion of women complaining of 'pain' and therefore classified as 'worse' both in the 'Terminated' and 'Not terminated' categories. Perhaps the noteworthy finding under this heading is that this is a more important feature following second trimester termination by saline injection and hysterotomy (see Table 2:18).

Leucorrhoea

An increase in vaginal discharge at the time of the follow-up examination was thought to be present by a large proportion of the women, whether the pregnancy had been terminated or not (see Table 2:14). Not one subject felt that the pregnancy had caused any reduction in vaginal secretion. The method of termination used (see Table 2:19) appears to have been immaterial so far as the incidence of leucorrhoea is concerned.

Urinary symptoms

Although the number of women who developed urinary symptoms after pregnancy termination was small (Table 2:15), the incidence of urinary symptoms at the time of the follow-up examination was significantly higher in those terminated compared with those whose pregnancy progressed. Whether these residual urinary symptoms were due to the catheterisation done in most cases of termination, whatever method was used, is impossible to state, but the fact that urinary symptoms were less common following termination done by saline injection (see Table 2:20) suggests that this may be so. In any case, in all termination cases, women should be warned about the possibility of subsequent urinary symptoms, and about the need to have these investigated and treated.

General health

Finally, the women were asked whether they were, in general terms, feeling better, worse or unchanged as the result of their recent pregnancy. Very few thought that their health had changed in any way (Table 2:16). In the few cases where there was a change, it was, however, always for the worse. It was the multiparae whose pregnancy had been terminated, rather than the young nulliparae, who more often admitted to some deterioration in their general health. The method of termination (Table 2:21) did not appear to be an important factor.

Conclusion

This assessment of physical well-being after termination of pregnancy is limited by being a single assessment in one point of time only. Had it not been carried out with a number of 'control' subjects, who were also pregnant, but whose pregnancy was not terminated, the conclusion that pregnancy termination causes ill health in a large proportion of cases would have been inescapable. In this study the changes in symptomatology appear to have been due to the fact that the subject has recently been pregnant rather than that she has had a pregnancy terminated. The two exceptions to this generalisation appear to have been that in approximately 6 per cent of pregnancy terminations significant urinary symptoms were present; and that menstruation frequently deteriorated following hysterotomy and sterilisation in the elderly multiparous woman.

REFERENCES

1 The Abortion Act, 1967: Findings of an Inquiry into the First Year's Working of the Act conducted by the Royal College of Obstetricians and Gynaecologists, *Brit. med. J.*, 1970, **2**, 529.
2 Rhodes, P. (1966). In *Abortion in Britain*, proceedings of a conference held by the Family Planning Association at the University of London Union, Pitman Medical Publishing Co. Ltd., London.
3 MacGillivray, I. (1964). 'The clinical features of procured abortion', *Medicine, Science and the Law*, July, p. 175.
4 Diggory, P., Peel, J., Potts, M. (1970). 'Preliminary assessment of the 1967 Abortion Act in practice', *Lancet*, **1**, 287–91. Reference to the basis of the estimate is made in W. H. James, 'The incidence of illegal abortion', *Population Studies*, 1971, XXV, 2, 327.
5 MacGillivray (1964).
6 Stallworthy, A. S., Moolgaoker, A. S., Walsh, J. J. (1971). 'Legal abortion: a critical assessment of its risks', *Lancet*, **2**, 1245.
7 Good, S. V. (1971). 'Some operative and post-operative hazards of legal termination of pregnancy', *Brit. med. J.*, **4**, 270.

TABLE 2:1. *Referrals to consultants: proportion done, refused, not done for other reasons: 1963–70 combined*

			Number			Per cent		
		Total	Done	Refused	NDOR†	Done	Refused	NDOR†
Conservatives	(a)	126	57	51	18	45.2	40.5	14.3
	(b)	321	164	128	29	51.1	39.9	9.0
	(c)	216	119	77	20	55.1	35.6	9.3
Ultra-liberal	(d)	95	84	4	7	88.4	4.2	7.4
Liberals	(e)	246	176	40	30	71.5	16.3	12.2
	(f)	305	210	65	30	68.9	21.3	9.8
	(g)	302	217	53	32	71.9	17.5	10.6
	(h)	336	250	60	26	74.4	17.9	7.7

† Not done, other reasons.

TABLE 2:2. *Refusal rates of 'liberal' and 'conservative' gynaecologists: 1963–70*

	All years			1963–4			1965–6			1967–8			1969–70		
	Total	Refused	%	Total	Refused	%	Total	Refused	%	Total	Refused	%	Total	Refused	%
Liberals	1287	223	17.3	132	24	18.2	185	17	9.2	426	85	19.9	544	97	17.8
Conservatives	663	256	38.6	74	20	27.0	101	41	40.6	180	80	44.4	308	115	37.3

TABLE 2:3. *Indications for referral by year, and per cent terminated: 1963–9*

Indications	Total referred	Per cent referred	Per cent referred by year					Per cent terminated
			1963–4	1965–6	1967	1968	1969	
Medical	118	7.1	11.3	9.2	7.3	5.7	4.3	67.8
Social	421	25.2	18.5	21.1	30.0	31.4	23.8	37.5
Eugenic	58	3.5	8.1	1.9	0.7	3.0	4.1	72.4
Socio-psychiatric	169	10.1	11.7	12.9	8.1	10.3	8.4	69.8
Medico-psychiatric	103	6.2	10.9	9.2	7.7	3.8	2.6	77.7
Medical/social	143	8.5	11.7	8.5	9.2	8.7	6.5	70.0
Socio-psychiatric/social	544	32.5	20.6	30.0	25.3	32.5	45.0	73.9
Medico-psychiatric/social	92	5.5	6.4	6.6	9.5	3.5	3.4	84.8
Not classified	23	1.4	0.8	0.6	2.2	1.1	1.9	47.9
Total†	1671	100.0	100.0	100.0	100.0	100.0	100.0	63.8
			(248)	(317)	(273)	(369)	(464)	

† *N* in parentheses.

TABLE 2:4. *Refusal rates of 'liberal' and 'conservative' gynaecologists by indications: 1967, 1968 and 1969 combined*

Indications	Liberals			Conservatives			Others†		
	Total	Refused	%	Total	Refused	%	Total	Refused	%
Medical	28	2	7.1	27	8	29.6	8	2	25.0
Social	182	74	40.7	87	64	73.6	37	17	45.9
Eugenic	21	1	5.0	7	0	0.0	4	0	0.0
Socio-psychiatric	67	9	13.4	22	6	27.3	9	4	44.4
Socio-psychiatric/social	266	32	12.0	98	32	32.6	32	6	18.7
Medico-psychiatric	22	2	9.1	19	3	15.8	5	0	0.0
Medical/social	52	6	11.5	31	9	29.0	5	1	20.0
Medico-psychiatric/social	38	2	5.3	13	3	23.1	3	0	0.0
NS	11	5	45.4	3	0	0.0	0	0	0.0
Total	687	133	19.3	307	125	40.7	103	30	29.1

† These are mostly registrars and other non-consultants and a few consultants who were not on the staff of the Aberdeen hospitals for the whole or a major part of the study period.

TABLE 2:5. *Method of termination: 1963–9*

	1963–4		1965–6		1967		1968		1969		Total	
Hysterotomy	4	2.5%	11	5.2%	10	5.7%	21	10.0%	7	2.2%	53	4.9%
H & S	71	45.2%	57	27.0%	63	36.0%	68	32.1%	56	18.0%	315	29.5%
D & C	30	19.1%	54	25.5%	40	22.9%	27	12.7%	50	16.0%	201	18.9%
Hysterectomy	20	12.7%	17	8.0%	3	1.7%	1	0.4%	4	1.3%	45	4.2%
Saline	30	19.1%	70	33.0%	40	22.9%	41	19.3%	47	15.1%	228	21.3%
Suction					14	8.0%	47	22.2%	116	37.2%	177	16.5%
D & C/sterilisation	1	0.6%	2	0.9%	3	1.7%	5	2.4%	4	1.2%	15	1.5%
Suction/sterilisation	—		—		2	1.1%	2	0.9%	27	8.7%	31	3.0%
Saline/sterilisation	—		1	0.4%	—		—		—		1	0.1%
NS	1	0.6%	—		—		—		1	0.3%	2	0.2%
Total	157	100%	212	100%	175	100%	212	100%	312	100%	1068	100%

TABLE 2:6. *Gestation at operation*

Gestation (weeks)	All pregnancies				
	1963–4	1965–6	1967	1968	1969
<8	1.9	3.3	0.6	0.5	1.3
8 and <13	36.0	31.1	34.3	39.6	47.7
13 and <18	38.0	35.9	34.8	34.9	41.0
18+	22.8	28.8	30.3	24.5	9.0
NS	1.3	0.9	0.0	0.5	1.0
	100.0	100.0	100.0	100.0	100.0
	N = 158	212	175	212	312

Gestation (weeks)	Legitimate pregnancies				
	1963–4	1965–6	1967	1968	1969
<8	1.6	3.6	0.0	0.0	1.5
8 and <13	36.9	35.1	36.3	47.9	45.5
13 and <18	40.2	38.7	38.5	39.4	44.7
18+	20.5	21.6	25.3	11.7	6.8
NS	0.8	0.9	0.0	1.1	1.5
	100.0	99.9	100.1	100.1	100.0

Gestation (weeks)	Illegitimate pregnancies				
	1963–4	1965–6	1967	1968	1969
<8	2.8	3.0	1.2	0.8	1.1
8 and <13	33.2	26.7	32.1	33.1	49.4
13 and <18	30.6	32.7	31.0	31.4	38.3
18+	30.6	36.6	35.7	34.7	10.6
NS	2.8	1.0	0.0	0.0	0.6
	100.0	100.0	100.0	100.0	100.0

TABLE 2:7. *Average numbers on waiting list, N.E. of Scotland region: 1965–71*

	Major abdominals	Major vaginals	All majors	Minors	Total
1965	138	220	358	249	607
1966	203	334	537	313	850
1967	304	363	667	310	977
1968	187	387	574	232	806
1969	191	291	482	270	752
1970	253	318	571	373	944
1971	446†	336	782	323	1105

† Includes 222 for sterilisation.

TABLE 2:8. *Obstetric and gynaecological beds required for terminations of pregnancy in the N.E. of Scotland region: 1967–71*

	Obstetric beds			Gynaecological beds			Total		
	Patients	Bed days	Average bed days	Patients	Bed days	Average bed days	Patients	Bed days	Average bed days
1967	30	284	9.7	254	2549	10.0	284	2833	10.0
1968	37	356	9.6	312	2560	8.2	349	2916	8.3
1969	178	677	3.8	332	2298	6.9	510	2975	5.8
1970	181	647	3.6	370	2677	7.2	551	3324	6.0
1971	161	482	3.0	552	3336	6.0	713	3818	5.3

TABLE 2:9. *Obstetrical and gynaecological beds required for termination of pregnancy of Aberdeen city patients: 1968–71*

	Obstetric beds		Gynaecological beds		Total	
	Patients	Bed days	Patients	Bed days	Patients	Bed days
1968						
Suction or curettage	3	15	78	364	81	379
Saline	5	35	37	178	42	213
Abdominal operation	9	131	80	948	89	1079
	17	181	195	1490	212	1671
1969						
Suction or curettage	80	221	116	507	196	728
Saline	33	153	15	68	48	221
Abdominal operation	5	65	62	658	67	723
	118	439	193	1233	311	1672
1970						
Suction or curettage	88	235	122	468	210	703
Saline	39	178	4	22	43	200
Abdominal operation	4	27	93	1032	97	1059
	131	440	217	1522	350	1962
1971						
Suction or curettage	68	149	186	633	254	782
Saline	33	142	0	0	33	142
Abdominal operation	0	0	94	997	94	997
	101	291	280	1630	381	1921

TABLE 2:10. *Days in hospital for terminations: single and ever-married Aberdeen city patients, 1968–71*

	Single			Ever-married		
	Patients	Days	Average bed days	Patients	Days	Average bed days
1968	96	577	6.0	116	1094	9.4
1969	155	600	3.9	157	1072	6.8
1970	168	725	4.3	186	1240	6.7
1971	174	622	3.6	207	1299	6.3

TABLE 2:11. *Days in hospital for terminations with and without sterilisation: ever-married Aberdeen city patients, 1968–71*

	With sterilisation			Without sterilisation		
	Patients	Bed days	Average bed days	Patients	Bed days	Average bed days
1968	75	896	11.9	41	198	4.8
1969	90	829	9.2	67	243	3.6
1970	107	948	8.9	78	292	3.7
1971	117	968	8.3	90	331	3.7

TABLE 2:12. *Gynaecological symptoms at follow-up: menstruation*

	Same	Better	Worse	Not stated	No.	
Terminated						
Nulliparae	54.0%	25.8%	20.2%	—	124	100%
Multiparae	49.5%	14.6%	31.6%	4.4%	206	100%
Not terminated						
Nulliparae	35.1%	35.1%	29.7%	—	37	100%
Multiparae	46.9%	24.7%	28.4%	—	81	100%

TABLE 2:13. *Gynaecological symptoms at follow-up: pain*

	Same	Better	Worse	Not stated	No.	
Terminated						
Nulliparae	68.5%	4.8%	26.6%	—	124	100%
Multiparae	57.7%	1.5%	40.8%	—	206	100%
Not terminated						
Nulliparae	43.2%	8.1%	48.6%	—	37	100%
Multiparae	59.3%	3.7%	37.0%	—	81	100%

TABLE 2:14. *Gynaecological symptoms at follow-up: leucorrhoea*

	Same	Better	Worse	Not stated	No.	
Terminated						
Nulliparae	72.6%	—	27.4%	—	124	100%
Multiparae	57.8%	—	42.2%	—	206	100%
Not terminated						
Nulliparae	62.2%	—	37.8%	—	37	100%
Multiparae	71.6%	—	28.4%	—	81	100%

TABLE 2:15. *Gynaecological symptoms at follow-up: urinary*

	Same	Better	Worse	Not stated	No.	
Terminated						
Nulliparae	94.4%	—	5.6%	—	124	100%
Multiparae	93.2%	—	6.8%	—	206	100%
Not terminated						
Nulliparae	100%	—	—	—	37	100%
Multiparae	98.8%	—	1.2%	—	81	100%

TABLE 2:16. *General health at follow-up*

	Same	Better	Worse	Not stated	No.	
Terminated						
Nulliparae	94.4%	—	5.6%	—	124	100%
Multiparae	89.8%	—	10.2%	—	206	100%
Not terminated						
Nulliparae	97.3%	—	2.7%	—	37	100%
Multiparae	95.1%	—	4.9%	—	81	100%

TABLE 2:17. *Symptoms by method of termination: menstruation*

	Same	Better	Worse	No.	
Dilatation and curettage	37.7%	24.5%	37.7%	53	100%
Suction	60.0%	18.7%	21.3%	75	100%
Saline	53.8%	25.0%	21.2%	52	100%
Hysterotomy	76.2%	9.5%	14.3%	21	100%
Hysterotomy and sterilisation	53.6%	3.6%	42.8%	28	100%

TABLE 2:18. *Symptoms by method of termination: pain*

	Same	Better	Worse	No.	
Dilatation and curettage	64.1%	7.5%	28.3%	53	100%
Suction	68.0%	—	32.0%	75	100%
Saline	53.8%	1.9%	44.2%	52	100%
Hysterotomy	52.4%	4.8%	42.8%	21	100%
Hysterotomy and sterilisation	60.7%	3.6%	35.7%	28	100%

TABLE 2:19. *Symptoms by method of termination: leucorrhoea*

	Same	Better	Worse	No.	
Dilatation and curettage	56.6%	—	43.4%	53	100%
Suction	60.0%	—	40.0%	75	100%
Saline	65.4%	—	34.6%	52	100%
Hysterotomy	61.9%	—	38.1%	21	100%
Hysterotomy and sterilisation	71.4%	—	28.6%	28	100%

TABLE 2:20. *Symptoms by method of termination: urinary*

	Same	Better	Worse	No.	
Dilatation and curettage	94.3%	—	5.7%	53	100%
Suction	93.3%	—	6.7%	75	100%
Saline	96.2%	—	3.8%	52	100%
Hysterotomy	90.5%	—	9.5%	21	100%
Hysterotomy and sterilisation	100%	—	—	28	100%

TABLE 2:21. *General health by method of termination*

	Same	Better	Worse	No.	
Dilatation and curettage	92.5%	—	7.5%	53	100%
Suction	90.7%	—	9.3%	75	100%
Saline	96.2%	—	3.8%	52	100%
Hysterotomy	85.7%	—	14.3%	21	100%
Hysterotomy and sterilisation	100%	—	—	28	100%

3 THE WOMAN'S STORY: MARRIED WOMEN

Jean Aitken-Swan

Between September 1968 and June 1969, 342 Aberdeen women applied for an abortion through the usual national health service channels. This part of the study refers to 167 of them; the rest, allocated randomly, were interviewed by Colin Farmer in furtherance of his study of decision-making. The two groups were not dissimilar as regards marital state, age and broad social class distribution and these results are assumed to be representative of all the women referred about abortion at that time, except private patients.

On applying for an abortion the patient's first contact, after her general practitioner, was with the research worker, the interview usually taking place a day or two before the appointment with the consultant. The patient was seen in a comfortable, private consulting room and the interview was held in an unhurried and relaxed atmosphere. She was encouraged to talk about her problem in a semi-structured type of interview. Before seeing the patient, consultants received a factual report of her circumstances and reasons for wanting an abortion, which saved the patient repetition, and the consultant time if the general practitioner's letter of referral had been uninformative. It also made some return for the interference with usual administrative procedures necessitated by the study and, in fact, created a demand for the continuation of the reports when the research project ended. Care was taken that the report did no more than present the facts as given by the patient.

Interviewing of patients began about a year before the interviews of the 342 research subjects began. During this year, different schedules were tried out and the time taken shortened to an average of one hour. Married women generally talked more freely than single women, but the latter sometimes found it a relief to be drawn into this preliminary

96

discussion of their problems, especially if they had felt unable to confide in any relative or friend. However, contact with the patient was inevitably superficial, the research worker being neither the doctor making the decision nor the social worker getting to know the family through offering continuing help and visiting the home. The social worker is perhaps the best person, apart from the patient's general practitioner, to understand the total situation, but obvious problems arise if helping and research roles are combined.

How accurate are the facts given? Patients saw the interview as relevant to their application. They cannot be expected to be objective about their situation if they are desperate to have the pregnancy terminated, and in these circumstances facts are understandably more likely to be embroidered. The patient has only a short time in which to make an impression on an unknown doctor whose decision on her behalf will affect her life for the foreseeable future. In the stress of the moment she may underestimate as well as exaggerate her symptoms. Tredgold[1] thought that underestimation was a far commoner risk – a patient might minimise her symptoms because she had been led to think that abortion was probable. It would be true to say that few in the present series were confident about the outcome of their application, and any bias would be likely to be the other way. It would be unrealistic to expect the full facts to be stated, but the very variety of the details given and the fact that a later interview seldom revealed discrepancies in the original story suggest that the accounts given by at any rate the married women are probably broadly correct. The truth of the single women's stories of deserting boyfriends and unsympathetic parents is more difficult to assess; in the case of students at least the more abortions done the more the grapevine makes them aware of the 'best' way to present their case. Some distortion of fact is inevitable and follow-up interviews have given some indication of it. Other facts are less liable to bias, such as use of contraception in relation to earlier pregnancies, knowledge of abortion, etc., and there is no reason why these data should not be as accurate as memory allows.

Practical considerations determined the place and time of the sociological–gynaecological follow-up interviews. It was thought necessary to see the women, whether terminated or not, at approximately the same interval after conception. This could not be too long an interval as the 1968–9 patients were seen nearer to the time limit set for the completion of the study than the pilot group first seen in 1967–8 who were followed up by the psychiatrists. Although told at first interview that they would be asked to come again, and nearly all agreed to do so, patients were not particularly motivated to return, especially if they had not been accepted for termination. Home visiting by the sociologist might have raised problems, especially in the case of single women, and would have entailed the loss of the gynaecological assessment. It seemed that the best response would be achieved if patients *who had not had their pregnancy terminated* were interviewed when they would be attending the hospital anyway. This happens at the 34th week of pregnancy, one of the stages at which women getting their ante-natal care at a peripheral clinic or through the combined general practitioner–hospital scheme routinely attend hospital to be seen by an obstetrician. Those who *had had an abortion* were asked to come again at what would have been the 34th week had their pregnancy continued. This usually worked out at about four or five months after their first attendance.

This is a very short interval, and in the case of those going on with their pregnancy meant that they were seen near to the time of their confinement, eliciting a perhaps temporarily more contented reaction than might have been obtained if seen at an earlier or later date. On the other hand, if the pregnancy had been terminated, follow-up at such a short interval has something to be said for it, in that the abortion and the feelings and circumstances surrounding it are close enough to be recalled vividly and there has been less time for other events to intervene to blur the picture. In any case, this follow-up is only a supplement to the longer term psychiatric follow-up in depth of the other but similar group of women who comprise Dr Olley's and Dr McCance's study.

The distribution of the interviewed group by marital state at the time of the first interview and legitimacy of the pregnancy is shown below:

	Total	Legitimate	Illegitimate
Currently married	71	68	3
Separated, divorced	14	0	14
Single	82	0	82
Total	167	68	99

MARRIED WOMEN

In Aberdeen, women seeking abortion through the national health service are more often wives of manual workers than of non-manual workers. A few, predominantly married to men in professional or managerial work, prefer to have their pregnancy terminated in a private ward, but their numbers are not large and they were not interviewed. Their omission means however that the married women's story is biassed towards the working class woman's problems, the non-manual group being represented by 16 of the 85 interviews.

There is seldom one aspect of the woman's situation which can be picked out as the precipitating factor causing her to seek abortion. Contact with rubella early in pregnancy is one and the fear that the baby might be defective as a result. In most cases the presenting problems are varied and difficult to categorise but an attempt is made below to do so. There is obviously some overlapping but the situations have been described according to the emphasis the women themselves put on the different aspects of their story. All the pregnancies are legitimate except those in category 6.

1 *Marital troubles*: husband drinks, gambles, won't work (she maybe has to work): impending or recent breakdown of marriage (with which the pregnancy may have had something to do); if they have parted, there may be financial and accommodation problems for herself and the existing children.   16

2 *Financial troubles*: but family united. Includes associated problems such as poor and inadequate housing, overcrowding, etc.   16

3 *Too old*: there is a group aged 35 or more, some already grandmothers, tired, anxious about pregnancy, whose last child was born many years before, who cannot face the prospect of starting again at their age.   14

4 *Family complete*: these women, all under 35, do not want any more children; their way of life is settled; they may be working and have financial commitments or plans for the family which depend on two wage-packets coming in.   10

5 *Eugenic*: contact with rubella early in pregnancy.   6

6 *Pregnancy illegitimate*: 7 of these women were divorced, 7 separated from their husbands (including 2 cohabiting) and 3 were married and living with their husbands. Although the problems of these women could be properly described under some of the above headings, illegitimacy is an additional complication and the group is shown separately.   17

7 *Miscellaneous*   6

Among these interrelated social circumstances, it is striking what a large part marital troubles play in this group of women seeking abortion. If the 14 women in category 6 who are divorced or separated from their husbands are added, the unplanned pregnancy had occurred in the context of a broken or unstable marital relationship in 30 of the 85 cases.

Marital troubles (16)

This is a shifting, unreliable area but the problems and stresses may be very real, making the coming of another child an intolerable burden on the woman and a risk to the existing children. This is particularly so when the family has split up and the woman is virtually homeless, living with her children in one room with relatives, or when the children are in care and she has to go to work to support the family. This was the situation in 5 of the 16 cases. In the remainder the couple were still together, but alleged alcoholism, gambling or violence on the husband's part made an unhappy home and the wife did not want to bring another child into it. Some were working to give themselves an independent source of income, and some were waiting until the youngest child was old enough, before they left their husband. In only 2 of the 16 cases did the follow-up give any reason to doubt the truth of the patient's account. Dr Olley has also noted a particularly high incidence of unhappy or broken marriage in his group of wives of semi-skilled and unskilled workers applying for abortion compared with the upper socioeconomic groups (Chapter 5).

All 16 were married to men in manual occupations, mostly semiskilled or unskilled. Ten of the 16 had their pregnancies terminated.

Financial troubles (16)

In this group, mostly wives of manual workers, multiparity and financial troubles were associated. Thirteen of the 16 had between 3 and 9 children. Low wages, insecurity of income and the burden of debt made the thought of an addition to the family a last straw. In many of the cases there was overcrowding, and the accommodation was unsuitable (a room up three flights of stairs) or substandard. There were medical and psychiatric indications for termination of pregnancy in over half the cases, asthma, debility, depression, severe varicose veins, etc. One patient changed her mind about having an abortion; of the other 15, 13 had their pregnancy terminated.

Too old (14)

The majority of wives of the non-manual workers in the group comes into this category. Half the 14 patients were aged 35 to 39 and half between 40 and 46. Patients felt they would be unable to cope with a baby so late in life and several feared the actual confinement or recurrence of previous complications of pregnancy. Medical and psychiatric indications were considered to be present in 9 of the 14 cases. Two turned out not to be pregnant and 7 of the 12 others had their pregnancy terminated.

Family complete (10)

The 10 women in this category, wives of manual workers, were positive that they wanted no more children, not because of their age (all were under 35) but because they had other plans and commitments which they wished to fulfil. These included working to help keep the family while the husband took a professional training or 'to give the children their chance' of further education, or simply to maintain the family's living standards. Some wanted no more children for health reasons and nearly all hoped to be sterilised. Medical and psychiatric indications were considered to be present in 9 of the 10 cases. Only 4 of the 10 in this group had their pregnancy terminated.

Eugenic (6)

In 3 of these 6 cases of contact with rubella (2 first pregnancies and a second) the pregnancy had been intentional. The other 3, third and fourth pregnancies, were unplanned. All 6 were aborted.

Pregnancy illegitimate (17)

The widowed, divorced or separated woman is in a particularly vulnerable position if she becomes pregnant. The single woman, however reluctant she may be to tell her parents of her pregnancy, usually does have them to depend on. They do not often 'turn her out', although she sometimes uses this threat as an argument for abortion. The ever-married woman, on the other hand, may have several young children dependent on her, and the pregnancy, if it continued, could adversely affect them as well as the mother, who has to cope both domestically and financially. Parents often help a daughter having marital troubles by giving her a room in their own home for herself and the children, despite the resulting overcrowding. Apart from anything else they may feel about her illegitimate pregnancy, another child would add to the overcrowding, and the arrangement, sometimes of advantage to both parties, breaks down so that these mothers do run the risk of being turned out with nowhere else to go. In this event, children who are minded by grandparents while their mother works are also the losers.

The 14 women away from their husbands had 38 children between them, nearly half of them under school age. Only 5 women regularly received maintenance payments for them from the children's father and in 6 cases maintenance had never been paid. The general pattern was that if they were living in a parent's house, the mother went out to work, mostly full-time. If they had a council house of their own, they were living on social security benefit. In either case, an addition to the family could only add to the mother's difficulties and spread more thinly her means of looking after and providing for the children. Why then did she become pregnant? Some of the women are still hoping for a stable marriage and run the risks which figure in the stories of the single girls – men friends who desert them or who turn out to be already married. Others are wary of marriage if the putative father drinks heavily or does not get on with the children, and a few are not free to marry. Most of them, however, are young and lonely and at risk of casual relationships.

Where husband and wife are separated decision-making is made difficult because doctors are uncertain of the possible legal consequences of aborting a pregnancy without the husband's consent. For this reason women in anomalous marital situations may have less chance of having an illegitimate pregnancy terminated than other women in stressful situations. In this group 10 of the 17 had their pregnancy terminated.

Miscellaneous (6)

Two of these patients were atypical in that they did not want an abortion unless it was medically necessary. Both were Roman Catholics and in neither case was abortion recommended. Four others were afraid of further pregnancy on health grounds, because of previous obstetrical complications or because a handicapped child in the family might suffer through the claims of a new infant. All 4 had the pregnancy terminated.

The 85 married women defined their problems in terms of one or other of these categories. Circumstances differed, but the constellation of factors which stood out are multiparity, instability of family life and poor socio-economic circumstances. There is nothing special in many of the situations described that would provide grounds for abortion unless the social stress had a direct bearing on the woman's health and ability to continue the pregnancy successfully. The doctors did not find undue physical or emotional stress in 26 of the 85 cases and thought the patient's reaction to the pregnancy was in proportion to the effects of the unfavourable environment. In the majority of cases, however, associated medical conditions, adverse personality factors or psychiatric indications were also considered to be present.

Whatever the doctor thought about the stress suffered by the women, most of the women themselves were quite clear in their minds that another child in their circumstances would be a disaster. Eighteen (21 per cent) admitted to having tried to abort themselves but usually with 'old wives'' remedies. One would expect motivation to avoid pregnancy to be high in the group but unfortunately multiparity, instability of family life and poor socio-economic circumstances are also characteristic of poor family planning.

FAMILY PLANNING AND USE OF CONTRACEPTION

Many of the patients interviewed for this study had started their families in the years before the contraceptive pill became generally available, when the most effective methods of contraception were the condom and vaginal diaphragm. Previous studies of family growth in Aberdeen have shown that few women, particularly in the lower socio-economic groups, used these methods regularly and that with each pregnancy the proportion 'unintended' increased. Since then oral contraception has replaced the vaginal diaphragm as the method of choice of the family planning clinics, especially for younger women. An Aberdeen study in 1969[2] suggested that women in the non-manual classes, who had been the chief users of the vaginal diaphragm, were then changing to the pill, as were women in the lower socio-economic groups, many of whom had previously relied on coitus interruptus. The popularity of the pill has continued, despite a setback in 1969 resulting from publicity given to a statement linking pills of high oestrogen content to an increased risk of thromboembolism.

In the present study the degree of planning of pregnancies throughout the patient's married life was investigated by a series of questions, including:

(a) Before your (first, second, etc.) pregnancy, were you using any method of birth control?

(b) Did you get advice on birth control from anywhere?

(c) Did you mean to have your (first, second, etc.) pregnancy when you did?

I have tried to distinguish 'intended' from 'unintended' pregnancies. Where there was no positive planning but readiness to accept a pregnancy if it came, this is counted as 'intended'. An 'unintended' pregnancy is one which the patient did not plan and would rather not have had, at any rate at that time.

According to this definition, 43 per cent of all births, including pre-nuptial conception, to the 68 women whose pregnancies were legitimate, had been 'unintended'. The proportion rose from 23 per cent in the non-manual and 38 per cent in the skilled, to 56 per cent in the semi-skilled and unskilled manual group. If pre-nuptial conceptions are omitted, still 11 per cent of first births were unintended, increasing sixfold when it comes to fourth or later births.

	Total	Unintended pregnancies	
		No.	%
First births (excluding pre-nuptial conceptions)	37	4	11
Second births	50	14	28
Third births	34	12	35
Fourth or later births	26	18	69

The wives of non-manual workers were older and most had been married longer than the wives of skilled and unskilled manual workers, which affects their contraceptive practice, i.e. younger women are more likely to be on the pill. None in the non-manual group was under age 25 at the time of referral, whereas a quarter of the skilled and over half the unskilled were under 25. Most of the wives of non-manual workers first began to use contraception after the first pregnancy while in the unskilled group it was not unusual to begin after the third, fourth or even later pregnancy.

Eight of the 68 women, all wives of manual workers, had used no method of contraception other than coitus interruptus during their married life. Three of the 8 were having their first pregnancy and in 2 of these contact with rubella was the only reason for considering termination. Forty-four of the remaining 60 had used a method in their own control, most often the pill, but also the diaphragm or IUD or more than one of these methods. Many of these couples had also at some time used the condom; in only 16 cases had nothing but the condom been used throughout married life. One-third of the women had had no professional advice on contraception and family planning. The other two-thirds had been advised by family planning clinics (28), practitioners (15) and obstetricians (2).

With increasing numbers attending the family planning clinics and with effective means of contraception available to all in Aberdeen (free to those requiring it on medical grounds who could not afford to pay), it might seem that the time is getting nearer when it should be possible to prevent unwanted pregnancies rather than abort them. But the contraceptive practice of the 68 women interviewed in 1968–9 shows that there is still a long way to go. Two-thirds had either not been using a reliable method when they became unintentionally pregnant or had not been using it regularly. Some who blamed the failure of the appliance or pill may not have been using it correctly and a few had difficulties over timing when to take the pill (Table 3:1).

Some of the women thought they were too old, or sexual intercourse was too infrequent, for them to get pregnant. Others had stopped taking the pill temporarily on medical advice or on their own initiative and took no other effective precautions. In a few cases the husband was absent from home for long enough for contraceptive measures to lapse and they were not resumed in time. Ambivalence as well as mistakes and carelessness lie behind some of the failures of contraception. While a woman knows in the rational part of her mind that a pregnancy would cause untold difficulties, she may still unconsciously desire to be at risk of pregnancy and feel less pleasure in sexual intercourse without the risk. Being largely unconscious these feelings may not be recognised or, if the women do recognise them, they might not want to appear irrational by discussing them. In considering why many still become unintentionally pregnant in these days when efficient contraception is potentially available probably not enough weight is given to the complexity of women's attitudes to getting pregnant. It is perhaps too readily assumed that overburdened married women and single women having sexual relationships 'naturally' want to avoid pregnancy. Even among the present small group one woman was able to explain in a confused way that although she did not want any more pregnancies she felt it would be 'cheating' to go on the pill. She preferred the diaphragm, apparently because she felt it did not entirely eliminate risk.

Many of the Aberdeen women were afraid of what they had read or heard from others about the pill, and some who started taking it gave up without seeking further advice when they put on weight, became depressed or had other symptoms which they attributed to the pill. The diaphragm was disliked by some, and found difficult to use by others who described overcrowded living conditions and dark, outside toilets. Lack of communication between husband and wife and fatalism about family size was not uncommon. The wife of a skilled manual worker said: 'The family was never planned or spoken about – it's a thing I think you just accept.'

Some idea has been given why at the present time when contraceptive methods are more available and more reliable than ever before some Aberdeen married women still get unintentionally pregnant and become candidates for therapeutic abortion. Forty-seven of the 68 women were either using no contraceptive method or an unreliable method or a reliable method but not regularly. The 17 patients whose pregnancies were illegitimate were no more efficient in the use of contraception than the rest of the married women in their socio-economic group but in what are sometimes unstable and temporary relationships this is understandable. Twelve had taken no reliable precautions and 5 had used the condom or pill but only occasionally. Numerous surveys have confirmed these poor results. Ann Cartwright in her recent study of family planning services in England and Wales[3] shows that about a third of those mothers' pregnancies were unintended and just under half the failures arose when the women were not attempting to use any method of birth control. The high proportion of failures in the present group is not necessarily typical of Aberdeen married women, as the falling legitimate birth rate shows. But although the practice of birth control is now widespread, motivation is variable and may be subject to unconscious emotional blockages, however rationalised. Many women are not capable of the sustained vigilance needed for success. How to help those most in need of help is a problem which faces all who attempt to provide a preventive medical service, but family planning is also up against moral and social attitudes particularly slow to change. Abortion also arouses strong feelings, but it is a remedy for a catastrophe that has already happened and not merely a precaution against something that with any luck might not happen.

Nearly three-quarters of the 68 women with legitimate pregnancies hoped that the pregnancy they wished terminated would be their last. Nineteen thought they would want another later on, or were undecided. These were cases where the marriage was on the point of breaking up or contact with rubella was the only reason for termination, or a handicapped child needed special care which the mother felt she would be unable to give if she were caring for a new infant. Half the 49 women who wanted no more pregnancies hoped to be sterilised. Their views on future contraceptive measures are summarised below:

Would like to be sterilised	24
Will do whatever the doctor advises	11
Pill	7
Pill or sterilisation	2
Afraid of sterilisation; would use cap or pill	2
Will continue to rely on coitus interruptus	1
Not sure	2
	49

In 13 of the 68 cases the question of sterilisation had been raised before by the patient or doctor after a previous pregnancy. Seven of these mothers, each with between 4 and 12 children, were afraid of sterilisation, having heard alarming stories about its supposed effects from relatives, and had not had it done. Three patients with smaller families had wished it done but the doctor had not recommended it, and in the other 3 cases arrangements for sterilisation had fallen through for various reasons.

Since the 1950s tubal ligation has played an increasing part in family limitation in Aberdeen, mainly benefiting older, multiparous women who were unable to prevent pregnancies by other means. Between 1963 and 1971 an average of 60 per cent of ever-married women having a pregnancy terminated were sterilised at the same time. Over the years the age of women offered sterilisation has fallen and also their average family size, from 7 or more in the 1950s to 4 or even 3 if the mother is certain that her family is complete and she does not want to take the pill indefinitely. Careful consideration is given to all the circumstances, present and foreseen. Previous follow-up of sterilised women has shown that not all react well to sterilisation, some blaming it for their physical ills, depression or loss of libido. That half the women in the present study who wanted no more children were hoping to be sterilised suggests that by 1968–9 there was less fear of the operation. Some of those who had refused it before were now willing to have it done. The introduction of laparoscopic sterilisation in Aberdeen in 1969 may have made the procedure more acceptable than it had been. Women could then be sterilised by a simple method with low post-operative morbidity, and without having to be away from home for several days, an added inducement to those with large families.

KNOWLEDGE OF ABORTION

It might be supposed that in a city with a 'liberal' policy towards abortion information would soon get around and more women would know about it as the numbers sent to hospital increase. However, although over 1000 women in Aberdeen have been referred in the last three years and abortion has been frequently in the news, there seems little general knowledge of it, at least among married women.

Several questions were asked in the interview to try to find out what the 85 married women knew about abortion, what they had read or heard about it, if they had known anyone who had had a pregnancy terminated and how they first came to think of getting it done. Interviewing had begun four months after the Abortion Act came into operation, with all its attendant publicity, but over a third of the women were unable to say when the last law on abortion had been passed.

Do you know anything about the law on abortion – for instance, when was the last law passed?

	Total	Non-manual	Skilled	Unskilled
Knows accurately or fairly accurately	43	10	13	20
Knows vaguely†	10	2	5	3
Does not know	32	4	15	13
	85	16	33	36

† I.e. 'within the last year or two'.

Few could mention any of the circumstances in which a doctor is allowed to terminate a pregnancy and 90 per cent seemed unaware that Aberdeen is regarded as one of the more 'liberal' centres as regards abortion. Their ignorance appeared perfectly genuine.

Do you think you are more likely or less likely to get an abortion if you live in Aberdeen than if you lived in some other place, or does it make no difference where you live?

	Total	Non-manual	Skilled	Unskilled
More likely	6	3	3	—
Less likely	3	—	1	2
No difference	32	9	6	17
Does not know	44	4	23	17
	85	16	33	36

Considering the wide reporting of the abortion controversy by the news media and later the publicity given to inequalities in the availability of abortion in different parts of the country, these answers reflect how little impact it made in the long run on the general public of Aberdeen. Only 33 of the 85 married women claimed to have seen a television programme on abortion or to have read anything about it in papers or magazines. They gave the impression that so long as it did not concern them personally they did not pay much attention, and they could only remember vaguely what they had read or seen. The impact was obviously greater if it came at a time when a woman was worrying about an unwelcome pregnancy, but on the whole newspaper and television publicity played only a small part in stimulating this group of 85 Aberdeen women to seek an abortion, and in one case had the opposite effect. This woman, having seen a hysterotomy performed on television just before her first appointment at hospital, changed her mind about having an abortion. Nevertheless, the news media may indeed have contributed to the rise in the number of referrals of married women since 1967 but through their effect on general practitioners rather than on the woman herself. Attitudes to abortion were changing and because of this doctors may have felt freer to refer patients whom before they might have discouraged from seeking a second opinion.

Only 12 of the 85 women said they had been motivated by something they had read or seen on television to seek an abortion. On the other hand, such publicity sometimes produced inquiries from outside the region from women who were having difficulty in obtaining an abortion elsewhere, but as a general rule hospitals do not accept patients from outside their own catchment area.

In view of the increasing number of abortions being performed, it is perhaps surprising that few of the women knew anyone who had had it done.

(a) *Have you known anyone personally who has had a pregnancy terminated, or who has tried to have it done?*

(b) *Have you heard of anyone?*

	Total	Non-manual	Skilled	Unskilled
Knows someone personally	13	3	6	4
Does not know anyone personally but has heard of someone	22	3	12	7
Knows no one, has heard of no one	50	10	15	25
	85	16	33	36

The figures suggest that married women who have an abortion do not speak of it very much to others, perhaps for fear of disapproval. This is not the impression, however, given by the women interviewed at their first attendance and follow-up. According to them, there is certainly less talk of it at the time they are considering having an abortion than there is after the event. At first interview 30 per cent of the married women had talked of it to their husbands only, but by the time those who had their pregnancies terminated were followed up this proportion had fallen to 18 per cent. Mothers are generally told but mothers-in-law sometimes take their place as confidante if the patient's own mother is elderly or unwell or if it is thought she would disapprove of abortion. Disapproval is sometimes anticipated if the patient's mother had had a big family herself. According to patients, it is rare for anyone with whom they discussed the abortion to disapprove of it. Nearly all are reported to have agreed that it was the best thing in the circumstances or at least that 'it's up to yourself'. This may be due to careful selection of confidantes or to the fact that those who discuss their intentions with people who disapprove may be persuaded not to apply.

Women who had had their pregnancies terminated were asked if any of the other patients in their ward had known what they were in hospital for and who among their friends and relations knew that they had had an abortion. Half the women had spoken of it to others in the ward. 'I didn't mind them knowing – I've nothing to hide', was the view of this group, but they were sometimes advised by fellow-patients or nurses to be discreet. Several mentioned the moral support they derived from knowing that someone else was in for the same thing. At follow-up, most of the women had discussed their experience with close relatives besides their husband and a few (18 per cent) with a wider circle, such as 'all my relations and the neighbours in the tenement'.

The majority of the women said that they themselves had been the first to raise the subject of abortion with their doctor, but there is no one answer to how the patient came to think of having it done. Some factors will have more weight than others while some will not be mentioned at all. In 16 of the 85 cases it was not possible to say what had motivated them. Of the other 69, the largest group (18) said they had not thought of it until their own doctor had mentioned the possibility, but this cannot be taken at its face value, although it is consistent with what has been said about Aberdeen married women's ignorance of abortion. Apart from the exceptional case, the doctor would be unlikely to mention abortion if the patient had not given him an obvious opening to do so. Some patients described such an indirect approach on their part. 'I implied it but I didn't actually suggest it – well, I couldn't very well ask the doctor to do something' – i.e. the doctor–patient relationship as seen by some women precludes their initiating a course of action just as they would feel it inappropriate to suggest a course of treatment. On the other hand, to put the onus for suggesting an abortion on their doctor might seem an obvious way of relieving any moral doubts they might feel about abortion.

The next largest group (15) said that they had known or heard of someone who had had an abortion and this had encouraged them to apply. As already mentioned, 12 more applied as a result of abortion publicity on television or in papers. The remaining 24 were motivated in a variety of ways; some had made a previous application, some were referred by doctors from the family planning or other clinics and some were already attending their doctor when the pregnancy was discovered. Several more were advised by a health visitor or other nurse and others had nursing experience of their own which had made them aware of the possibility of abortion. In a few cases the patient's mother had taken the initiative and had discussed abortion with the doctor on the patient's behalf.

If these married women seem unexpectedly unknowledgeable about abortion considering Aberdeen's 'liberal' reputation in gynaecological circles, this may have something to do with the type of area it is. Aberdeen is a city with its roots in the country, a fairly stable, settled community, not particularly affluent or socially mobile and without marked extremes in living standards. It may be a little isolated from the pressures of social change that beset the more militant south. There is a good deal of talk about abortion in some groups, but on the whole the procedure attracts very little public attention. Married women applying for abortion through the national health service are still uncertain in what circumstances their application will succeed and their approach to abortion is tentative. If it is not recommended, the great majority acquiesce in continuing the pregnancy, as shown in Table 1:17 (p. 46 above). 'There's nothing else I can do, is there?', expresses the usual attitude. The consultants they see are the same consultants who will be seeing them throughout their pregnancy and sometimes the offer of post-partum sterilisation is enough to encourage a patient to continue. They are mostly ignorant of any alternative. Aberdeen's geographical remoteness also contributes to acceptance of the consultant's decision. Even if they thought of it, a journey to London would be a very unusual and too costly step for many women in north-east Scotland.

AFTER THE ABORTION

When seen again four or five months after their abortion the majority of the 50 married women who had had it done reported no change in their social circumstances, as might be expected. The abortion alone is unlikely to effect an improvement in overcrowded living conditions or in domestic or financial troubles, but at least these problems had not been made worse by the advent of another child. Other events besides the abortion had been happening since the patient had first been interviewed which could have affected her circumstances and state of mind when seen again. The group which most consistently described an improvement in their situation were those who had been classified as having marital troubles, and the improvement was usually attributed to a change in their husband's attitude. A change might be due to the removal of the threat of a pregnancy which the husband had not wanted or perhaps to a more conciliatory attitude on his wife's part out of relief at having the pregnancy terminated or being sterilised. Several of the men who had left home returned, and in one case plans for a legal separation which had been started were cancelled. In other cases, the husband's excessive drinking was said to have lessened, with a general improvement in their financial circumstances and relationship. Two women who had been sterilised following their abortion described the change: 'We're happier now than we've ever been', and 'We've come a bit closer – more like when we were first married.' How long the improvement lasted and whether the same problem recurred later on cannot be answered by the short-term follow-up.

Almost all the patients were surprised at how easy the abortion had been in comparison with their expectations. Only 5 described pain or thought the experience worse than they had expected. These were 3 of the 19 who had had a hysterotomy and sterilisation, one of the 5 who had had a saline termination and one who had had a suction termination, right oophorectomy and Pomeroy sterilisation. Post-operative pain and discomfort is to be expected when the abdomen has been opened and it is of note that so many dismissed it as of little account. This is not the place to consider the justification for the complaints of the 5 but in this small number of cases the patients who complained of pain or discomfort were usually those who said they did not feel so well at follow-up as they had before and who expressed some reservations about having had an abortion, indicative, perhaps, of guilt feelings rather than of specific post-operative symptoms. One patient regarded the 'agony' she was in after the operation as the penalty for having her illegitimate pregnancy terminated and spoke of the 'morbid dreams' she had had at the time.

Their experience in hospital had been made pleasanter by the evidently unexpected kindness of the nurses and other ward staff. Recent publicity has suggested that nursing staff dislike the termination of pregnancy and are becoming increasingly reluctant to take part in the care of these patients. If they feel strongly about it, it might be difficult to hide their feelings from the patient who would sense an atmosphere of disapproval. To encourage discussion of this aspect, the women were asked: 'Did you get any impression that you were treated differently by the ward staff because you were in to have an abortion?' Only 2 of the 50 patients had any adverse comment to make and one of these did not concern a nurse. They seemed surprised by the sympathy and kindness they met with as in some cases friends, and even a patient's doctor, had warned them of the negative attitude of some hospital staff to the termination of pregnancy. Nurses' attitudes to abortion are liable to be influenced by the prevailing medical opinion of a particular centre and the way the subject is treated in the clinical and teaching situation. It would be surprising in a centre with a liberal tradition if the consultants could not take the nursing staff along with them on this issue.

After an abortion, the question of contraceptive precautions for the future becomes a matter of urgency. In the present group of 50, over half the women (28) had been sterilised at the time of their abortion, and all but 4 were satisfied or even delighted about the benefits of the procedure. They said: 'It's made a terrible difference and I'd recommend it to any woman in my situation.' 'I've never felt better. If I canna have bairns I've no problems.' This successful outcome is confirmed by a follow-up study of sterilised women in Aberdeen by Thompson and Baird,[4] who found the vast majority were satisfied with the operation and were enthusiastic advocates of sterilisation. Their satisfaction might be due to the careful selection of patients to whom sterilisation was offered. Eight of the 186 women they followed up regretted for various reasons having been sterilised, sometimes because of changes in their circumstances. In the present study, the interval between sterilisation and follow-up was considerably shorter than in the other study, so that there was less time for circumstances to change and also less time in which to adjust to the idea of being unable to have any more family. Four of the 28 had regrets or vaguer feelings of disappointment about having been sterilised, one (para. 7+) being described by the consultant as 'at least moderately psychiatrically disturbed' at follow-up. The other 3 had had time to think they they might have wanted another child after all. For example, a patient with four children, who had gladly accepted the doctor's offer of sterilisation, said at follow-up: 'I don't know how I'd feel about it if I could choose again. The children are all growing up and soon I'll have nobody. My husband says you'll be able to enjoy yourself, but being a mother you don't feel like that.'

Thompson and Baird's results showed that women were more likely to be satisfied if they had post-partum sterilisation. All in the present group were sterilised in association with the termination of a pregnancy and this could make it a more disturbing procedure.

While 28 of the 50 women had had their contraceptive problems solved by sterilisation, 22 were still at risk. They were almost equally divided into those who were on the pill, those relying on the condom and those taking no precautions for various reasons (i.e. not associating with any man, ready to get pregnant again at any time or already pregnant by intention). Only one woman in the 22 seemed to be running the same risk of an unwanted pregnancy that had led to her abortion. She would not like to be sterilised, was 'allergic to Durex' and did not 'believe in' the pill. According to her, her own doctor had not discussed contraception with her after the abortion. She was relying on infrequent intercourse, and on her husband being 'careful'. General practitioners are playing a larger part than before in giving advice on birth control to their patients but, as Ann Cartwright comments: 'The limited time they have or are prepared to give to discussion of family planning precludes them from persuading hesitant family planners to become effective ones.' Certainly after an abortion is a time when women might be most receptive to advice.

The vital question of whether there were any ill-effects on the woman's physical health or emotional equilibrium from the abortion is discussed in the sections of this report dealing with the gynaecological and psychiatric follow-up. In the present group of 50 (and 2 more who had obtained their abortion elsewhere) short-term reactions were canvassed on a more superficial level. The final questions of the interview tried to elicit the patient's feelings about the abortion in a standardised way by asking her to select from a printed card whichever of three sentences most closely represented her own point of view at that moment:

(a) I have no doubt at all that to terminate the pregnancy was the right thing to do.

(b) It seemed the best solution at the time, but now I'm not so sure that it was.

(c) If I could decide again, I would not have it done.

Those who chose (a) were further asked: 'Although it was necessary in your case, have you felt in any way sad or regretful at having had the pregnancy terminated?' If they chose (b) or (c) they were asked: 'Could you say something about why you feel like this?' The respondent's own words were taken down at this point.

Put in this way, 48 of the 52 women had no doubt at all that to terminate the pregnancy had been the right thing to do. Their comments suggested that they could accept an abortion without regret if it was done early enough in the pregnancy, if it was not suggested to them that they should feel guilty about it, if their existing children were of the desired sex, if, in the case of an illegitimate pregnancy, they had no particular feelings for the father, and so on. Both the patients who had obtained an abortion of an illegitimate pregnancy privately elsewhere were certain that it had been the right thing to do. One said with evident sincerity: 'It was less to me than having a tooth out.'

Other comments were:

'I think maybe if it had been four or five months on and I'd felt movements it would have been different and I'd really have thought twice, but to me it was just a – nothingness. I've never regretted it, no.'

'No, but when I hear St John Stevas or someone talking on TV, I think what have I done for a moment. But I don't regret it. When I think I might have a baby now to look after, I'm thankful I got it done.'

'Yes, I do feel sad – well, any mother would, it's not a thing you do lightly. I've had no ill-effects. It's just natural to feel like that, isn't it?'

A patient whose pregnancy had been illegitimate said:

'If I felt anything towards the man I might have felt differently but in the circumstances I didn't feel anything at all about getting it done. I'm very glad I did.'

Taken at its face value, 48 out of 52 who considered on looking back that they had done the right thing is a high rate of satisfaction, but not unexpected in view of the results of our present psychiatric study and of some other studies. Speaking of psychiatric disturbance, Pare and Raven[5] found remarkably little provided that the patient herself wanted the operation, and adverse reactions were rare among the women in their series who were refused but who had obtained an abortion by one means or another. Clark et al.[6] asked 118 women for their reaction to the termination of their pregnancy six months after the event, and report that 108 were wholly satisfied, 3 acquiescent, 3 more dissatisfied and in 4 cases their reaction was unknown. In Ekblad's group[7] 25 per cent of the women felt some degree of 'self-reproach', 11 per cent feeling serious self-reproaches or regret, but more than half the women in his study had manifested symptoms of chronic neurosis or abnormal personality before the pregnancy and all were terminated on psychiatric grounds. McCoy[8] was doubtful about the probable outcome of termination in patients with genuine psychiatric disturbances but found that if pregnancy was socially untenable abortion was rarely regretted. In the present series none was dissatisfied to the extent of choosing the statement 'If I could decide again, I would not have it done.' The view of 4 was that abortion had seemed the best solution at the time, but now they were not so sure that it was. It is worth looking at this less satisfied group in some detail. In 2 cases, there had been a change in the patient's marital situation.

1 This patient had requested termination of her pregnancy because of the break-up of her marriage, her uncertain financial situation, overcrowded living conditions and her recent confinement. At follow-up she had had to leave the room she was in. She was successful in obtaining a house for herself and her children from the housing department, and her husband had returned to her. Although she chose (b) she was only minimally regretful about the abortion. 'I sometimes think it might have been better to continue with the pregnancy', she said, 'but then I think it is better to wait and see how things turn out.'

2 At first interview this patient was cohabiting in overcrowded conditions and already had several children, the youngest only a few months old when she got pregnant again. At the time of follow-up, marriage had become possible and was planned for the near future. She said: '(b) expresses it exactly. I expect he [the doctor] was thinking of the children and how I'd cope if I was having another – I think he took all that into consideration when he decided to do it. Well, it's all right for me to talk now that I'm feeling OK but at the time it seemed best and I was in an awful state.' 'I don't really blame myself for being selfish', she added, 'for I was only thinking of myself. When you're upset you put it on, but my troubles don't seem to have been so very great now, looking back.' This patient also regretted having been sterilised.

Doctors can only make up their minds on the facts presented at the time and changes in circumstances are a possibility which the patient as well as the doctor must take into account when asking for an abortion. 'When you're upset you put it on.' All doctors know this, and some feel that patients can be helped through this phase without abortion.

Professor McLaren claims that admission to an appraisal ward where the patient can relax away from home pressures while her problem is sorted out often results in a quite dramatic improvement in her outlook.[9] This is to be expected, especially as the pregnancy progresses, and in Aberdeen too, in doubtful cases, patients are admitted for assessment of their true wishes and the best way of handling the situation. Nothing takes the place of careful assessment but meantime doctors' and social workers' time is being taken up and the pregnancy is progressing. Unless the outcome is almost invariably that abortion is not recommended, a certain amount has to be taken on trust at the first few interviews and the decision made on the situation as it then is.

3 The third patient was in a different category. She and a large family, all boys, and an unsupportive husband lived in overcrowded accommodation and she depended on her part-time work to keep things going. She asked for the termination of her pregnancy and to be sterilised at the same time. 'Although', she said, at the first interview, 'if I thought I was destroying a little girl, I would regret it.' Sure enough, she did regret it and had thought of changing her mind at the time she was admitted to hospital. At follow-up, she chose (b) and said: 'I wish now I'd had the baby and got sterilised after. I keep thinking it might have been a girl and my husband keeps saying to the children you might have had a sister by now.'

4 The fourth patient who chose statement (b) was also a multiparous married woman with an unsupportive husband and depended largely on her own earnings. Although at follow-up she was ambivalent about the abortion she was positive that it had been necessary. 'I would have gone off my head if I hadn't got it done.' After a lot of thought she said her view was 'between (b) and (c)'. She said: 'The sterilisation is hurting me more than the termination.'

The finality of sterilisation rather than the abortion seems to have been the cause of regretful feelings on the part of these two women. Both were wives of unskilled workers. Sterilisation had not been undertaken without good reason for they had 17 pregnancies (13 live-born children) between them. This illustrates the unrealistic attitude of some women to the question of family size and the problems posed by the production of babies long after the point at which the family is able to maintain them. Family planning is not characteristic of this group and it is difficult to reach them with educational and preventive services. Sterilisation, if they will accept it, offers them the safest means of contraception.

One advantage of admission to an 'appraisal' ward is that it gives the patient time to change her mind, although it is possible that women who would be most helped by getting away from heavy family responsibilities might be the very ones who would be too worried about what was happening at home to avail themselves of the opportunity. However there is time to reconsider in the interval before the first appointment with the consultant and again before admission to hospital. It has already been shown (p. 31) that over the nine years of the study 137 women (14 per cent of all referred for consideration of abortion, including single women) changed their minds. The further on the pregnancy of course the more likely this is. The doctors commented:

'Much more settled in her mind and thinks she would like to proceed with pregnancy.'

'Took a very mild line indeed and was quite content with suggestion of PPS.'

'Has only come along so that an opinion could be given that would satisfy her husband. Would be very upset if termination recommended.'

'Patient unreliable and often changes her mind. Today absolutely definite she wants to keep the baby.'

'Only wants abortion if it's twins.'

The interviews showed that other women had felt inclined to change their minds but had not done so for various reasons. Women who had had their pregnancies terminated were asked: 'Did you at any time between then [being told that the pregnancy would be terminated] and coming in to hospital feel like changing your mind about having it done?' Thirty-eight of the 50 patients answered with an unqualified no, but 12 described various degrees of uncertainty up to the night before the operation. Five were evidently prepared to change their mind if their husband had changed his, but he had not.

'He said that's what you've come in for.' (What if he had suggested you going on with it?) 'I suppose I would have. It's a matter of agreement, isn't it, and if he'd wanted it too I'd probably just have had it.'

'I felt rather guilty – just a slight twinge. I talked to my husband but he seemed adamant.' (And if he had not been adamant?) 'I don't think I'd have changed my mind. Well, I might have changed it several times.'

A third patient said: 'If I had felt the baby it might have been different and I might have changed my mind but I felt nothing. If my husband had said to go on with it, I think I would have. I asked him on Sunday night if he still felt the same about the termination and he said yes, it would be best.'

Another patient was in hospital for termination of pregnancy and sterilisation when it was found that her husband had not signed the necessary form of consent to the operation. He had said he would come to see her the night before the operation. She said that if he had not come she had meant to leave hospital and not have it done. Asked why she felt like this, she said: 'You've time to think in hospital – it was just the thought that I'd never have another bairn.'

Such examples hint at the pressures for and against abortion that some of the women experienced, and at the part played by husbands in stiffening their resolve. In spite of these doubts, 10 of the 12 patients who had felt at some point like changing their minds were certain that abortion had been the right thing when they were followed up four or five months later. The other 2, though regretful, would not have wanted a different outcome.

ABORTION NOT DONE

In a few of the 25 cases where the abortion was not done the patient had changed her mind about wanting the pregnancy terminated, had aborted spontaneously while her case was being considered or was prepared to go on with the pregnancy if the consultant thought it was safe to do so, which he did. The majority (18), however, went on with the pregnancy because the consultant did not feel justified in terminating it. Most of the patients accepted this decision without demur; at follow-up they did not question the doctor's explanation that termination would involve too much risk, that the pregnancy was too far on or that the indications for doing it were inadequate. A few were dissatisfied or resentful but had taken no further steps to obtain an abortion.

Three of the 18 did not accept the doctor's decision. One made a serious but unsuccessful attempt to abort herself and was admitted to hospital as an emergency, and the 2 others obtained legal abortions elsewhere. In none of the 18 cases did the patient obtain an illegal abortion. In comparison, Clark *et al.*,[6] describing the outcome of pregnancy in 93 cases out of 109 refused abortion in London, found that 32 had obtained an abortion elsewhere (12 legally and 20 illegally). Several Aberdeen patients mentioned people they said they had been told might help them if they were not accepted for a hospital abortion, but this was probably more in the nature of a threat, or perhaps the unknowledgeable Aberdeen married woman may not be so persistent in following up such leads. At any rate, these 2 are the only patients among the 366 unsuccessful ever-married applicants for a hospital abortion known to have obtained one elsewhere (Table 1:17), which confirms the impression in Aberdeen that resort to back-street abortionists is uncommon.

Early in the referral procedure 4 of the 25 patients changed their minds about wanting an abortion. Two had been uncertain from the start and in both cases their change of mind was associated with an improvement in their relationship with their husbands. Another had applied for an abortion in an initial state of shock at a late unexpected pregnancy but after supportive sessions with the consultants she felt better physically and mentally and decided to continue. The pregnancy in the fourth case presented a serious financial problem to an already overburdened family, but the patient said she changed her mind as a result of a suggestion that she might later on regret having had it terminated. This seems to have confirmed her own thoughts, suggesting that perhaps pressure from members of her family had been responsible for her initial request. In all 4 cases the patient's ambivalence was discernible when first seen. All 4 went on with their pregnancies and at follow-up none regretted the decision.

It is not surprising to find that when the 18 patients who were not recommended for abortion were seen again at about the 34th week of their pregnancy most had settled down and accepted the situation. Their reaction was tested in the same way as in the other group but the statements reading:

(*a*) I still think it would have been better if the pregnancy had been terminated and I still don't feel happy about having the baby.

(*b*) I still think it would have been best if the pregnancy had been terminated, but I'm beginning to feel happier about having the baby.

(c) I'm glad I didn't have the pregnancy terminated.

Ten of the 18 chose the statement 'I'm glad I didn't have the pregnancy terminated.' The other 8 still thought abortion would have been best, but 7 of these were beginning to feel happier about having the baby.

It would have been surprising if women so near the time of their confinement had not forgotten some of their initial worries in looking forward to the new baby. Because these 'natural' maternal feelings usually assert themselves is not to say that abortion is rarely justified. A contented confinement is a happy outcome for a woman with an unwanted pregnancy and the doctor's responsibilities stop there or soon after. The implications for the mother, however, and for the child itself, are longer term and the future holds greater risk than in the case of a wanted child, as Forssman and Thuwe have dramatically shown for Sweden.[10] The one patient who chose the statement 'I still think it would have been better if the pregnancy had been terminated and I still don't feel happy about having the baby' seemed to be thinking of the uncertain future.

She had been treated for some years by her doctor for 'nerves' and had asked for the termination of her fourth pregnancy on the grounds of her husband's drinking and violence. The existing children were already suffering from this, despite police intervention. She hoped to leave him when the youngest child was older but could not do so if she had another baby. She felt it would be wrong to bring another child into such a home.

At follow-up the situation was unchanged. She had hoped for a miscarriage. She said: 'I'd still ask for it to be done, but there's nothing I can do now but accept it, is there?' She was still depressed. 'I seem to settle down but it flares up again.' She was looking forward to being sterilised.

The other 7 women who would still have preferred an abortion were beginning to feel happier about having the baby when they were followed up.

One, an older woman, had had her last child many years before, was tired out and sometimes depressed. Her husband's excessive drinking made things unhappy at home and 'they always seem to get worse when you're pregnant', she said.

At follow-up she still thought she should have been allowed an abortion, and she would still ask for it to be done if she could. Now that the pregnancy had continued so far she was accepting the situation, though with reluctance. 'If I'd had the money', she said, 'I could have gone to London and got it done.' (Would you have?) 'Yes, I would.' She had seen a television programme about the possibilities there.

Three final examples describe some of the 10 patients who chose the statement 'I'm glad I didn't have the pregnancy terminated.'

A young woman with 3 boys asked for abortion because she could not afford another child on a labourer's wage. Five of them were living on less than £12 per week. In addition, she was not getting on with her husband who had been in trouble with the police; she said they only stuck together for the sake of the children. She was 'perfectly certain' she wanted an abortion, so much so that when this was not recommended she sought a second opinion which was also negative.

At follow-up she was affable and contented. 'If I get my quinie [girl] I'm not really worrying now', she said. In explanation, she said: 'I think it would have been on my mind if I'd had an abortion – you know, on my conscience.' Asked how much she had really wanted it in the first place, she said: 'I wasn't really worrying if I had it or not.'

The consultant's prior knowledge of this second patient, an emotionally unstable woman, helped him to reach a negative decision. When seen again she had had the baby, and although she had pressed for abortion with earnestness and determination, she seemed very content. 'We've got a son now', she said, 'and we love him and we're happy.' She said that none of the statements expressed her views exactly. 'I can't say I wish the pregnancy had been terminated. I'm very glad it wasn't now we've got him.' She said later: 'I feel much more fulfilled than if I'd had it terminated and I'd never ask for a termination again. I see it from a completely different point of view now.'

The final example is of another woman in an unhappy family situation in which the children were suffering from the violence of both parents and the general marital discord. She felt that with her 'nerves' she could not stand the noise of another baby and feared she would have even less control of herself. Her husband took no responsibility but she herself was a Roman Catholic and was clearly ambivalent about abortion.

At follow-up she was glad the pregnancy had not been terminated as she said she really thought of abortion as murder. She still thought it would have been best, however. Complaining of her husband's indifference, she said rather interestingly that it might have been that she had wanted to punish him by having the pregnancy terminated so that she could blame him for her feelings of guilt.

All the three Roman Catholics who were not recommended abortion chose the statement 'I'm glad I didn't have the pregnancy terminated.' However, abortions were performed on 3 Catholics and on 4 others whose husbands were Catholics, and only one of the 7 expressed any reservations at follow-up. All 7 chose the statement 'I have no doubt at all that to terminate the pregnancy was the right thing to do.'

CONCLUSIONS

The group of 85 women described here is thought to be representative of Aberdeen ever-married women referred for consideration of abortion with the exception of the small group of private patients. It is clear that the majority seek abortion because of serious social and psychological pressures created by predominantly socio-economic difficulties. Unhappy marital relationships (in which excessive drinking, a chronic problem in Scotland, often seems to play a part), financial troubles (not uncommon in an area of high unemployment) and an illegitimate pregnancy to a woman who is the family breadwinner, are the circumstances most frequently mentioned. Many of the women already have large families and are clearly unable to practice effective birth control. Forty-three per cent of all the legitimate pregnancies had been unintended and over a third of the couples had used no method of contraception throughout their married life except the condom or coitus interruptus. At the time of conception of the pregnancy they wished aborted two-thirds of the women were using nothing or no reliable method although some of these said they used a reliable method occasionally.

These findings are very similar to the findings of other studies and make it clear why there is a continuing demand for abortion. Oral contraception does not suit all women, some do not like it, the use of other forms of contraception may be less reliable, mistakes occur and advice on family planning still does not reach many of the women most in need of it. In 1949 the Royal Commission on Population considered that it was initially the family doctor's duty to give advice on contraception to his patients but not all see this as their role. Little has been done to prepare them for it and studies of the attitudes of general practitioners have shown that many still prefer to follow their patient's lead rather than take the initiative themselves for giving advice on birth control for non-clinical indications. This of course is not enough where some women are too ignorant, indifferent or shy to bring the matter up. The increasing numbers of abortions being applied for throughout the country is a measure of the failure of contraceptive services to reach effectively many of the women at risk. Requests for abortion in Aberdeen have been increasing concurrently with a considerable expansion of the work of Aberdeen's family planning service, 1970 being their busiest year since the service was founded in 1946. The great number of abortions in Britain has at least had the effect of stimulating the government to give greater priority to the family planning services, and in 1971 plans were announced to help local authorities to triple their expenditure on these services and to promote research into the best way of bringing them to all sections of the population. The private member's bill of 1972 to provide vasectomy on the national health service is another effort to substitute birth control for abortion.

It seems that in a city such as Aberdeen legal abortions can be performed quietly for many years without a demand for abortion being created and indeed without the general population knowing very much about it. The study suggests that generally Aberdeen married women do not know if they qualify for an abortion or not, but better education, higher expectations from life and the stirrings of independence lead some to question what before seemed inevitable. They were not often motivated to apply by what they had read or seen on television but if they knew anyone who had had an abortion this encouraged some to ask their doctor if they too could be considered. If the consultant thought there were no adequate grounds for abortion married patients generally continued the pregnancy and did not go outside the area for it. Some were content with the offer of post-partum sterilisation. Their attitude may have resulted from ignorance of any alternative and lack of financial resources but may also indicate uncertainty in their own minds about abortion (6 per cent of all ever-married women referred changed their minds and withdrew their application for abortion). A follow-up of the records of ever-married women who had not been accepted for abortion (1963–71) showed that only 0.5 per cent had the pregnancy terminated legally elsewhere (both were illegitimate pregnancies), while the great majority continued their pregnancy and were confined in Aberdeen. This supports the impression that women in Aberdeen do not commonly seek a private legal abortion or resort to illegal abortion if they do not get it done through the national health service.

The suggestion that social support should be given as an alternative to abortion requested on primarily social grounds is not entirely realistic in the more chronic situations. Constructive help might entail rehousing a family, ensuring that a married woman has the security of some income in her own control, seeing that maintenance grants are actually received or making far better provision for help with child care than at present exists. It is hardly necessary to say that denial of abortion does not entitle the overburdened woman to special consideration of this kind and she is left to manage her increased family as best she can. It is as well to be clear about the reality of the 'social help' so easily invoked. Without improvements in the conditions under which married women are expected to function the demand for abortion on primarily socio-economic grounds is not likely to be reduced.

The examples have been chosen to illustrate not only the kind of situations that drive married women in Aberdeen to seek abortions but also the problems facing doctors in deciding if the continuation of the pregnancy involves more risk to the woman's physical or mental health than its termination. The doctor knows best the contra-indications and risks involved in the procedure, but he does not speak with the same authority on the stress created by her home circumstances which the law now allows her to ask to be taken into consideration. Health service consultants find decision-making difficult and onerous in this intangible area but if medical autonomy is to be preserved in regard to abortion this self-imposed responsibility cannot be avoided. It may be however that new developments in the techniques of birth control will relieve them of it in the not too distant future.

The examples quoted suggest that if abortion were available on the woman's initial request some might subsequently regret their decision. Ten of the 18 women who were refused abortion said later that they were glad it had not been done. As they were within a month or two of their confinement when they said it their feelings are understandable, but this gives more weight to the reaction of the other 8 who had been refused and who still thought it would have been best if the pregnancy had been terminated.

While 8 of the 18 *refused abortion* were not happy with the decision but were making the best of it, the great majority of the 52 women who *had had an abortion* said they were glad it had been done. Only 4 expressed regret, their regret being associated with a change in their marital situation or, somewhat unrealistically in their circumstances, with having been sterilised at the same time. Some spoke of temporary depression on their return from hospital. Interview at a deeper level and at a later stage would be needed to try to assess the success of the decision in the long run in these cases. Dr Olley's longer term psychiatric follow-up described elsewhere also shows for his group that the aborted women were generally more satisfied with the result than those who had carried the pregnancy to term.

If abortion through the national health service were 'on demand' husbands and wives would have to accept greater responsibility than they do at present for the outcome of their decisions as they have to do in the private sector where an 'on demand' situation virtually exists. As it is, in Aberdeen if abortion is offered it is almost invariably accepted, if refused this is more often than not accepted – in either case the real decision is out of the mother's hands. (This may be inevitable if she is backward or mentally disturbed.) In the group interviewed whatever decision was reached by the doctors in the great majority of cases the patients had adjusted to it when seen four or five months later, though those refused abortion were less satisfied than those who had been aborted. These results were not achieved by granting abortion 'on demand' but by careful time-consuming assessment in many cases, sometimes reinforced by social workers' reports and psychiatric opinions. This kind of care is surely necessary if the doctor is to take over the decision on so important a matter on his patient's behalf, but as the number of referrals continues to rise it becomes increasingly difficult to make time for it.

The abortion problem might be contained if married women only were concerned. It is not easy to project oneself imaginatively into the domestic pressures and mental processes of others but at least the problems of the married state are universal and can be recognised. The married woman is always at risk of unwanted conception. Contraceptives may fail and the most motivated couples may not be constantly vigilant. Many are careless in their sexual relationships, 'taking a chance' which is so much a part of life in other contexts. Social workers are aware that despite the improvement in the position of women in the lower socio-economic groups the situation deplored by the Church Assembly Board for Social Responsibility as 'the sexual exploitation by man of woman within marriage' is not entirely a thing of the past. In some relationships there is little mutuality and no communication between the partners on matters of importance to each, such as birth control. The problems of married women of limited education, over-burdened with domestic cares and unable to practise efficient contra-ception, are generally appreciated. The illegitimate pregnancy, however, arouses different feelings. The following chapter concerns the pregnant single woman and attempts to show the circumstances that bring some of them to seek abortion in Aberdeen.

REFERENCES

1 Tredgold, R. F. (1964). 'Psychiatric indications for termination of pregnancy', *Lancet*, **2**, 251–4.
2 Thompson, B., Durno, D., MacGregor, J. E., McGregor, M. S. M. (1969). 'Some aspects of oral contraception and married women', *Med. Officer*, cxxi, **8**, 93–6.
3 Cartwright, A. (1970). *Parents and Family Planning Services*, Routledge and Kegan Paul, London.
4 Thompson, B., Baird, D. (1968). 'Follow-up of 186 sterilised women', *Lancet*, **1**, 1023–7.
5 Pare, C. M. B., Raven, H. (1970). 'Follow-up of patients referred for termination of pregnancy', *Lancet*, **1**, 635–8.
6 Clark, M., Forstner, I., Pond, D. A., Tredgold, R. F. (1968). 'Sequels of unwanted pregnancy', *Lancet*, **2**, 501–3.
7 Ekblad, M. (1955). 'Induced abortion on psychiatric grounds', *Acta psychiat. neurol. scand.*, Suppl. 99.
8 McCoy, D. R. (1968). 'The emotional reaction of women to therapeutic abortion and sterilisation', *J. Obs. Gynaec. Brit. Comm.*, **75**, 10, 1054–7.
9 McLaren, H. (1969). 'Abortion or modern obstetrics?', *Brit. J. hosp. Med.*, **2**, 607–12.
10 Forssman, H., Thuwe, I. (1965). 'One hundred and twenty children born after application for therapeutic abortion refused', *Acta psychiat. scand.*, **41**, 71–88.

TABLE 3:1. *Use of contraception at time of becoming pregnant*

	Total	Non-manual	Skilled	Semi- and Unskilled
Nothing used or nothing reliable being used	26	3	12	11
Reliable method but not used regularly	21	5	5	11
Failure of contraceptive method blamed	14	3	6	5
Difficulties with timing when to take pill	3	—	2	1
Pregnancy intended	4	—	2	2
	68	11	27	30

4 THE WOMAN'S STORY: SINGLE WOMEN

Jean Aitken-Swan

So far abortion has been discussed in relation to married women only but they are not the main problem to the doctors at the present time. The rise in the number of illegitimate pregnancies and the increasing number of women in the higher occupational groups led to a growing demand for abortion from single women. The Abortion Act came into operation at a time when attitudes to sex and sexual morality were undergoing a periodical upheaval and when young people were forcing the pace of change by opting out of accepted social conventions which seemed irrelevant to their preferred way of life. In every generation youth challenges authority and tries to create the kind of world it wants to live in. Now working class youth, at last emancipated by better health, education and greatly improved material conditions of life, made their values part of the new ethos, for instance, pleasure now rather than the postponement of pleasure. They produced a youth culture, which was different, anti-establishment and which through commercial promotion became attractive to young people everywhere.

Some people saw in this a spirit of hopefulness, the promise of a healthier, less class-conscious, franker, freer, more sexually equalitarian type of society, but the pace of change and some of the consequences of permissiveness worried many. Negative aspects could not be ignored nor their impact on the most vulnerable sections of society, the immature and unstable. Too often these young people were the victims of the new addictions, the illegitimate pregnancies and venereal disease. They were educated enough to be dissatisfied with their opportunities in life and attracted by what appeared to be exciting new freedoms but their education had not prepared them for these dangers. The adult world, feeling in some way responsible, was alarmed but did not seem to know how to help.

Aberdeen no less than centres further south reflected these stresses. Pregnancies to single women increased from 151 in 1963 to 453 in 1971. Sixty of these were to girls of 15 or less and 75 to girls still at school. Women who might be thought to have too much to lose by getting illegitimately pregnant, professional women, students, nurses, etc., were getting pregnant in increasing numbers. Many of these were unwilling or unable to bring up a baby themselves or to consider adoption. They asked for abortion. The rise in the rate of abortions and the numbers occurring in much publicised sub-groups such as students or girls under 16 years of age attract attention and arouse emotion without very much being known of what lies behind the figures, the motivations and perceptions of the individual woman, why she got pregnant, what happened and how things turned out for her. This narrower focus provides a background to the statistics and helps in understanding the problems of the single woman seeking abortion. Between September 1968 and June 1969 82 single women were interviewed, nearly half the total applying. Their story is told here.

As already shown (Table 1:10, p. 40) single women referred for consideration of abortion are not typical of all pregnant single women; the former tend to be younger and at the higher end of the scale of women's occupations. The 82 follow this pattern, half of them being teenagers (the youngest 14), and nearly three-quarters being students, nurses or clerical workers (Table 4:1).

In Table 4:2 the father's or guardian's occupation is used to indicate the socio-economic group of the family.

The professional–managerial category contains 4 professional men. Together with farmers, shown separately, the two groups comprise the Registrar General's social classes I and II. The proportion of women in this category (one-third of the total) is higher than would be expected from their numbers in the population, which is merely to confirm that referral for abortion is more often arranged for single women whose fathers' occupations, as well as their own, are at the upper end of the scale. At the same time, the high proportion of applications from a semi-skilled or unskilled working class background is interesting as women who are themselves in this type of work are the least likely to be referred (Table 1:10). Associates at work may have suggested the possibility of abortion to them or it may be that the same initiative that led them to take up skilled or clerical work, nursing or further education, led them to seek abortion when they became pregnant rather than following the traditional patterns of getting married or producing an illegitimate baby.

In this group the incidence of 'broken homes' is very much lower than it was at the time Thompson made her study of illegitimate maternities in Aberdeen in 1949–52.[1] Then 40 per cent of unmarried women having a baby came from a broken home (i.e. had lost a parent through death, separation or divorce before the minimum school-leaving age). Despite a considerable increase in divorce since those days, only 12 per cent of the present group came from a broken home. This may indicate the change that has taken place in the social characteristics of women getting illegitimately pregnant, but there is also a selection factor here in that broken homes are more usual in the lowest occupational groups, who are the least likely to be referred for consideration of abortion.

It is usual for girls to have boyfriends older than themselves and this group was no exception. In most cases the difference was one or two years only but 20 of the putative fathers were between 5 and 28 years older than the girl – these were mostly married men or men who had been married. Where the difference in age was most extreme the girls themselves tended to be older. The man's occupation usually fell in the same, or a higher, socio-economic group as that of the girl's father. The boyfriends of students and girls still at school were often fellow-students or schoolmates (Table 4:3).

More than half the women (47) had an apparently serious relationship with their man friend. A few were engaged or had made their marriage plans but most were 'going steady'. The relationship in 31 other cases seems to have been essentially friendly only; marriage had not been contemplated or pregnancy had resulted from a casual encounter. These two groups, which account for 78 of the 82 women, are described in more detail in Table 4:4. The stories of 3 who alleged unwilling intercourse may be true – 2 were very young. The truth of the account given by one woman was seriously questioned and is here included under 'indeterminate'.

Engaged, marriage plans made, going steady (47)

Although 47 of the 82 women thought they had a serious relationship with their man friend which was leading to marriage, 13 of them were 'going steady' with a man who was not free to marry. In some cases this was only found out when the pregnancy was discussed; in others, the man was separated from his wife and had said he was in process of obtaining a divorce. Another 10 men, although free to marry, did not want to do so on hearing of the pregnancy – some of these had disappeared. In 4 cases the parents of young girls opposed any question of marriage and asked for abortion of the pregnancy. Two other pregnancies would have continued and the couple would have brought forward the date of their marriage had not the question of termination arisen as a result of early contact with rubella. The remaining 18 couples could not, or did not want, to marry then for a variety of practical reasons – they were not yet in a financial position to do so, they had to complete their studies or they had mutually broken off their engagement or friendship before the pregnancy had been discovered. In some cases the woman herself had broken off the relationship on discovering that her man friend was unreliable or in trouble with the police. Several were unwilling to prejudice the success of their marriage by marrying when pregnant.

Some relationships were therefore not strong enough to stand the test of a pre-marital pregnancy and in other cases it was only prudent not to marry. There can be little new in the situations in which young women seeking marriage partners find themselves. What is new, at any rate for some groups in society, is that the restraints which formerly inhibited many of them from having pre-marital intercourse have been so weakened that it is now almost taken for granted that a developing friendship may become a sexual relationship, given the changing and in some respects uncertain standards of behaviour of the present day.

Friendly or casual only (31)

It is a sidelight on the changing times that 31 of the 82 women had little hesitation in describing the casual nature of their association with the putative father, and that they felt free to do so gives confidence in the general truth of their story. Twelve, mostly aged between 19 and 21, were having a casual affair without expecting or wanting it to lead to marriage. Sometimes the relationship appeared to be drifting, or a steady relationship had been broken off but the couple were still occasionally seeing each other. Girls away from home and not in a position, or wanting, to get married became involved in affairs with men who similarly did not want to marry. Several had broken off the relationship before realising they were pregnant.

Eight rather younger women claimed that the pregnancy had resulted from an unpremeditated incident, usually after a party at which they had had too much to drink. Their boyfriends were about the same age as themselves and the climate of some teenage parties gives no reason to doubt this part of the story although the frequency of intercourse may be understated.

Five of the 31 young women could be described as emotionally disturbed. They gave a history of depression, suicidal gestures, emotional troubles and disturbed home backgrounds. Four very young girls were evidently experimenting with sex, in 3 cases with boys as young as themselves. The 2 remaining women in the group who had temporary relationships came from different cultural backgrounds abroad.

It is conventional to insist that young women should not enjoy sexual pleasure outside the married state, although with the coming of really efficient contraceptive techniques the double standard may require new justification. It is, however, quite wrong that they should become unintentionally pregnant. Previous studies have established that young unmarried people are not very knowledgeable about contraception and do not use it when they should, perhaps not surprisingly in view of the difficulties put in their way. The fear of pregnancy is still valued as a deterrent to a girl having pre-marital intercourse, and there is no consensus of opinion as to whether she is behaving badly or responsibly if she seeks contraceptive advice. While it may be agreed that contraception should be discussed in sex education lectures at school or elsewhere this is not the same as teaching young people that if they must have pre-marital sexual relationships it is their duty and responsibility to see that an unwanted pregnancy does not occur, and making the means available without embarrassment to them. The impression is sometimes given that were contraception made freely available to single women there would be a ready (and undesirable) demand for it, but this suggests a rationality and purpose not very evident in the thinking of many of the young women in the present study.

CONTRACEPTION

'I'm afraid it was the furthest thing from my mind at the time.'

'He said he knew what he was doing. I trusted him, I suppose. It never entered my head' [about the risk of pregnancy].

'I didn't worry about it because he didn't worry. He said if you get pregnant I'll get my divorce.'

These three typical comments show that the thinking of the present group has not advanced very far since Schofield described attitudes to birth control in his study of the sexual behaviour of young people in the early 1960s.[2] Then two-thirds of the girls having sexual intercourse were at risk, the majority neither taking precautions themselves nor insisting that their partners should do so. Nearly all the girls left the matter to their partners. Yet the replies of the boys showed that 29 per cent of them exhibited a lack of concern and disinclination to think about birth control best classified under the category 'don't care'. Schofield's data indicated that 56 per cent of boys and 49 per cent of girls had very little interest in birth control and would be slow to profit from instruction in the use of contraception. If this is so, and the findings for the present rather older and pregnant group support it, the problem is not whether single women should have access to contraceptive facilities but rather how they can be persuaded to make use of them.

In the present group intercourse was often unpremeditated and possible consequences were forgotten, the girl assuming that what risk there was would be taken care of by her older, more experienced boyfriend. In all only 5 of the 82 couples had used an effective method of contraception regularly and 23 occasionally. Forty-four used nothing except perhaps coitus interruptus. A contraceptive method was used more often when the couple were engaged or 'going steady' than when the relationship was merely friendly but the latter group contained many who claimed that intercourse was unpremeditated and occurred once only (Table 4:5).

Sexually experienced young women tended more frequently to have used a contraceptive method than women who said they had had no other sexual partners, but again the former did not use it regularly. Condoms are not always available, intercourse is often unplanned or infrequent and the respondents seemed to feel that to take contraception seriously or to 'go on the pill' would change the relationship with their boyfriend in a way that neither of them wished. They valued spontaneity and seemed to regard effective precautions as calculating.

Only 12 of the 82 single women had sought advice on contraception, 7 from their own doctors, 2 from student health services, one from a medical student friend and 2 from books. They were either too late and were already pregnant or for various reasons they had stopped taking the pill which had been prescribed. In another 3 cases in which the doctor had offered advice after a previous pregnancy or negative pregnancy test, none of the young women had acted on the advice given. One professed to be 'quite shocked' at an unmarried friend of hers who was on the pill. The second was away from her home town and the general practitioner who had advised her, and her precautions lapsed; the third thought that if she went on the pill it would only encourage her to go back to her boyfriend, with whom she was trying to break.

The doctors consulted by 9 of the 12 single women who wanted contraceptive advice were all willing to prescribe for them or to refer them to an appropriate clinic. However it was generally thought that contraceptive advice would not be given to unmarried women or at least that they would be criticised for asking for it, and this was given by some as a reason for taking no action. The women seemed to see an illegitimate pregnancy as the result of bad luck rather than bad management and an abortion as less 'immoral' than being in a state of pre-paredness for sex. Typical attitudes are expressed in these replies to a question on whether or not they had sought advice on contraception:

'I didn't know I could get any. Although I did know one or two girls on the pill but they were engaged or going steady. I didn't think of asking for it as I wasn't serious about him.'

'I could never have discussed the pill with my doctor – it's too cold-blooded an approach to sex.'

Another girl did not approve of an unmarried friend obtaining contraceptives from a family planning clinic. She said: 'It makes it seem so premeditated. I think your moral standards would begin to go and it's better not.'

It is not surprising to find in a group referred for consideration of abortion many who have been unsuccessful or careless about contra-ception, but there are signs of the stirrings of a more responsible attitude among single women. An analysis by Dr Thompson of new attenders at the Aberdeen family planning clinic during the first quarter of each year from 1964 to 1970 showed a marked increase in the number of unmarried women attending, from 2 in 1964 to 97 in 1970. A striking change has been that up to 1967 nearly all these women were seeking advice on contraception prior to their marriage which had already been arranged, but from 1967 onwards the proportion of new attenders whose marriage was already arranged was falling. Presumably women having a sexual relationship not leading to marriage in the near future were beginning to ask for contraceptive advice, a promising trend given the sexual freedom of the present day. Their interest in contraception has been encouraged by the increasing use and popularity of the 'pill', which was the method prescribed for nearly all the unmarried women attending the clinic. The provision is part of Aberdeen's excellent comprehensive family planning service which since 1968 has been made available to all women referred to it, regardless of marital state. Students, particularly university students, predominate among the new attenders, with teachers, other professional women, nurses and clerical workers making up most of the remainder. There is little sign yet that contraceptive advice is being sought to any great extent by single women in the lower occupational groups.

The male partners, to whom was left the major share of the responsibility for contraception, were not always unsuccessful in preventing pregnancy. Sixteen of the 82 single women had had between one and six previous sexual partners without becoming pregnant and this may have encouraged them in their happy-go-lucky or trustful attitude. Nineteen others had been pregnant before (the same proportion of second or later pregnancies noted in Table 1:13 for all Aberdeen single women pregnant in 1968 and 1969). What happened the first time and how pregnancy occurred a second time is considered in some detail in these 19 cases.

MORE THAN ONE ILLEGITIMATE PREGNANCY

Although parents and society may excuse a first pregnancy in a single girl on the grounds of youthful inexperience, it is harder to understand or tolerate a second. Many young women illegitimately pregnant marry before the birth of the baby and do not get pregnant again outside marriage. Others do not or cannot marry and continue at risk of another illegitimate pregnancy to which, judging from psychiatric evidence, some are predisposed through personality characteristics of immaturity and emotional instability. Young women having a second or later illegitimate pregnancy often come from disturbed and broken homes and may have attended psychiatric clinics, compensating perhaps through maternity for their own poor family relationships and lack of opportunity. Some are not highly motivated to avoid pregnancy and seem to drift into the same relationships, i.e. with married men, which let them down before. What happened at the time of the first pregnancy may have a bearing on the occurrence of the second. Pressure from parents, boyfriends or others to have an abortion or to have the baby adopted could be emotionally traumatic to a girl who in getting pregnant is perhaps seeking some kind of fulfilment she cannot find elsewhere. The timing of the second pregnancy in relation to the first seems to agree with the theory of the compulsive nature of many second pregnancies. In the present small group whose first pregnancy ended in the birth of a baby which they kept, the interval before they got pregnant again was usually longer (between 1 and 5 years) than when the first pregnancy had ended in an abortion, neonatal death or adoption of the baby, when almost all were pregnant again between 3 and 11 months later. However, this could be due to the restricted opportunities of the mother of an infant to get about and meet people, or equally likely to be a function of the small number of cases.

The outcome of the previous and present pregnancies is shown in Table 4:6, whether to the same or a different man and the interval of time between them.

Women in skilled, semi-skilled or unskilled manual work ('all other occupations' in Table 4:6) are over-represented in the group, no fewer than 42 per cent of them having had a previous pregnancy compared with only 16 per cent of the combined students, nurses and clerical workers. This accords with what has already been said about pregnancy-repeating (Chapter 1, p. 25). The social composition of the 19 reflects the selection criteria of the referring doctors and it would seem that women in manual occupations are more likely to be referred if they are having a second or later pregnancy than if it is their first. For one thing, most of the manual workers had kept their first baby and a second illegitimate pregnancy could present considerable practical difficulties besides jeopardising the girl's relationship with her parents.

The reasons why the 5 women who had more than one pregnancy to the same man did not marry him are the usual reasons for not marrying the putative father: a steady relationship breaking up, economic difficulties, a divorce not yet absolute (or not applied for). More interesting are the reasons why these women who had already had an illegitimate pregnancy had allowed themselves to become pregnant again, as if the experience had taught them nothing. Their contraceptive practice before the first and subsequent pregnancy is shown in Table 4:7.

The 3 women who had had more than one previous illegitimate pregnancy appear to have been equally unconcerned about contraception. Two had taken no precautions before either pregnancy and the third had taken the pill erratically so that she was unprepared when her man friend came out of prison.

The statements seem to indicate that these young women were psychologically unwilling to protect themselves against the risk of pregnancy. It may be thought that this lack of concern is a natural consequence of the present availability of abortion and weakening of sanctions against illegitimate pregnancy. But Leontine Young described much the same lack of concern nearly twenty years ago among her neurotic unmarried mothers when she spoke of the girls being conspicuously disinterested in the use of any protective devices to prevent pregnancy. 'Questioning of a large number of girls as to whether they had considered the use of contraceptives brought always the same response, an expression of flat astonishment and bewilderment and the answer "no".'[3] The motivation of the present young women and what meaning pregnancy had for them cannot nowadays be explained narrowly in terms of the neurotic needs of the mother, although neurotic traits are present, as Dr Olley has shown, particularly in the girls who had experienced a previous pregnancy. Perhaps they manifest the same psychological denial sometimes perceived when what people want to believe (in this case, that they will not get pregnant) conflicts with what they know theoretically to be true (that they are likely to get pregnant if they have uncontracepted intercourse). Their apparent indifference to the practical difficulties which a further pregnancy would bring suggests a degree of emotional disturbance in some cases; in others the second pregnancy may have been precipitated by the same environmental influences which had brought about the first.

McCance and Hall[4] in their study of Aberdeen university students found that girls who had been pregnant in the past were the most careful with their contraception afterwards. Certainly the proportion of single women who had other pregnancies besides the one they wished aborted was lower among the students referred than in any other occupational group, but even so 11 per cent of students (of all types) had been pregnant before or became pregnant again after referral (up to 1970). About half were university students. Psychiatric indications for abortion were considered to be present in the great majority of cases.

Apart from the question of psychiatric instability, many more women than before are now having pre-marital sexual intercourse and this does not necessarily stop on having had a first pregnancy. Feelings about contraception are often mixed particularly in the lower occupational groups, to whom the majority of second illegitimate pregnancies occur, and they are slow to seek advice. Practitioners are perhaps still too slow to offer it to unmarried women. There is clearly a need for counselling and careful follow-up of young women after an illegitimate pregnancy.

REACTIONS OF PUTATIVE FATHER AND PARENTS

Usually the first person told about the pregnancy was the putative father. Sometimes he was not told at all, particularly if the relationship had been of a transitory nature; then most of the young women confided first in a girlfriend or flatmate. Parents were seldom the first consulted, and then only by girls living at home, mostly in the younger age groups. Some of the older single women had discussed the matter with no one prior to their interview at hospital except the doctor who had referred them.

The putative father's views are seldom heard at first hand although he shares responsibility for the occurrence of every aborted pregnancy and his reaction to it (if a fiancé or steady boyfriend) often determines whether or not an abortion is applied for. As the person at risk (and also the most under pressure to co-operate), attention in studies of illegitimate pregnancy and abortion is concentrated on the young woman, her attitudes and behaviour. It is almost customary to accept that the male partner is ineducable in matters of sexual responsibility and that his side of things would add little to knowledge of the problem of illegitimate pregnancy. It is the young woman who in becoming pregnant is considered deviant, not the man for making her so. Male interviewers, including many doctors, generally lack interest in overcoming the barriers to communication with other men on sexual matters (on a serious level, at any rate) and might find such an interview uncongenial, although the recent report on sociological research[5] into the American 'tearoom trade' (fellatio in public lavatories) shows that, given the will, anything is possible. It would be interesting to know, for instance, if the putative father's view of the relationship was the same as that of his girlfriend, to what extent he felt implicated, what consideration, if any, was given to his wishes in regard to the pregnancy, what his influence had been on the girl's decision to seek an abortion, if there was anything in his own background or personality which made unmarried fatherhood attractive to him, if men feel less responsible towards women as sexual partners now that equality is the watchword and oral contraception is available, if they regard abortion as an ethical issue that concerns them at all.

However, the single woman has to speak for both of them. According to her at the first interview, more than half the fiancés and steady boy-friends who knew of the pregnancy were repudiating responsibility, were leaving matters to her or had deserted her. Where the relationship had been friendly or casual only, only 5 of the 31 putative fathers accepted responsibility and were trying to help (Table 4:8).

The boyfriends were often as young as the girls and, not unnaturally, in many cases the first consideration is to avoid involvement. Their repudiation of responsibility could be an immediate shock reaction to a pregnancy of which they had only recently heard. Apart from the engaged girls, several of whom were bitter about the break-up of their marriage plans, few of the girls expressed resentment at their boy-friends' attitude towards them. They were usually quite realistic about what was to be expected from them.

In a third of the cases the girl described her boyfriend as standing by her and trying to help. But her reaction, too, to the shock of pregnancy was sometimes to turn against him and to reject any suggestion of marriage, whether the offer was realistic or not. 'Becoming pregnant made me realise just how much I didn't want to marry him.' Marriage was not seen as the acceptable solution it once was to the problem of the illegitimate pregnancy. If it did not seem to promise emotional satisfaction, it was not wanted. These young people did not feel it necessary to marry in haste. One said: 'We feel it impossible to know just yet how marriage would work out. A broken marriage would shatter both of us as well as the child.'

In most cases the situation they described four or five months later followed on logically from what they had said about their relationship with their boyfriend in the first instance (see p. 133 above). In very few cases was there any suggestion that the story of desertion was used without justification to influence the decision on abortion.

In this group the young woman's boyfriend and peer group played a more important part than her parents in helping her to decide what to do about the pregnancy, unless she was very young and living at home. At the time of their application for abortion, over half the young women said that their parents did not yet know of their pregnancy. Girls who lived at home had usually told their parents while those living away from home had not. Such a confession is difficult for anyone even if she has a stable and supportive family but some of the young women had specific reasons for not wishing their parents to know. Illness and nervous troubles at home, narrow religious views, mother widowed, elderly, parents abroad or separated – the truth of these assertions is not known. It suggests lack of interest as well as lack of rapport between the daughter and her parents when 7 of the girls living at home were able to have an abortion without their parents being aware of their pregnancy or, in some cases, of the fact that they had been in hospital at all. Whether the young women eventually told their parents or not almost invariably depended on whether they were successful in obtaining an abortion. If successful, they saw little point in upsetting their parents about it or simply wished to avoid unpleasantness.

Fear of their parents' reaction to news of the pregnancy was often expressed, but the young women themselves were not always good judges of this. Hardly any who told their parents of their pregnancy were 'thrown out', as they sometimes prophesied. Even girls fearful of divulging a second illegitimate pregnancy reported unexpectedly mild reactions. One said of her mother: 'I think she was upset in her own way, but she didn't get in a temper like the last time.' At follow-up many considered that their relationship with their parents had improved as a result of the crisis. 'I'm closer to my mother now', one girl said. 'Before we couldn't speak about things but now it's quite different.' Another said: 'They take me more seriously now. I can talk to them more easily because they treat me differently. I've more experience.' A third said: 'They've more respect for me as a person.' A girl's need to give her parents convincing proof that she is no longer a child could have been an underlying factor in her getting pregnant in the first place.

KNOWLEDGE OF ABORTION

The subject of abortion was given considerable newspaper and television publicity at the time the Medical Termination of Pregnancy Bill was being debated by parliament, but it made no lasting impression on the women interviewed for the present study. Although interviewed soon after the bill became law, few of the single women could state, except in the broadest terms, any of the grounds for terminating a pregnancy and they had only a hazy idea of what the procedure entailed. 'It's only now that I've really thought about it', as one young woman explained. Nearly half the single women could not say when the Abortion Act was passed, although students and nurses were less ignorant on this point than the rest.

Do you know anything about the law on abortion – for instance, when was the last law passed?

	Total	Students, nurses	Clerical	All other
Knows accurately or fairly accurately	43	25	12	6
Knows vaguely†	1	1	—	—
Does not know	38	2	11	25
	82	28	23	31

† I.e. 'within the last year or two'.

The vagueness of their answers to questions about abortion suggests that they were not seeking abortion simply because they thought the new Act now legally entitled them to do so. Like the married women, they were not sure what indications would be acceptable, although as time went on students probably began to exchange information and experiences. The close contacts and easy communication of communal living could also account for the higher proportion of students and nurses who had known someone personally or who had heard of someone who had had an abortion.

(a) *Have you known anyone personally who has had a pregnancy terminated, or who has tried to have it done?*
(b) *Have you heard of anyone?*

	Total	Students, nurses	Clerical	All other
Knows someone personally	16	9	3	4
Does not know anyone personally, but has heard of someone	32	13	11	8
Knows no one, has heard of no one	34	6	9	19
	82	28	23	31

Students were also more aware than other single women of Aberdeen's reputation as a comparatively liberal area for therapeutic abortion
and some of the nurses knew of it through their experience in the wards.
Very few single women, apart from students, nurses and clerical
workers, thought they would be more likely to get an abortion if they
lived in Aberdeen than if they lived in some other area.

*Do you think you are more likely or less likely to get an abortion if you
live in Aberdeen than if you lived in some other place, or does it make no
difference where you live?*

	Total	Students, nurses	Clerical	All other
More likely	20	11	6	3
Less likely	1	—	1	—
No difference	22	7	6	9
Does not know	37	10	9	18
NS	2	—	1	1
	82	28	23	31

Although 20 of the single women compared with only 6 of about the
same number of married women thought abortion more likely in
Aberdeen, the number who thought it made no difference or did not
know is surprisingly high. The point is of interest because it shows how a
liberal abortion policy can operate under the national health service
for years in a city such as Aberdeen with the fact hardly known to the
local population.

AFTER THE ABORTION

Some of the single women had left Aberdeen by the time for follow-up and although several wrote giving a general impression of how they were they are not included in these results. Fifty of the 56 who had had their pregnancies terminated were interviewed four or five months later.

Girls who had been living with their parents were still at home when seen again, with 2 exceptions (one working elsewhere and one who as a result of her pregnancy had been told by her stepfather to leave home and had not returned). Only 13 of the 50 were still associating with the putative father, 2 being married to him and 2 about to be married (Table 4:9). In 2 of these cases the relationship described by the young woman at the first interview had been friendly or casual only and the putative father had not been told of the pregnancy or proposed abortion. Marriage appears to have been initiated by him at some later stage after he had heard of what happened. In the other 2 cases marriage had been intended but delay in divorce proceedings in one case, and contact with rubella early in pregnancy in the other, were factors in the referral for consideration of abortion.

Where at first interview the putative father had been said to be taking no responsibility or to be deserting her (28 cases), in almost all (26) the relationship had ended at the time of follow-up and many of the young women said they had a new boyfriend. Where the putative father had accepted responsibility and tried to help (12 cases) 7 couples were still together at follow-up and only 2 among the 12 girls had a new boyfriend. The preponderance of women whose relationship with their partner was not serious or lasting is not surprising in a group seeking abortion if, as appears likely, the single women who seek contraceptive advice tend to be those with stable relationships. The question of contraception for the future was, however, of practical concern to many in the present group but when seen again about half of those potentially at risk were taking no precautions. There was a tendency to think 'it could never happen again'.

Some said they had been offered contraception by their doctor but did not want it or felt it would be unnecessary. In other cases no advice had been offered. One doctor was said to have disapproved of the abortion and would not advise on contraception after it. In the 5 cases where the relationship had broken up and the young women had no new boyfriends, the pill appears to have been given as a precautionary measure, 3 of the 5 having had previous illegitimate pregnancies.

Apart from the women's own doctors, efforts are made at hospital level to ensure that no unmarried woman having had a baby or an abortion goes away without knowing how to prevent further unwanted conceptions. It is still possible, however, that some do not get advice if, for instance, they default from attending the post-natal clinics, and apart from the giving of advice, aftercare is needed to encourage the girl to act upon it.

Single women, like the married, seldom found the abortion procedure upsetting or frightening in any way and 45 of the 50 thought it had been no worse than expected (Table 4:10). None found the procedure upsetting when the abortion was performed by the suction method or by dilatation and curettage. 'There was nothing to it.' 'It wasn't painful at all – I was surprised.' 'I felt so much better immediately afterwards. It was like having been sick – you know, such a feeling of relief. I expected more pain. There seemed so little to it.' A few (3) had had pain or bleeding after they had returned home but this had cleared up spontaneously. Five of the 17 women whose pregnancy had been terminated by the intra-amniotic injection of hypertonic saline or by abdominal hysterotomy had found the experience upsetting. 'If someone had asked about it soon after, I'd have advised them to have the baby rather than go through that – but you forget.' A young woman who had already had a baby said: 'I thought it canna be as bad as having a right bairn but I'd rather have my boy again than have an abortion.' (Why do you say that?) 'There's no needles. Then the afterbirth wouldn't come away and the doctor had to press on my stomach and that was agony.' Some very young girls were among those who denied that they had found a saline termination upsetting. One had been 'very scared of what it would be like but they froze my stomach and I didn't feel a thing'. This girl thought it would have been more painful to have delivered a full-term baby. A young girl whose second pregnancy was terminated by saline said that 'The actual birth was not painful but when the fluid went in the labour pains were worse than when I had the baby. But they weren't all that bad.' Another said: 'I was so exhausted with anxiety and worry about whether I'd get it done or not I went through it without much alarm. The doctor explained what he was doing but I couldn't concentrate – I just said yes, I understood. It wasn't really too bad.'

Although in retrospect the abortion was not generally regarded as an ordeal it is regettable that in no less than a third of the cases the maturity of the pregnancy necessitated the more radical procedures. It is known that women with illegitimate pregnancies are liable to delay seeking ante-natal care, with consequent risk to the mother and possible ill effects on the baby. There is similar delay by many of those seeking abortion yet speed is particularly important if the risks of abortion and perhaps of emotional damage are to be reduced. Despite the liberal appearance of the times, concealment of pregnancy because of fear of social attitudes and parental disapproval was common in this group.

As abortion patients single women are more lonely than married women in the ward situation as few feel they can share their worries with other patients for fear of censure. They are particularly sensitive to the attitudes of ward staff towards them and sometimes see slights where none may be intended. One admitted that she might have been 'a bit paranoid' at the time and another also saw that her own feelings could have had something to do with the 'atmosphere of unfriendliness' she sensed around her. Nothing more tangible than this and 'queer looks' were mentioned and 46 of the 50 were surprised and relieved to find the ward staff as understanding as they were.

Single women no less than married women, and in the same proportion (92 per cent), were predominantly satisfied that they had done the right thing in having had the pregnancy terminated. They were asked to select from a card the one of three statements which most closely corresponded to their own opinion at that moment:

	No.
(a) I have no doubt at all that to terminate the pregnancy was the right thing to do;	46
(b) It seemed the best solution at the time but now I'm not so sure that it was;	0
(c) If I could decide again, I would not have it done.	4
	50

Two nurses and 2 clerical workers wished that they had not had the abortion although at the first interview 3 of the 4 had been certain that this was what they wanted. In 2 of the cases there had been a change of circumstances:

1 A girl, having her second pregnancy, had not told her boyfriend of it for, she said, intercourse had only occurred on one occasion and marriage had not been intended. She did not want to be in the

position of 'being forced to marry'. Now her boyfriend had got to hear of it and wanted to marry her. She regretted having had the abortion and wished she could have foreseen what would happen. (On the other hand, she did not know if the young man would have offered marriage had she remained pregnant.)

2 In a similar case in which a change in circumstances made the young woman regret having had the pregnancy terminated, the couple were waiting for the man to obtain his divorce. Circumstances made it impossible for her to return home pregnant. Some months after the abortion, they were to be married, and she regretted having had it done. 'After all, it's our first pregnancy', she said. 'We want another as soon as possible.'

A different type of problem arose in the case of the other 2 women who said that if they could decide again they would not have the abortion:

3 Marriage had not been intended either by this nurse or her friend. Although plans for her career would have suffered had the pregnancy continued her main anxiety was the state of health of her mother, a serious chronic invalid. At follow-up she said she would never have another abortion. She supposed she felt guilty about it – 'it's a life, after all'. She had seen hysterotomies performed and 'thought if awful' and had been impressed by the completeness of a 12-week-old foetus seen in the laboratory. Had it not been for her mother's health she felt she would just have had the baby.

4 This couple had broken off their engagement before they knew of the pregnancy. The young woman refused a renewed offer of marriage when the pregnancy was confirmed on the grounds that her boyfriend was unsettled and would not work and their prospective living conditions were inadequate. There were psychiatric problems at home and poor family relationships, but she was undecided whether or not to ask for an abortion. At follow-up she was clearly sad about it. She felt however that it would not have been fair to ask her mother to look after a baby, and 'to have it adopted would have hurt me more than an abortion'.

Although she chose the statement 'If I could decide again I would not have it done', this last patient may not be regretting having had the abortion so much as the circumstances which made it necessary. Some of the 46 women who chose (*a*) regretted the abortion but did not doubt it had been the right thing to do.

At follow-up 29 of the 50 women who had had their pregnancy terminated gave no indication that they had not adjusted to the situation. They were young, resilient and quite practical. One who had expected to feel guilty about the abortion 'because of the pressure of opinion about this sort of thing' had not done so and said she did not think about it now. Another said: 'I look at it like this. I was in a mess and it got me out of the mess. Selfish, I suppose, but that's how I felt. I'm glad it was done.' This girl said she had expected 'to feel awful about it' every time she saw a baby but had not done so. A girl who said she was 'rebuilding her life' after her abortion tried not to think of it. 'It is not an operation I approve of but in my circumstances it was best. I sometimes believe in God and sometimes I don't, and it's when I do that I feel it was wrong – but it would have been worse to go on with it.'

The 21 others described feelings of sadness or guilt, were unhappy if they saw a baby, had periods of depression and generally did not appear to have recovered from the experience as fully as the others.

1 An introspective girl who had had an unhappy home life was rejected by her stepmother and alcoholic father when she became pregnant. Her boyfriend's reaction was to become engaged to someone else. She considered the three statements for a long time before saying: 'I fully agree with (*a*). If I'd had it it would just have been another child for adoption.' She spoke of the abortion (by saline injection) as 'an extremely enlightening experience'. 'The tragedy was it was so far on. It was my own fault it was left so long.' Afterwards, she said, 'it had felt dead, a very empty, strange feeling. It made such a great impression on me, being so far on, but don't think for a minute I regret it.'

2 A young woman who described herself as 'a terribly nervous person' and her parents as 'terribly narrow-minded' had concealed her first pregnancy for over seven months. She would have kept the baby had her parents supported her in this but she was sent away from home and the baby was placed for adoption on their insistence. When she returned the incident was never referred to again. She would not attend a post-natal clinic and her doctor could not persuade her to come to see him. She was pregnant again in a few

months' time. This pregnancy was aborted and for about two weeks afterwards she said she had felt 'terribly depressed' and wished she had not had it done. 'However, it was a passing feeling and I haven't thought of it since. I just feel completely different.' She had a new boyfriend but felt there would be no risk of another pregnancy as she was 'just not interested in sex'. 'I feel a lot older now and I'll be able to cope with him', she said.

3 A young woman who had already had one pregnancy to the same man (ending in spontaneous abortion) sought termination of her second pregnancy on the grounds of the break-up of her marriage plans to him. At follow-up she and the man were as close as ever. She said she did not think she would have been strong enough to go through with the abortion if it had not been for him but he did not let her change her mind. It had occurred to her that his threat of desertion could have been intended to bring pressure on her to agree to abortion and to strengthen her case. She herself took motherhood seriously and would not want to have a baby when unprepared for it financially and domestically. She said: I think about it sometimes but I don't brood on it. I really don't have any regrets taking everything into consideration.

In this group of 50 young women who had had an abortion there was no one who expressed feelings of guilt or regret on a more profound level than this. Women can readily be made to feel guilty in matters affecting their biological function of motherhood (their vulnerability to attack on this score has been played on for years). The impression gained from a careful but superficial interview four or five months after the abortion is that many young women have temporary doubts, depression and guilt feelings after the abortion but these fade in most cases with the pressure of other events, new relationships and the passing of time. If the girl had been psychologically disturbed in the first place, and this includes many of those who become pregnancy-repeaters, an abortion is not likely to solve the underlying difficulty and might be followed by psycho-pathological problems. Drs McCance and Olley, following up another group assumed to be a similar sample of Aberdeen single women seeking abortion, were able to study them again a year or more after their abortion and to assess the psychiatric effects in greater depth (Chapters 6 and 7).

ABORTION NOT DONE

Twenty-six of the 82 single women did not have their pregnancy terminated, at least in Aberdeen. Three changed their minds and 3 aborted spontaneously, but in the majority of cases (20) the consultant had considered the grounds for the request inadequate or the pregnancy too far advanced (between 16 and 24 weeks gestation in 8 of the 26 cases). The majority of the single women accepted the consultant's decision and took no further action. Only 2 sought a second opinion, and 2 others obtained a legal abortion elsewhere. The readiness of some to be diverted from their intention suggests ambivalence in the first place or an underlying fear of the abortion or its consequences. Their lack of forcefulness may have had some influence on the consultant's decision.

'The doctor said it was like ending a life so I just decided to go on with it.'

'You can't really discuss it – there were other doctors and nurses present. Even if there hadn't been I wouldn't have argued about it.' A different general practitioner in another town had tried to arrange for her to have a further opinion but despite efforts on his part she 'didn't bother'. (Why not?) 'I thought Aberdeen was further on with these things and if Aberdeen couldn't do it, I wouldn't bother.' With the passing of time this patient had probably become reconciled to continuing the pregnancy.

A young woman having a second pregnancy to the same man, and who regarded the likelihood of marriage to him with some scepticism, said of the doctor's decision not to terminate the pregnancy: 'Come easy go easy is how I look at it. If you can't have it done you have to make up your mind to it, that's all there is to it.'

What happened to the 26 applicants who did not have their pregnancy terminated in Aberdeen is summarised below:

Remained unmarried and had the baby in Aberdeen (12) or elsewhere (2)	14
Married putative father and had the baby	5
Spontaneous abortion	3
Therapeutic abortion elsewhere	2
Left town, outcome not known	2
	26

Women who do not succeed in their application for abortion are perhaps less motivated than others to co-operate in follow-up inquiries and are difficult to approach direct for fear of causing trouble at home. A few had left Aberdeen by the time they were due to be seen again. In all, 20 of the 26 were followed up, most of them around the 34th week of pregnancy, the same interval being used for those who continued the pregnancy as for those who did not.

Remained unmarried and had the baby (12 interviewed)

Nine of these were not recommended abortion and 3 had changed their minds about having it done. The changes of mind had occurred between discussion with the general practitioner and the first appointment with the consultant. Acceptance of the pregnancy by the girl's family probably accounted for the withdrawal of her request in 2 of the 3 cases; both families were supportive and after the initial upset were prepared to welcome the baby. In the third case the change of mind occurred in the context of a stable relationship leading to marriage after the baby's birth.

When seen again 9 of the 12 young women were no longer associating with the father of the pregnancy. In 2 of the 3 cases where they were still together they could not marry because the man was already married. In the other case, the putative father, a student, was financially unable to support a family but as a result of the pregnancy they became engaged to marry whenever he had qualified in his profession. Half the young women in this group of 12 intended to keep their baby and half planned adoption.

Married putative father and had the baby (5 interviewed)

These 5 showed different reactions to the consultant's advice to continue the pregnancy. Two, both 16-year-old shop assistants, were happy to do so as the decision put pressure on their parents to agree to their marriage, hitherto opposed on the grounds of their youth. The other 3 were less happy. All were students, ambitious for their careers. One, however, a Catholic, 'was glad the doctor had made up her mind for her', and she did not press the matter of abortion. The other 2 seem to have succumbed to pressure from their family or boyfriend to marry.

Had an abortion, spontaneous or therapeutic (3 interviewed)

Three pregnancies ended in spontaneous abortion. None would appear to have been self-induced as in 2 cases abortion occurred before a decision had been reached and in the other after the girl had been accepted for termination. The 2 young women who had had their pregnancies terminated elsewhere had hinted at this possibility at their first interview. Their boyfriends were active in the arrangements and in neither case did the girl's parents know of the pregnancy or abortion.

At four or five months distance it is not easy to elicit the events and pressures that led the girl to follow one path rather than another after she had been refused abortion. They are not usually referred for social work help unless there is seen to be a particular problem and the girl, her family and the family doctor generally have to work out the next step themselves. This may present no difficulty and the girl turns up at the ante-natal clinic in due course, not linked to the previous request for abortion. Where the mother is keeping the baby or marrying the father it is sometimes assumed that no problems exist, yet at this stage decisions are made that can be all-important to the future welfare of the mother and child. Marriage is as serious a step as abortion, adoption needs to be considered well in advance, practical problems have to be decided. Unless followed through this phase only the outcome of the decisions is discovered four or five months later rather than the process by which they were arrived at. However, the young woman's reactions to the situation as it then is can be obtained.

As in the case of married women, the single women continuing their pregnancy were asked to select from a card the statement which most closely represented their own point of view at the time of follow-up. By then 5 of the young women were married and one married soon after the baby's birth.

	Remained single	Had married
(a) I still think it would have been better if the pregnancy had been terminated, and I still don't feel happy about having the baby;	2	0
(b) I still think it would have been better if the pregnancy had been terminated, but I'm beginning to feel happier about having the baby;	6	2
(c) I'm glad I didn't have the pregnancy terminated.	4	3
	12	5

Ten of the 17, including 2 who had married, were still of the opinion that it would have been better if the pregnancy had been terminated, although when seen most of them were beginning to look forward to the baby. Only 2 of the 17 appeared from their choice of statement (*a*) not to have adjusted to the situation. One girl from a broken home said she would have been feeling happier about having the baby if she had not resolved on having it adopted. The other, whose parents were on the point of separating and had done so by the time of follow-up, had broken off the relationship with her boyfriend and was positive she would have the baby adopted. She felt 'very depressed' at follow-up and said that statement (*a*) ('I still think it would have been better if the pregnancy had been terminated and I still don't feel happy about having the baby') expressed her view exactly.

A motherless teenage girl who chose the less positive statement (*b*) said: 'The doctor said he thought I should just go through with it and never mind about abortion – there was no cause for doing it. So I just made up my mind to go on with it.' Her father had told her she need not come home if she were pregnant. Asked about his reaction to her failure to obtain an abortion, she said: 'He said, ah well, you learn by experience. Why don't you adopt it – it's only your first.' Shortly after her application she had seen a television programme on abortion which had made an unpleasant impression on her. She said: 'I'd never ask for an abortion again.'

Seven of the young women including 3 16-year-olds chose statement (*c*): 'I'm glad I didn't have the pregnancy terminated.' Three of these had changed their minds so only 4 would have had it done had the doctor agreed. On being refused, 3 had married the father and the fourth, whose family had rallied round, became reconciled to continuing the pregnancy and eventually was glad she had done so.

Two of the girls who had changed their minds did so in the interval between seeing their own doctor and first attending hospital. One denied that she had ever thought of abortion but this did not agree with what her doctor wrote. The mother of another had recently had a baby and the family felt it would be 'unfair' to expect their daughter to have an abortion. The girl herself, on seeing her mother's baby, was keen to continue and the situation was accepted. The third young woman who changed her mind only wished an abortion by an impossibly simple method and when the procedure was explained she decided she did not want it and that she would marry the father when he was free. The marriage was unsuccessful for reasons unconnected with the pregnancy.

The evidence from this small group of single women followed up a few months after their abortion or after their request for abortion had been turned down suggests that in the great majority of cases those who were successful in obtaining an abortion did not regret having had it done. The majority of those who continued their pregnancy would still have preferred an abortion but at that stage many of them were becoming reconciled to having the baby. This supports Dr Olley's findings described in Chapter 6. In a clinical assessment of the group of single women followed up by him after a longer interval he found single aborted women to be less depressed than single non-aborted women, and a significantly greater proportion both of total regrets and of severe regrets among those who were not aborted.

CONCLUSIONS

The increased demand for abortion from single women has created ethical and practical problems for gynaecologists everywhere and has added to the emotionalism which discussion of abortion often arouses. Those who dislike the new licence fear a situation in which the unmarried woman feels safe to follow her own sexual inclinations and becomes promiscuous; women are thought to be the natural guardians of conventional sexual morality. Abortion like contraception for unmarried women seems to threaten familiar beliefs which have been unquestioned by the majority of people for a long time – that women are 'naturally' chaste, monogamous by nature, too vulnerable emotionally to be happy with casual affairs, that it is in their best interests to forgo sexual experience until they are married. The stresses and strains which a restrictive morality imposed upon the individual were accepted; they bore most hardly on women. The present rejection of these beliefs by the young and their readiness to experiment with new patterns of companionship have created different stresses for themselves and for society. It is difficult for an older generation born in the conditions of the 1920s and 1930s to understand young people who have grown up in times quite different from their own, who mature earlier physically, who are better off and more widely educated by school and television than they themselves were. The young look to each other rather than to their parents for guidance, assuming that adults will not understand or be in sympathy with their problems. Parental authority is unfashionable and self-expression is of more concern than adherence to any external code of behaviour. The tolerant outlook of the present day puts a burden of responsibility on the young and inexperienced that many of them are not ready for. The problem is how best to help the casualties of this time of transition. There is little doubt that if abortion is available it will be expected and asked for increasingly by unmarried women and their men friends. Foetal life will be devalued and the use of effective contraception will seem less important. It is clear however that if abortion is denied them they will still run the risk of pregnancy and the child will be exposed to all the risks of the illegitimate state.

Although today attitudes towards illegitimacy are more humane than they used to be the handicaps suffered by illegitimate children have by no means disappeared. Two recent studies[6,7] have drawn attention to the extent of the illegitimate child's legal, educational, financial and emotional disadvantages especially where they are brought up by their own mothers. The effects of deprivation and unwantedness are felt not only by the child who may become neurotic and maladjusted but in the long term by society which may suffer from his anti-social behaviour.

At a time when in England and Wales over 50,000 children are received into care, and of these nearly 20,000 are 'unwanted' or lacking adequate parental care (i.e. deserted, homeless or abandoned) no one can be unconcerned about children born to unmarried mothers. If they survive the hazards of the neo-natal period (in Scotland in 1970 the neo-natal mortality rate for illegitimate infants was 17.4 per thousand live-births compared with 12.4 for legitimate infants) they have a less than one in three chance of adoption. Others will be brought up by foster-parents, sometimes by a series of foster-parents, in homes or by their own mothers, whose pay reflects the assumption that single women have no dependants. The worst-off illegitimate children from the financial point of view are those who are being brought up by their own mothers, and more mothers than before are trying to do this.

For some reason there is more concern about the possible feelings of regret or guilt a woman may have afterwards if she has her pregnancy terminated than if she has her baby adopted. The long-term effects of adoption on the natural mother are less often studied. To give her baby away to be brought up by another woman unknown to her and never to see it again might be thought to be quite as likely to cause depression, guilt feelings and serious psychiatric sequelae as the termination of a pregnancy which has hardly acquired a separate identity in the mother's eyes. Now that young people are forcing a change in punitive attitudes to illegitimate pregnancy, single women (at least, those in Aberdeen, and they are unlikely to lead the way) are saying plainly that they regard producing a baby, if they are not in a position to bring it up themselves, as more 'immoral' than having the pregnancy terminated.

While the unmarried mother is not allowed to think that she is performing a social service, the fears sometimes expressed about the effect of the increasing number of abortions on the supply of children for adoption might almost suggest that she is. The efficient use of contraception by single women might be opposed for the same reason. The number of adoptions in Scotland in 1970 has shown a fall for the first time in ten years, which supports the suggestion that the young women who would previously have surrendered their baby for adoption are those who are now most frequently accepted for abortion. The future may look bleak for would-be adoptive parents but there are signs that it may become more hopeful for the less attractive children who have hitherto been denied an adoptive home.

Many of the single women interviewed for this study became pregnant in the course of a serious relationship with their boyfriend. Given the greater expectations of today they did not assume that the event would ruin their prospects or force them to marry. They were concerned about the moral aspect but in a different way from their elders. They agreed that it was wrong that an unmarried girl should make use of contraception but some were beginning to see that it might be right for her to protect herself in advance from the risk of pregnancy in a steady relationship. Neither they nor anyone else have yet solved the dilemma of premeditation posed by present methods of contraception. There is a long way to go educationally before Aberdeen girls and their parents are persuaded, if it is so, that the use of contraception is less morally reprehensible than risking an unwanted pregnancy. Unwanted pregnancies are therefore bound to occur and it would be more realistic to face the probability than to hope that pre-marital sex is not going to become an accepted part of growing up among some young people.

The high proportion of boyfriends who did not see the pregnancy as anything to do with them shows that the new freedoms are still attended by the old risks despite the modern feeling for greater mutuality in sexual relationships. But this feeling is not yet shared by all classes. The young women themselves, apart from those who were engaged or about to marry, seemed to accept their boyfriends' repudiation of responsibility and saw the pregnancy as their own problem, one that did not even concern their parents if possible. The putative father's view point has been almost entirely neglected in the flood of research on illegitimate pregnancy and abortion, yet it is probably wrong to assume that there is nothing to be learnt from him. He has a considerable influence on the abortion rates as we have seen. The Working Party of the Royal College of Obstetricians and Gynaecologists[8] reports that the most important effect of the Abortion Act on men has been to encourage them to persuade the woman to seek abortion. They also influence the rates by their decision to stand by her or to desert her. We do not know enough about why they follow either course or how they see their responsibilities in a time when more young women than before are prepared to engage in pre-marital intercourse and when the most reliable of the present means of contraception is in her own hands, theoretically at any rate. However, deserting boyfriends are over-represented in any study of women seeking abortion and a less biased impression of them is seen when the outcome of all pre-marital conceptions is considered, whether abortion, illegitimate birth or birth following marriage. In Aberdeen in 1970, of 574 conceptions occurring before marriage well over half the couples (56 per cent) had married before the birth of the baby.

Follow-up was an essential part of this study but it is difficult to evaluate objectively the outcome of the decisions made in terms of human happiness. When a pregnancy is terminated the young woman has only her own feelings to consider. If she has no physical or emotional ill effects the abortion has at least done no harm, except to the unborn foetus (this fortunately has no way of knowing what happened to it so the question of whether it would 'prefer' to have been born only troubles the happily alive). When abortion is refused the effects are more difficult to assess because the decision has wider repercussions and it is not easy to know which are due to the failure to abort and which to other causes. If a young woman feels obliged to marry because of continuing the pregnancy and the marriage turns out badly, or if the child is still unwanted when born and suffers in consequence, was the decision the right one? Even the most careful doctor cannot take responsibility for such long-term eventualities nor does he usually even know of them to help to guide him in future decisions. He has merely failed to intervene in a process initiated by the young woman for whatever reason of her own (pregnancy), and once he is away from the firm ground of medical indications the decision is inevitably a fairly arbitrary one.

REFERENCES

1 Thompson, B. (1956). 'Social study of illegitimate maternities', *Brit. J. prev. soc. Med.*, **10**, 75–87.
2 Schofield, M. (1965). *Sexual Behaviour of Young People*, Longmans, London.
3 Young, L. (1954). *Out of Wedlock*, McGraw-Hill Book Co. Inc., New York.
4 McCance, C., Hall, D. J. (1972). 'Sexual behaviour and contraceptive practice of unmarried female undergraduates at Aberdeen University', *Brit. med. J.*, **2**, 694–700.
5 Humphreys, L. (1970). *Tearoom Trade*, Duckworth & Co. Ltd., London.
6 Weir, S. (1970). 'A study of unmarried mothers and their children in Scotland', *Scottish Health Service Studies*, no. 13, Scottish Home and Health Department.
7 Crellin, E., Pringle, M. L. K., West, P. (1971). 'Born illegitimate', National Foundation for Educational Research in England and Wales.
8 Working Party of Royal College of Obstetricians and Gynaecologists (1972). 'Unplanned pregnancy'.

TABLE 4:1. *Age, by occupation*

Age group	Total		Occupation			
		Students	Nurses	Clerical workers	School-girls	All other occupations
14–15	4	—	—	1	2	1
16–17	13	1	1	4	3	4
18–19	24	4	5	8	—	7
20–24	34	13	3	9	—	9
25 and over	7	—	1	1	—	5
Total	82	18	10	23	5	26

TABLE 4:2. *Father's socio-economic group by own occupation*

Father's socio-economic group	Total	Own occupation				
		Students	Nurses	Clerical	School	All other
Professional, managerial	20	11	1	4	1	3
Farmers	6	—	1	2	—	3
Non-manual, clerical, police, etc.	11	3	—	3	2	3
Skilled manual workers	22	2	5	7	1	7
Semi-skilled or unskilled workers	23	2	3	7	1	10
Total	82	18	10	23	5	26

TABLE 4:3. *Own occupation by putative father's socio-economic group*

Own occupation	Total	Putative father's socio-economic group					
		Students	Non-manual	Skilled	Semi- and unskilled	School	NK
Students	18	15	3	—	—	—	—
Nurses	10	1	5	1	3	—	—
Clerical	23	3	5	4	9	1	1
School	5	—	—	3	—	2	—
All other	26	2	3	9	7	1	4
Total	82	21	16	17	19	4	5

TABLE 4:4. *Relationship with putative father by own occupation*

Relationship with putative father	Own occupation					
	Total	Students	Nurses	Clerical	All other	School
Engaged, marriage plans made	9	—	2	4	2	1
Apparently serious, going steady	38	8	4	13	11	2
Friendly only, marriage not contemplated	31	10	3	6	11	1
Unwilling intercourse alleged	3	—	1	—	1	1
Indeterminate	1	—	—	—	1	—
Total	82	18	10	23	26	5

TABLE 4:5. *Use of contraception by relationship with putative father*

Use of contraception	Relationship with putative father					
	Total	Engaged	Going steady	Friendly, casual	Unwilling	Indeterminate
Regular use: pill	1	—	1	—	—	—
condom	2	—	—	2	—	—
condom, pill	1	—	1	—	—	—
pessary	1	—	—	1	—	—
Occasional use: pill (2) condom (21)	23	2	15	6	—	—
Regularity not known: condom	3	—	2	1	—	—
Natural method only	7	1	1	5	—	—
Nothing used, except perhaps c.i.	44	6	18	16	3	1
Total	82	9	38	31	3	1

TABLE 4:6. *Outcome of present and previous pregnancies of single women*

	Pregnancies				Interval from:			Same fathers?
	First	Second	Third	Fourth	1st to 2nd	2nd to 3rd	3rd to 4th	
Students, nurses and clerical workers								
1	Terminated	Terminated			6 mths			Yes
2	Baby adopted	Baby adopted			Not known			Not known
3	Spontaneous abortion	Terminated			3 mths			Yes
4	Spontaneous abortion	Terminated			3 mths			No
5	Kept baby	Terminated			4 yrs			No
6	Kept baby	Terminated			5 yrs			No
7	Kept baby	Terminated			14 mths			No
8	Baby died	Baby adopted			14 mths			No
All other occupations								
9	Baby adopted	Terminated			7 mths	—	—	No
10	Baby died	Terminated			11 mths	—	—	No
11	Kept baby	Terminated			6 mths	—	—	No
12	Kept baby	Terminated			1 yr	—	—	Yes
13	Kept baby	Terminated			14 mths	—	—	No
14	Kept baby	Terminated			14 mths	—	—	No
15	Kept baby	Baby adopted			13 mths	—	—	Yes
16	Kept baby	Kept baby			15 mths	—	—	No
17	Kept baby	Spontaneous abortion	Terminated		6 yrs	5 yrs	—	
18	Kept baby	Terminated	Baby adopted		9 mths	14 mths	—	No
19	Kept baby	Kept baby	Kept baby	Terminated	19 mths	17 mths	3 yrs	Yes

TABLE 4:7. *Contraceptive practice before first and present pregnancy*

Before first pregnancy	Before present pregnancy
Students, nurses and clerical workers	
1 Safe period only (RC)	Pill had been suggested but no action. 'Is sure' PF used a condom.
2 Not known	Coitus interruptus only. 'Contraception is the last thing you think of.'
3 Safe period. 'It was fool-proof for six months so you get complacent.'	Pill and at times condom. Knows condom failed once.
4 Nothing. Intercourse after a party and unprepared	Alleges unwilling intercourse. No contraception.
5 Nothing (aged 16 at the time)	Nothing. Says intercourse occurred once only. 'We talked of taking a chance.'
6 Nothing	Thinks PF used a condom but cannot remember exactly. 'I just never expected it to happen.'
7 Nothing. 'I never thought about it – I wanted the baby and I thought he wanted it, too.' (Pregnant to steady boyfriend.)	'I didn't worry about it [risk of pregnancy] because he didn't worry. He said "if you get pregnant I'll get my divorce".'
8 Nothing	Condom used but not regularly. Did not like to ask her doctor for advice.
All other occupations	
9 Nothing	Did not attend clinic or GP post-natally, despite her doctor urging her to attend. Risk of pregnancy not discussed with new friend. 'I can't speak to people – I get too embarrassed – even my own doctor.'
10 Nothing	GP in another town advised her to take pill but nothing done. Neither she nor PF took precautions although she said she did worry about the risk of pregnancy.
11 'He promised I wouldn't get pregnant and he tried to be careful.'	'He said he did [use condom] but I don't know.' Had meant to consult GP about the pill but had not got round to it.
12 Nothing. RC but did not know about safe period	After her confinement asked GP for the pill. Had side effects, stopped taking it, started again, forgot, etc.
13 Nothing	No attempt at contraception and can say nothing about what she thought of the risk of pregnancy.
14 Nothing. 'It sounds silly but I never thought it could happen.'	Avoided GP after confinement as she did not want to be examined. Felt she did not need contraceptive advice as 'I didn't think I'd be so stupid again.'
15 'He told me he was careful – I just believed him.'	Intercourse once with an acquaintance. 'Afterwards I asked if he'd been careful. He said he had but I didn't believe him.'
16 Nothing	She had never asked her doctor but says she thought he would not give advice to the single. 'I left it to [PF] to be careful and we never went the whole way.'

TABLE 4:8. *Putative father's reaction to the pregnancy by type of relationship*

Putative father's reaction	Total	Engaged	Going steady	Friendly, casual	Other
Leaving matters to her, deserting her	42	3	19	18	2
Accepts responsibility, trying to help	24	4	15	5	—
At school, parents coping	3	—	1	2	—
Indeterminate	2	1	—	—	1
Not told about pregnancy	11	1	3	6	1
Total	82	9	38	31	4

Relationship (header spanning Engaged, Going steady, Friendly casual, Other)

TABLE 4:9. *Relationship with putative father at follow-up by use of contraception at follow-up*

Relationship with putative father at follow-up	Total	No contraception being used	Pill
Had discontinued relationship with putative father and has no new boyfriend	18	13	5
Still in touch with putative father	9	4	5
Has a new steady boyfriend	19	12	7
Married, or about to be married to putative father	4	—	4
	50	29	21

Use of contraception at follow-up (header spanning No contraception being used, Pill)

TABLE 4:10. *Method of abortion by how patient found the procedure*

Method of termination	Total	No worse than expected	Painful or upsetting
Suction	18	18	—
D & C	15	15	—
Saline	14	10	4
Hysterotomy	3	2	1
Total	50	45	5

How patient found the procedure (header spanning No worse than expected, Painful or upsetting)

5 SOCIAL AND PSYCHOLOGICAL CHARACTERISTICS AT REFERRAL

Peter C. Olley

INTRODUCTION

The rights and wrongs of therapeutic abortion and its supposed long-term effects continue to provide abundant fuel for controversy, prejudice and speculation. Though dogmatic opinions proliferate, the amount of factual material on which firm conclusions can be based remains strictly limited. Many key questions about abortion and particularly its psychological aspects remain without satisfactory answers.

Psychiatric grounds for abortion were included in the Abortion Act of 1967 which came into operation in England, Wales and Scotland in April 1968. The relevant clause for legal abortion on psychiatric grounds required that two registered medical practitioners state in good faith that the risk of injury to the woman's mental health or to that of her existing children would be greater if the pregnancy were continued than if it were terminated. A social dimension was also introduced in that her actual or reasonably foreseeable environment could be taken into account in making this decision. These clauses give considerable scope for different interpretations of what for example is 'injury', 'mental health', or 'reasonably foreseeable environment'.

A certain amount of confusion prevails. The concept of psychiatric grounds for abortion has itself been called into question by some psychiatrists. One writer saw the problem mainly in terms of the presence or risk of major mental illness such as schizophrenia or psychotic depression and contended that such patients could be successfully supported through the pregnancy and post-partum period.[1] On the other hand, the BMA Committee on Therapeutic Abortion considered severe reactive depression, especially where there is a risk of suicide, certain obsessional states, schizophrenia and mental subnormality as possible, though not absolute, indications for termination.[2] However, many psychiatrists would maintain that the main problem of psychiatric ill health among abortion applicants lay in the realm of the so-called minor mental disorders – the neurotic and personality disorders. These conditions, intimately bound up with social and environmental stress, can further disrupt family relationships and affect the quality of maternal care. Such patients, often barely coping with their ordinary life situation and making a precarious adjustment to their family and environment, are liable to break down with overt psychiatric symptoms under the extra stress of an unwanted pregnancy and the subsequent tasks and responsibilities of child-rearing.[3]

Medical practitioners are called upon to make predictions about the likely course of events and the woman's future behaviour, often on the basis of relatively restricted information. Complex and momentous decisions must be made though few reliable guide-lines are available for weighing up the multiple factors that often operate in any individual case. It is unlikely (and in one sense probably undesirable) that hard and fast rules can be laid down to deal precisely with every situation. To some extent there are unique factors operating in each woman's web of circumstances. Nevertheless some general principles might provide a useful framework for decision-making which can then be modified to take account of certain individual features. In establishing these principles, answers are required to certain key questions: what is the risk of psychiatric morbidity after abortion? and the important complementary topic, what is the risk of psychiatric morbidity after continuing an unwanted pregnancy to term? Supplementary questions include: are there certain groups of women at special risk in these circumstances? and, do certain grounds for abortion and certain techniques for abortion carry greater risk of unfavourable sequelae?

A number of previous studies on these topics have produced contradictory results. Simon and Senturia in their comprehensive review of the literature on psychiatric sequelae of abortion for the period 1935–64 commented on a number of fundamental defects in the methodology of many studies which raised serious doubts about the accuracy and relevance of their findings.[4] Major shortcomings centred mainly on the use of small and unrepresentative populations of abortion candidates, retrospective research designs, vague criteria for assessing outcome, absence of comparison groups of women continuing the pregnancy and inadequate periods of follow-up. Ekblad's study of 479 Swedish women who were aborted on psychiatric grounds was considered to be the most satisfactory of the studies that were reviewed and remains a classic in the field.[5] Even here, the data were collected post-abortion and there was no parallel study of women who were refused termination. Since the above review was published there have been a number of notable additions to the literature. These have included studies in North America, Scandinavia and Britain.[6-20]

Aberdeen, because of its relatively static population, and comprehensive and well-organised obstetric and psychiatric services, provided a particularly favourable situation for research into the late psychosocial effects of abortion, and the psychological study reported here sought to avoid many of the methodological defects of some earlier projects. It formed part of a wider inter-departmental study on abortion in Aberdeen with research workers drawn from the university departments of Obstetrics and Gynaecology, Mental Health, and the MRC Medical Sociology Unit.

SELECTION OF THE COHORTS

Many earlier studies were carried out with small, highly selected populations, yielding conclusions of very limited validity. It was important therefore to study a large and highly *representative* sample of abortion applicants. The present study aimed for the epidemiological ideal of complete enumeration and examination of all women referred for abortion from a defined community in a defined period of time. Women considered suitable for inclusion in the study were those who were:

(i) Referred for consideration of therapeutic abortion to the national health service facilities in Aberdeen city during the inclusive fourteen month period July 1967 – August 1968.

(ii) Considered on medical examination to be pregnant.

(iii) Normally resident in the city of Aberdeen or its suburban areas.

Visitors to the city seeking abortion were excluded, though students and temporary workers who spent the greater part of the year in Aberdeen but had homes elsewhere were eligible for the project.

Five women referred for termination and tested by the research workers were found not to be pregnant at gynaecological examination and were therefore omitted from the series.

The Aberdeen study was also *prospective* in nature. Women satisfying the above selection criteria were included in the cohorts *only* if they were

167

assessed by the researchers *prior* to the decision about the abortion being made. In some instances the researchers were unable to secure an interview before the decision-making clinicians. Such cases were not included in the study, though their basic social and medical characteristics were obtained later for comparison purposes. For these reasons, the epidemiological ideal was not attained, but nevertheless the referral cohorts comprised 370 women, 90 per cent of the city's NHS abortion applicants during the fourteen-month research period. It should be noted that private practice patients constituting less than 10 per cent of the total applicants in the period 1967–8 were not included in the investigation.

METHOD OF STUDY

The study divided logically into two parts – each attempting to answer different sets of questions about abortion practice in Aberdeen. Part I, the referral section, linked the basic social and medical characteristics of the applicants obtained by the medical sociologists with the initial psychological assessments carried out by the psychiatric personnel. Essentially it tackled the questions: What type of woman is referred for an abortion? What type of woman gets an abortion? The research material also allowed examination of psychological factors in contraceptive practice and in illegitimate pregnancy.

This sets the stage for Part II, the follow-up section. Active efforts were made to trace and re-assess as many as possible of the initial cohorts no matter whether they had aborted or had continued the pregnancy. The time interval between referral and follow-up exceeded one year in all cases and had a median value of 18 months. This period was considered sufficiently long for transient reactions to have remitted and most long-term effects related to the pregnancy to have become established. Criteria for defining an unfavourable outcome were laid down in advance of the follow-up study. Part II concentrated on the main research themes: what are the long-term effects on the applicants of abortion or of continuing an unwanted pregnancy to term? Similarly, what are the late psycho-social sequelae of sterilisation? what is the incidence of ill-effects after these procedures? The relationship of an unfavourable outcome to key variables such as marital status, social class, type of termination, psychological state at referral was also investigated.

As already noted the psychological study formed one part of a larger inter-departmental study of abortion in Aberdeen. A multi-disciplinary team approach, while conferring many advantages, may also impose limitations on the research design. In this instance the form of the initial psychological assessment was largely determined by the necessary division of labour and restricted time available.

Both the medical sociologists and psychiatrists were intent on studying the same group of applicants at the time of referral. Many of these applicants were quite distressed by their predicament and could be expected to cope with only a limited period of assessment – in the region of two hours. Approximately one hour was therefore allocated to the medical sociologist's interview which was particularly concerned with collecting data on the woman's social background and the circumstances of conception. Inevitably in the process of obtaining this information they had formed a social relationship with the applicant. To follow this immediately by another hour's interview with a psychiatrist, probably covering similar topics, would be confusing to the patient and probably counter-productive for the study. In the circumstances it was decided to confine psychiatric interviewing to the follow-up, at which time the medical sociologists were no longer studying this group of patients. Thus at the referral stage a clinical psychiatric interview was dispensed with and a battery of standardised psychological questionnaires following the medical sociologist's interview substituted. These tests were chosen to be measures of (a) the current mental state and (b) more enduring personality traits of the applicant.

TYPES OF TEST USED

1 The Beck Depression Inventory (BDI)

This is a widely used instrument which has been validated for American and British populations[21-23] and consists essentially of a list of descriptive statements about symptoms encountered in depressive illness. These are each graded in severity from absent or neutral to severe and scored accordingly 0 to 3. The total score can be used as a guide to the presence and severity of depression and is thus a measure of current mental state. Operational definitions consistent with the results of validation studies were used to grade the depression, viz. (total scores): 0–9, depression absent; 10–16, mild depression; 17–24, moderate depression; 25 +, severe depression.

Individual items such as the presence of suicidal thoughts or lack of sexual interest could also be picked out from the inventory for group comparison. The total score on the BDI is considered sensitive to changes in the mental state.

2 Fould's Hostility Scales

This questionnaire test consists of a selection of fifty-one statements from the MMPI (Minnesota Multiphasic Personality Inventory) which relate to aggressiveness, hostility and blame directed outwards towards other people, objects or ideas (extropunitiveness) or directed inwards towards the self (intropunitiveness). The patient has to choose whether each individual statement is 'on the whole' true or false and is scored 0 or 1 depending on the particular item and the particular response to it.

Items are grouped into five sub-scales: AH – the urge to act out hostility; CO – critical of others; DH – projected, delusional hostility representing outward hostility; SC – self-critical; DG – delusional guilt, for inner-directed hostility.

Since Fould's initial formulation there have been a number of modifications in the way sub-scale scores were combined though the items and sub-scales themselves have remained constant. One version is the HDHQ – Hostility and Direction of Hostility Questionnaire.[24] The form used in this study is that suggested by Philip.[25] In this scheme, the extropunitive score (Ex) is the sum AH + CO + DH and the intropunitive score (In) the sum SC + DG. (Ex) is interpreted more as a measure of personality disturbance akin to psychopathy while (In) is more an index of personal disturbance in the form of psychiatric symptoms.

Scores for normal and neurotic Aberdeen populations are available as are studies using versions of this test on such groups as hospitalised psychopaths, unmarried mothers and attempted suicides. (In) tends to be more variable with time than (Ex) and in normals lower than (Ex). In the psychiatrically ill there is a rise in intropunitiveness to approximate equality with the extropunitive score and a greater fall in the former with successful treatment. Hospitalised psychopaths tend to score high on both measures.

3 Fould's Personal Illness and Character Disorder Scales

The Personal Illness schedule PI is derived from part of the larger Symptom Sign Inventory (SSI).[24, 26] It is directed towards establishing the presence of symptoms that are common in neurotic patients. The occurrence of such symptoms however does not necessarily imply functional impairment. Combined with the PI schedule is Fould's Character Disorder Scale (CD), which is also selected from the SSI.[27] The Character Disorder Scale attempts to identify patients with long-standing inter-personal and adjustment difficulties often combined with shallow emotional reactivity and plaintiveness. While presenting frequently with neurotic symptomatology, such individuals are more accurately described as having a personality disorder, to which such diagnostic labels as 'immature', 'inadequate' or 'hysterical psychopath' may be applied.

The combined Personal Illness and Character Disorder questionnaire contains twenty-seven questions concerning the presence or absence of symptoms, and scores of 1 or 0 are assigned to each item accordingly. Scores of 4 or over on the CD scale are classified for women as character disorder.

Individuals with less than 4 are then graded on the Personal Illness Scale (PI). A score of 5 or more on the latter constitutes 'personal illness', 2, 3 or 4 'borderline personal illness', and 0, 1 as 'normal'. A number of studies using these scales on psychiatric patients, women attempting suicide and prisoners are available for comparison.[28, 29] This test was used in the study mainly as an estimate of personality disorder as a supplement to the 16 PF.

4 Cattell's 16 Personality Factor Test

16 PF (Form C) was the main personality measure used in the study. Cattell, in this extensively researched questionnaire test, describes the structure of adult personality in terms of sixteen basic dimensions or factors.[30, 31] Each factor has a high scoring (+) and a low scoring (−) pole representing the extremes of opposing personality traits. Scoring is on a standardised ten-point scale (1 to 10) in units called stens calibrated against a reference population with a mean of 5.5 and a standard deviation of 2 stens for each factor. Cattell's general population of non-student women[31] was the reference population used for converting raw scores in the study to stens.

The sixteen factors are identified by letters as in the following text table, and their (+) and (−) poles each have a descriptive title attached which roughly conveys the main features of the personality dimension.

Brief descriptions of personality factors in the 16 PF

Low score (−) pole	Factor	High score (+) pole
Reserved	A	Outgoing
Less intelligent	B	More intelligent
Emotional	C	Stable
Submissive	E	Dominant
Sober	F	Enthusiastic
Expedient	G	Conscientious
Shy	H	Venturesome
Tough-minded	I	Sensitive
Trusting	L	Suspicious
Practical	M	Self-absorbed
Forthright	N	Shrewd
Placid	O	Apprehensive
Conservative	Q_1	Radical
Group-dependent	Q_2	Self-sufficient
Uncontrolled	Q_3	Controlled
Relaxed	Q_4	Tense

The shorter version of the 16 PF – Form C – was used in the study. Despite its lower reliability compared to Forms A or B, Form C was considered more suitable for such diverse groups of women because of its simpler vocabulary, the limited time available for testing and the existence of norms in this version for a large group of Aberdeen nursing students.

Form C includes an extra Motivational Distortion Scale (MD). A high score on this indicates a tendency to distort answers in the direction of socially desirable personality traits. An extensive literature on the 16 PF includes personality profile results for special populations, e.g. psychiatric patients, certain occupational groups, aggressive criminals, motorists subject to repeated accidents.

TEST ADMINISTRATION

Verbal interaction with the patient was, as far as possible, deliberately restricted to a few remarks to help put her at ease, and a standard explanation of the test procedures. The standard instructions for the first test (16 PF Form C) contained the statement that the questions gave the applicant a chance to say what sort of a person she was and an opportunity to state her interests and attitudes. Most women appeared to accept this level of explanation and quickly settled down to complete the questionnaires. A few inquired further about the purposes of the tests and were told that the researchers were interested in understanding what kind of people applied for termination of pregnancy. It is possible that some women thought that the tests would influence the clinician's decision though, if they did, it was not expressed to the assessors. In fact the clinicians' judgements were made independently of the psychological test results as the latter were not communicated to the decision-makers.

A small number of women felt too distressed at referral to finish the whole battery of tests. Approximately 1 per cent of the Beck Depression Inventories and the 16 PF tests were uncompleted. Unfortunately it was not found possible to administer the Personal Illness and Character Disorder Scales to the first few applicants and only 96 per cent completed these schedules.

It might be worth while summarising briefly some of the advantages and disadvantages of self-report tests in psychological assessment.

Questionnaires provide a relatively standardised test situation compared with the usual unstructured psychiatric interview. Interaction between patient and assessor is likely to be less powerful and less distorting to evaluation. Also, highly trained personnel are not essential for the test administration. In the present study this was a decided advantage as notification of abortion applicants sometimes occurred at times quite inconvenient for a research worker with other extensive teaching and clinical commitments. Often it was imperative to complete the assessment within one or two days as interview with the clinician had already been arranged, time was short and the medical sociologist's schedule had also to be taken into account. In the event most of the tests were given by one of the psychiatrists (PCO) but their standardised nature allowed other workers who had been carefully instructed in their use to help out at certain times. At one period supervised final-year medical students on elective courses in psychiatry helped in the testing.

Statistical techniques can also be employed, norms constructed and comparisons made between individuals and groups. A well-constructed and validated test can allow a wide range of symptoms or personality traits to be evaluated in a limited period of time and in addition some individuals may be more candid in a questionnaire than in an interview situation.

Against these advantages, a number of criticisms may be levelled against the use of self-report tests compared with a psychiatric interview. It may be held that some questions will be misunderstood by certain patients and there is no opportunity for the assessor to realise this. The motivation to answer truthfully and correctly may be poor in some individuals. Thus, some may not bother to take account of the questions' content but answer in a haphazard manner and others may deliberately fake the answers to exaggerate their degree of impairment or present themselves in a more socially favourable light. Some tests (e.g. 16 PF Form C), however, employ Motivational Distortion Scales to detect such behaviour. Symptom checklists such as the Beck Depression Inventory (BDI) probably lend themselves to faking more readily than the 16 PF or Fould's Hostility Scales. The former have more obvious 'face validity', whereas the object of many questions in the latter is not so apparent. Personality tests may also be influenced to some extent by the current mental state and reflect the prevailing emotional situation rather than more enduring traits.[32, 33]

CONTROL GROUPS

Estimation of abnormal psychological features in the referred women required test data from normal populations. Many psychological tests and, especially, personality questionnaires are known to be age-, class- and culture-dependent, and, for instance, norms derived from a general American population of women with a mean age in the mid-thirties are likely to serve as poor comparisons for a group of Aberdeen teenagers. Also, pregnancy itself appears to increase 'neuroticism' scores in normal women.[34] Thus, published normative data on the tests was considered to be inadequate for comparison with the cohorts. Three control groups of Aberdeen women were therefore used in the study.

Eighty legitimately pregnant married women attending the Aberdeen Maternity Hospital ante-natal clinic completed the 16 PF (Form C) and other tests used in the cohort. They corresponded closely in period of gestation, age and social class distribution to the ever-married applicants with legitimate pregnancy. Women who had requested termination were of course excluded from the control group.

It was not found possible to test an adequate control group of pregnant single women who had not requested termination. *Faute de mieux* extensive 16 PF (Form C) test data completed by 619 female Aberdeen nursing students attending a routine course in psychology were made available by courtesy of Mrs C. Cordiner, Senior Clinical Psychologist, Ross Clinic, Aberdeen. A further 81 female nursing students completed the other tests in the battery. These two groups each had similar mean age (18.9 years) to the cohort of unmarried applicants and corresponded very closely in age to the 'student' group (see Tables 5:1 and 5:2).

COMMENT

The psychological tests were completed at the time of referral, a period of considerable stress. Ideally personality traits should have been measured before the crisis of the unwanted pregnancy. The 16 PF results were assumed to give a fair approximation to the basic personality characteristics, though it is conceded that anxiety factors may have been exaggerated.[30]

Clearly there are several drawbacks to the use of these comparatively crude instruments of psychological assessment, but alternative methods also have snags and inconsistencies. The tests used in this study had been validated and used in other related projects. On balance it was considered that their advantages in the context of the research 'situation' outweighed their disadvantages and they could afford useful clues to mental state and personality differences between groups.

THE COMPOSITION OF THE COHORTS

The referral cohorts were made up of 163 single and 207 'ever-married' women (see Tables 5:3 and 5:4). 'Ever-married' denoted those who had ever been married and included women living with their husbands and also those separated, divorced or widowed. Basic social and medical characteristics of those two groups however were radically different.

Ninety per cent of the *unmarried* applicants were less than 25 years of age and most were primigravidae, 131 (80.4 per cent) being pregnant for the first, 27 (16.6 per cent) for the second and 4 (2.5 per cent) for the third time. By contrast, 16.4 per cent of the *ever-married* were under 25 years and the majority (64.3 per cent) had 3 or more previous pregnancies. Only 5 (2.4 per cent) ever-married women were primigravidae and only a minority (17.9 per cent) were illegitimately pregnant.

Precise social class comparisons were not feasible because of the different definitions of social class that were employed. Single women were classified by their own occupation whereas ever-married women were assigned to the Registrar General's Scheme of Classification by their husband's occupation. Even so, certain major differences were apparent. The 'student' group formed a large proportion (38.1 per cent) of the single women's cohort, and fish-workers, semi-skilled and unskilled manual workers a comparatively small proportion (10.5 per cent). In this particular study 'student' referred to any woman continuing in full-time education and comprised 15 university students, 38 girls attending other colleges in Aberdeen and 9 schoolgirls. The small 'professional' group was composed entirely of teachers and trained nurses.

Jean Aitken-Swan's general findings on referral rates were also relevant to the period of this study (July 1967 – August 1968). Though about one-half of the pregnant unmarried women in Aberdeen were referred for an abortion, a pregnant 'student' or 'professional' was four times more likely to be referred than a semi-skilled or unskilled manual worker. The situation for pregnant ever-married women was quite different. About 7 per cent were referred for abortion and there were only minor disparities among the classes in referral rates. In this instance wives of semi-skilled and unskilled workers (classes IV and V) were rather more likely to be referred than the other classes.

The religious affiliation of the applicants in both cohorts was predominantly Church of Scotland. Only 11 single women (6.7 per cent) and 11 ever-married (5.3 per cent) were Roman Catholic.

Single women tended to be referred at a later stage of pregnancy than the ever-married group ($P < 0.001$). Only 98 (60.1 per cent) of the single but 161 (77.8 per cent) of the ever-married group were referred with a gestation period of less than 13 weeks. The two cohorts also differed in the types of main indication for abortion (see Chapter 2). Single women had a greater proportion with 'socio-psychiatric' and ever-married a greater proportion with main medical indications.

With such marked differences on a wide range of fundamental variables it seemed important to analyse the two cohorts separately and not amalgamate them. (The abbreviations CS for 'the cohort of single women' and CM for 'the cohort of ever-married women' are used in the text below where convenient.)

HOW REPRESENTATIVE WERE THE COHORTS?

To what degree did the study accurately portray the abortion scene in Aberdeen? In contrast to most research projects on termination of pregnancy it was carried out on a large and relatively unselected group of patients. In fact the study contained 90 per cent of the city's total population of applicants referred to NHS clinics during a specific fourteen-month period, 93.6 per cent of the 175 single and 87.8 per cent of the 236 ever-married referrals being included. Twelve single and 29 ever-married women who otherwise fulfilled the initial selection criteria were omitted from the study because they were not assessed prior to the clinician's abortion decision. The cohorts closely resembled the original applicant groups on a wide range of basic social and medical characteristics. However, 26 of the 29 ever-married women omitted from the study (an unusually high proportion) were subsequently aborted, and this group also contained a significant excess of women with a main medical indication and a class I socio-economic status. Many of these patients appear to have been lost to the study because of a particular mode of referral. They were referred directly from another hospital ward and accepted for abortion without having the usual out-patient assessment. The 'early warning' notification system for the research workers was principally geared to referrals from general practitioners via the outpatient clinics and inevitably functioned less efficiently for other routes of referral. Consequently notification sometimes occurred after the clinical decision had been taken and the patient was lost to the study. The small number of private practice applicants at this period was also excluded from the series, so, altogether, the study gave a somewhat distorted picture of the abortion situation for upper class married women as well as for those with clear medical reasons for termination. However, in other respects the study provided a representative overall view of an urban community's experience with abortion.

PETER C. OLLEY

PSYCHOLOGICAL ABNORMALITY IN ABORTION APPLICANTS

Are abortion applicants merely a psychological cross section of women of childbearing age in the community or do they possess unusual mental characteristics? Comparison of their test scores at referral with their controls highlighted a number of significant differences.

1 Unmarried applicants

Faced with the prospect of an illegitimate, unwanted pregnancy, the unmarried applicants, not surprisingly, rated as significantly more symptomatically depressed (BDI) and intropunitive (In) than the nursing student controls.† The applicants' high level of inner-directed hostility approximated to that of Philip's sample of Aberdeen 'neurotics' but greatly exceeded that of Weir's group of Scottish unmarried mothers.[35, 36] Single women in the cohort who continued the pregnancy were also more intropunitive than Weir's group. These results suggest that it was the more intropunitive and neurotic section of unmarried, pregnant women who were referred for abortion, a view consistent with Mayo's observation that marked intropunitiveness was associated with the presence of psychiatric symptomatology and a tendency to seek treatment.[37] However, this must be a qualified interpretation because of the diverse circumstances in which the three groups of women were tested. The abortion applicants were pregnant and in the middle of an acute crisis, the unmarried mothers were in the puerperium coping with their babies and the neurotic women were non-pregnant psychiatric outpatients. The cohort also were more character-disordered (CD > 3) than the nursing student controls.* In particular their 16 PF profile displayed a pattern of traits prominent in Cattell's 'neuroticism' cluster.[38] They were more emotionally unstable $C(-)$; sober and over-inhibited $F(-)$; dependent and overprotected $I(+)$; guilt-prone and apprehensive $O(+)$; tense and overwrought $Q_4(+)$. In addition to this 'neurotic' pattern they were more experimenting and free-thinking $Q_1(+)$ – a trait associated with critical attitudes to custom and tradi-

---

† Throughout the study two-tailed t tests or where appropriate chi square tests with a Yates correction were used for assessing significance. The 5% level was accepted as significant ($P < 0.05$). NS denoted 'not significant at the 5% level'. Tables are contained in the appendix on pp. 211–44. An asterisk (*) in the text denotes a reported significance test value either in a footnote or more usually in the appendix where it is cross-referenced by page and/or table number.

178

tion. Academically, they were duller B(−) than the nursing students, a finding that might be accounted for in two ways. Firstly, the cohort comprised women with quite diverse educational and social backgrounds compared to the comparatively homogeneous group of nursing students. Secondly, the performance on the reasoning items of the 16 PF was likely to be lowered by the emotional stress of an unwanted pregnancy. Perhaps the most distinctive difference was their tendency to be imaginative, Bohemian, absorbed in their own inner world M(+) (Tables 5:2 and 5:14).*

2 Ever-married applicants

Once again, depression and character disorder were marked features of the applicant's group at the time of referral (Table 5:13).* Compared to the group of legitimately pregnant controls they also showed certain 'neurotic' personality traits: emotional instability C(−); dependency I(+); tenseness Q_4(+); and submissiveness E(−). A high score on the imaginative M(+) dimension was in fact due to the sub-group of married women with illegitimate pregnancies (see later).

COMMENTS

Both cohorts contained a large proportion of women in a state of intense reactive depression reflected in high Beck and intropunitive scores. If it can be accepted that the Character Disorder Scales and the 16 PF were still adequate measures of basic personality traits under these stressful conditions, then the tests indicated a substantial proportion of applicants with abnormal, vulnerable personalities. A marked 'neurotic' pattern was evident in both groups, but the single women were also abnormally experimenting and self-absorbed. The proportions of character disordered women in the cohorts, 56.5 per cent single, 48.7 per cent married, approximated to the 58 per cent of women in Ekblad's study of abortion who had 'symptoms of chronic neurosis or deviating personalities', prior to the index pregnancy.[39] Ekblad's research concerned 479 Swedish women aborted on 'psychiatric grounds', which in practice also included women aborted for mixed psychiatric and social reasons – roughly equivalent to the non-medical indications in the Aberdeen study. Close parallels with Ekblad's results on abortion might be anticipated.

Another useful comparison study, in view of the suicidal threats occasionally made by abortion applicants, was Philip's Edinburgh series of men and women who had attempted suicide.[40] The same Personal Illness, Character Disorder and Hostility Scales were used in the Aberdeen project. A similar proportion (54 per cent) of Philip's sample of 50 women who had attempted suicide scored as character disordered (CD > 3) but they were much more extropunitive and intropunitive than the Aberdeen abortion applicants at the time of referral ($p < 0.001$). It might be inferred from the much lower hostility level that the Aberdeen women, though experiencing many personality problems, had a greatly reduced potential for suicidal attempts.

It must be re-emphasised at this point that the personality patterns described in the study are derived from group means and represent composite personality profiles. They do not imply that *all* the women in the relevant groups present these characteristics, indeed there are likely to be many exceptions and no one individual may have precisely this pattern. Instead, the profiles indicate general trends in personality functioning.

PREVIOUS PSYCHIATRIC HISTORY

Evidence of previous psychiatric maladjustment was obtained (a) from the medical sociologist's interview at referral and (b) from entries in N.E. Scotland Psychiatric Case Register. At interview some women gave a vague history of 'nervousness' and a tendency to react to stressful situations with excessive anxiety. Others reported being treated by their GP for similar symptoms – and a third group mentioned a definite referral to a psychiatrist. Some of this interview data was suspect, and may have been part of an attempt to secure an abortion by exaggerating vulnerability.

Case Register data are however of a 'harder' quality. The N.E. Scotland Regional Psychiatric Case Register which is located in the Department of Mental Health, University of Aberdeen, has been in operation since 1963. Comprehensive records of all patient contacts with the NHS psychiatric service in north-east Scotland are cumulated and computerised. These records were checked for contact prior to the index pregnancy and subsequent contact until the end of 1970.[41] (Figures in parentheses are percentage of respective cohorts.)

Type of previous psychiatric history

	Single	Ever-married
(a) Case Register evidence of psychiatric referral	10 (6.1%)	16 (7.7%)
(b) Psychiatric treatment from GP	10 (6.1%)	19 (9.2%)
(c) General complaints of psychiatric disability	10 (6.1%)	24 (11.6%)

A further 3 married women had been referred on a previous occasion specifically for an opinion on a termination of pregnancy. A great variety of diagnostic terms were used by the assessing psychiatrists but the majority implied the presence of neurotic symptoms of depression or anxiety with or without an underlying personality disorder. For instance, among the 10 single women previously examined by a psychiatrist, 4 were diagnosed as having neurotic depression, one a phobic anxiety state, 3 a personality disorder and one anorexia nervosa. In one case no psychiatric diagnosis was made. Two of these girls had made suicidal attempts but none had been psychiatric inpatients.

Slightly more serious mental illness was encountered among the 16 ever-married women previously referred to the psychiatric services. Six had been psychiatric inpatients. However the most frequent class of diagnosis was that of personality disorder, with or without co-existing symptoms of anxiety or depression (7 cases). A variety of diagnostic terms had been used to describe these personality deviations, e.g. reactive depression in an immature, inadequate personality, overdose in an hysterical psychopath, situational maladjustment in an hysterical personality. Many terms expressed 'acting out' or attention-seeking qualities. Three women had made suicidal attempts. Six others had presented with neurotic depression or anxiety states, and two of these subject to recurrent periods of depression had received ECT. Another patient was categorised as a barbiturate addict, another suffered from a puerperal depression and one woman had a paranoid state with delusions of jealousy concerning her husband, requiring treatment with phenothiazine drugs.

Compared with some other abortion series, few of the women had suffered in the past from major mental illness. Neurotic conditions and personality disorders predominated among the minority with previous psychiatric disturbance. This pattern was also confirmed among those referred for a psychiatric opinion for termination of the index pregnancy (see below).

PETER C. OLLEY

PROCESSES LEADING TO REFERRAL

Referral to a gynaecological clinic for a decision about abortion is often the culmination of a complex chain of events and decisions, of which four sets, distinct but related, can be distinguished:

(i) Events and causes leading to the conception, e.g. lack or failure of contraceptive precautions.

(ii) Reasons for the pregnancy being considered as 'unwanted', e.g. lack of support from the putative father.

(iii) Factors determining abortion rather than other measures, e.g. marriage or adoption as the solution of choice.

(iv) Circumstances leading to contact with the general practitioner and in turn to his decision to refer to the clinic.

Many social factors are bound up in the web of circumstances but what part if any does the woman's own personality and psychological motivation play in the sequence of events? The study provided an opportunity to examine certain personality aspects of contraceptive practice and of illegitimate pregnancy.

ILLEGITIMATE AND UNWANTED PREGNANCIES

Most of the women in the study, at referral, had a pregnancy which they defined as unwanted and unplanned, though a few had come for abortion under pressure from relatives, doctors or the putative father. The term 'unwanted' pregnancy has many pitfalls in its application. A pregnancy may be unwanted at one stage of pregnancy and wanted or adjusted to at a later stage. Some women changed their minds after interview with the clinicians and withdrew the application. Psychodynamic writers also comment on pregnancies being rejected at an 'unconscious' level while superficially they are wanted. It is pertinent to point out that the concepts illegitimate, unwanted and unplanned are not interchangeable, though many illegitimate pregnancies are also unwanted and unplanned.

These phenomena clearly complicate decision-making on abortion in any individual case and causative factors in the production of an illegitimate or an unwanted pregnancy are likely to be diverse, and multiple for any one woman. The occurrence of an unwanted or illegitimate pregnancy often seems to be the last event in a complex chain of circumstances.

Relationships and events in the family, social customs, particularly involving the peer group, lack of education on contraception, strength of sexual drives, economic circumstances – a wide variety of social, biological and psychological causes have been suggested. Ignorance of birth control techniques is a factor that is nowadays beginning to receive a lot of attention. Economic circumstances and a grossly disadvantaged social situation are more important in some areas than others in producing illegitimacy. The pattern in Great Britain has shown considerable changes in recent years, with illegitimate conceptions in single women being more widely distributed throughout the social classes.[42]

Apart from these external factors, to what extent are internal factors – e.g. the woman's own personality, implicated? Are there personality traits that might predispose a woman to become illegitimately pregnant in the conditions of our present-day society? Several writers have commented on psychological factors associated with illegitimate, unwanted or unplanned pregnancies. Aarons considered an unwanted pregnancy often to be the result of acting out an unresolved neurotic conflict leading to impulsive and risk-taking behaviour, while Patt *et al.* note in their study the large proportion of unwanted pregnancies occurring shortly after an unusually stressful event such as parental death or divorce.[43, 44] Biele described a 'depressive style' of life preceding unwanted pregnancy, and Bowlby stressed the neurotic background of unmarried mothers.[45, 46] Another study found that university students who became pregnant had a higher rate of GP consultation with psychiatric symptoms before conception than a control group of students, while Kaij *et al.* commented on the high incidence of unplanned pregnancies in women with psychiatric symptoms prior to conception.[47, 48] Dependency problems with their mothers and attempts to establish independence, doubts about femininity and the need to prove themselves, unresolved oedipal problems with absent fathers are discussed as factors causative of teenage pregnancy by Babikian and Goldman.[49]

It should also be pointed out however that other authors are sceptical of maternal domination, of illegitimate pregnancy being regarded as a psychiatric symptom and of the unmarried mothers being regarded as a homogeneous group.[50, 51]

The Aberdeen study yielded psychological test data on a large group of women with 'unwanted' and illegitimate pregnancies who had opted for abortion. As previously discussed, the social and demographic characteristics of single and ever-married women referred for abortion showed marked differences, and the changing trends of abortion referral were quite dissimilar for these two groups. Fundamentally different social processes would seem to be involved, legitimacy of pregnancy being a major discriminating dimension for the two groups, with 82.1 per cent of the ever-married applicants having legitimate pregnancies. In that illegitimate pregnancy in single women occurs mostly against a background of social sanction and parental disapproval it was postulated that there would be differences in personality structure with risk-taking and lack of awareness as prominent elements in the profile of the single women.

Significant differences were found on 9 personality factors when the 16 PF scores for the single women's cohort (CS) were compared with those of the 170 ever-married applicants with a legitimate pregnancy.

Unmarried applicants were distinguished from the married by being more imaginative and self-absorbed M(+); expedient G(−); uncontrolled Q_3(−); assertive E(+); group-dependent Q_2(−); shy H(−); intelligent B(+) (Tables 5:14 and 5:8).*

It is convenient at this point to describe in greater detail some of the complexities of these 16 PF factor poles.

(i) M(+) '*Self absorbed and imaginative*' is sometimes termed the 'Bohemian' trait. Such a woman tends to be unconventional, completely absorbed in her own ideas and easily swayed from practical judgements. Cattell described a placid disregard for practical matters alternating with periods of demanding, overwrought behaviour. A capacity for 'dissociation' is an important feature and the external world tends to be perceived in a distorted way conforming with their own wishes and fantasies.

(ii) G(−) implies an *expedient* and changeable quality as opposed to conscientiousness and perseverance. There is a lack of dependability and evasion of social rules. This trait contributes to emotional and impulsive behaviour and is often found in psychopathic and delinquent groups.

(iii) Q_3(−) *Uncontrolled*. Low scores on Q_3 are associated with a lack of self-identity and character stability.

(iv) E(+) '*Assertive*' is a dominant, attention-getting tendency in contrast to being humble and submissive.

(v) Q_2(−) denotes *group dependence* as opposed to self-sufficiency with heavy reliance on group approval. For the younger single woman the reference group is likely to be their peers and the teenage culture rather than society in general.

(vi) H($-$) represents a *shy*, timid trait in contrast to being socially venturesome. Low scores on the factor H correlate with difficulty in making social contacts, over-reacting to threatening situations and experiencing marked inferiority feelings.

(vii) B($+$) *More intelligent*. High scores on this factor suggest a high general ability, a quickness to learn and grasp ideas. It is a measure of general intelligence but also of academic sophistication.

The first four traits M($+$), G($-$), Q_3($-$), E($+$) have been noted as particularly prominent in personality profiles of individuals subject to repeated accidents, in the home or when driving motor-cars.[52, 53] That this pattern should be associated with 'accident proneness' is understandable when the individual traits are examined. M($+$) involves being absorbed in one's private world, and so cut off from outside checks or cues of danger. G($-$) represents a disregard for rules, Q_3($-$) a tendency to impulsiveness and the assertive, aggressive E($+$) trait favours risk-taking. By way of contrast, *ever-married* applicants with legitimate pregnancies were particularly guilt-prone and apprehensive O($+$), serious and over-inhibited F($-$) women.* O($+$) represents a trait of insecurity, worry, inadequacy and self-reproach with a trend to hypochondriasis. Cattell associates this factor pole with a tendency to suffer internal conflict rather than act out a problem. F($-$) indicates a sober, cautious tendency, introspective and full of care.

The composite picture derived from the 16 PF of the unmarried abortion applicant was that of an intelligent but fantasy-dominated girl, lacking in a clear self-identity, stubborn and impulsive, disregarding social rules, lacking self-sufficiency but relating poorly to others. This was a more psychopathic pattern than the evidently neurotic stereotype of the ever-married woman with a legitimate pregnancy, referred for termination – an insecure, apprehensive woman, weighed down with a load of care.

The greater expedience G($-$) and lack of control Q_3($-$) of the un-married applicants and the greater seriousness F($-$) of the legitimate pregnancy group may be a reflection of the ten-year age gap between these populations. Normal maturity processes tend to lead to greater emotional stability C($+$), seriousness F($-$), conscientiousness G($+$), tendency to experiment and be critical Q_1($+$) and control Q_3($+$) with increasing age.

Factors A, H, M, Q_2 of the 16 PF do not normally show age variation for women in the age range under consideration.[30] Age variation of test scores does not invalidate the existence of these personality differences, but may indicate that the group were less remarkable when compared to their peers. Students represent the least selected group of single women and thus give the closest available approximation to their pattern of illegitimacy.

When compared to their 'peers', the nursing student controls of similar age, the 62 referred 'students' exhibited a cluster of neurotic traits – emotional instability $C(-)$, sensitivity $I(+)$, tension $Q_4(+)$, seriousness $F(-)$ but also much of the pattern described above, scoring as significantly more expedient $G(-)$, self-absorbed and imaginative $M(+)$ and experimenting $Q_1(+)$ with a trend to lack of control $Q_3(-)$. Their lower intelligence scores $B(-)$ might be due to selective disruption of performance on reasoning items of the 16 PF by the stress of unwanted pregnancy (see Tables 5:2 and 5:11).*

When contrasted with the 25 married women aged 20–24 with a legitimate pregnancy, the 30 students in this age group still demonstrated the marked self-absorbed trait $M(+)$ but were also rather more expedient $G(-)$, uncontrolled $Q_3(-)$, sensitive $I(+)$, and aloof $A(-)$. Much of the 'illegitimacy pattern' noted above can still be recognised when age is controlled despite the small numbers involved.

EVER-MARRIED WOMEN WITH AN ILLEGITIMATE PREGNANCY

Another approach to illegitimacy is to study this situation among the ever-married women applying for abortion. Thirty-seven (17.9 per cent) of the ever-married group admitted at referral to being pregnant by a man other than their husband. Illegitimate pregnancy was more common (21.8 per cent) in the under 30 age group compared with the older women (14.2 per cent). Wives of skilled workers (class III) reported a significantly lower incidence (10.6 per cent) than the other social groups who all registered incidences near to 25 per cent.

Sixteen of the women had been separated, 8 divorced from their husbands and 6 widowed. Most had become pregnant to a man they could not or would not wish to marry, while a few had a steady relationship with the putative father and were waiting for a divorce to be confirmed before marrying him. The small group of widowed mostly had several children by their husband. Some had hoped for a second marriage but had been let down by their sexual partners. Several expressed considerable guilt and shame at the pregnancy. One young widow had coped well with her sexuality in marriage but had become illegitimately pregnant on two occasions since her husband died four years previously.

Seven women were still living with their husbands, and 5 made no complaint of marital disharmony and wished to preserve their marriage. Sexual intercourse had apparently occurred impulsively while husband was away on business or at sea, sometimes under the influence of alcohol after a party, and in several cases with a friend of the family. In one instance conception had occurred during a short period of estrangement from husband and, since then, reconciliation had taken place. Another woman's husband had been sterilised several years previously and she was now pregnant to one of his friends. A notable finding in the illegitimate group was the significantly high incidence of complete neglect of contraception (57.7 per cent) compared to 19.4 per cent for those with legitimate pregnancies.†

Ever-married women with illegitimate pregnancies were significantly more depressed and more hostile to others than the legitimate pregnancy group. They were also more self-absorbed $M(+)$, suspicious, jealous, difficult to get on with, and irritable $L(+)$ (see Tables 5:7 and 5:8). The legitimate group however scored as slightly more guilt-prone and apprehensive $O(+)$. In several other respects the personality profile of the married women with illegitimate index pregnancies resembled that of the single women rather than the profile of the ever-married, including trends to be more assertive $E(+)$ and group-dependent $Q_2(-)$.

Compared to the antenatal control group of married women with legitimate pregnancies they rated as significantly more emotionally unstable $C(-)$ and tense $Q_4(+)$ and in addition to these neurotic characteristics, particularly high on $M(+)$, the self-absorbed, imaginative, impractical trait.*

CONCLUSIONS ON PSYCHOLOGICAL FACTORS IN ILLEGITIMACY

A pattern of personality traits which has been noted in so-called 'accident prone' individuals was here associated with illegitimate pregnancies in women of different age and marital status applying for an abortion. It was not apparent in a group of abortion applicants with an 'unwanted' but legitimate pregnancy. The core of the illegitimacy

† Lack of contraception, illegitimate v. legitimate: $\chi^2 = 43.6$, d.f. $= 1$, $P < 0.001$.

pattern was the self-absorbed, imaginative, impractical 'Bohemian' trait named 'Autia' by Cattell.[30] Although it was possible to interpret these findings as personality changes secondary to the crisis, in view of the nature of the traits it was more likely that they were pre-existing and had predisposed to the illegitimate pregnancy. Psychological factors therefore would appear to play an important though probably not an exclusive part in the occurrence of many illegitimate conceptions.

AGE AND PSYCHOLOGICAL CHARACTERISTICS

About 10 per cent of the single cohort were over 25 years of age ranging up to 37 years. Many appeared to live rather lonely, restricted lives with widowed mothers to support, they regarded themselves as past marriage and generally saw themselves as unattractive persons.

They scored as more depressed and intropunitive than the younger groups and presented a more neurotic and introverted personality structure with a particularly high percentage (86.7 per cent) of character disorder. The 20–24 and the 15–19 age groups showed lesser degrees of character disturbance (60.0 per cent and 45.7 per cent respectively) and also lesser degress of depression and intropunitiveness. Five of the unmarried group (3.1 per cent) were 15 years of age and 7 (4.3 per cent) were 16 at the time of referral. A feature of these very young abortion applicants was their comparatively stable relationship with the putative father.

In the case of the ever-married women however it was the younger (under 30 years of age) rather than the older group who possessed the greater degrees of personality pathology. More frequently they had a background of an unstable or broken marriage and an illegitimate pregnancy. Many of the older women, on the other hand, got on well with their husbands but regarded their present family as complete.

SOCIAL CLASS AND THE ABORTION APPLICANTS

Are the implications of having an unwanted pregnancy different for upper and lower class women? Some clinicians maintain for instance that unmarried women of low socio-economic status are less threatened by an illegitimate pregnancy because a valuable and satisfying career is not at stake and a baby can be absorbed more readily into their parents' home. Whether or not this is true for the general population this hypothesis was certainly not confirmed for the *single women* who were referred for abortion in the Aberdeen study.

An increasing gradation of distress at referral was noted from the 'student' group through the clerical and distributive to the most disturbed group – the manual workers. The latter were significantly more depressed (BDI) and hostile, both towards others (Ex) and towards themselves (In) than the student group. Manual workers were more guilt-prone $O(+)$, rather more serious and over-inhibited $F(-)$ and generally more character disordered $(CD > 3)$ than the students, who by comparison were Intelligent $B(+)$, Expedient $G(-)$, uncontrolled $Q_3(-)$ and Experimenting $Q_1(+)$ (see Tables 5:9 and 5:11).*

Manual workers were an older group than the students, but a similar pattern was found for the clerical and distributive workers who had an equivalent age to the student group.

Only a small proportion of pregnant unmarried manual workers were referred for abortion in Aberdeen during 1967–8 (see Jean Aitken-Swan, Chapter 1). By contrast the 'referred' students were probably a largely unselected group and so it would appear that highly selected groups of unmarried applicants contained the most disturbed and vulnerable women. It is possible that in groups where referral for abortion is generally hindered, it is only the most psychologically distressed and unstable that find their way to the gynaecological clinics.

Differences in selection were less evident in the *ever-married* women, though the numbers in class I and II were likely to be an underestimate of the incidence of abortion referral because of private practice. Class III women scored as being the most stable and least depressed group at referral. Once more it was the lowest socio-economic group, class V, the wives of unskilled workers, who had the most distressed mental state at referral and the most 'deviating personalities'. The personality pattern in class V, the youngest group of married women, resembled that of the single women's cohort, with a cluster of 'accident prone' factor scores. They were significantly more assertive $E(+)$, expedient $G(-)$, uncontrolled $Q_3(-)$ and self-absorbed $M(+)$ compared to class III. In addition they were more suspicious $L(+)$ and exhibited two traits prominent in the 'neuroticism' cluster, emotional instability $C(-)$ and tension $Q_4(+)$. Classes I and II were very similar in test scores to III, and class IV wives of semi-skilled workers occupied an intermediate position between the extremes (Tables 5:10 and 5:12).*

PETER C. OLLEY

MARRIAGE AND THE ABORTION APPLICANTS

At the time of referral 170 (82.1 per cent) of the 207 ever-married applicants were living with their husbands. Thirty-eight (22.4 per cent) of the former group complained of a severely strained marital relationship, advancing it as one reason for termination. The remaining 132 women did not admit to serious disharmony, though it cannot be assumed that there were no strains in the marriage. These sub-groups are labelled below as 'disharmony' and 'no disharmony admitted'. Thirty-seven women, 17.9 per cent of the cohort, were 'parted' from their husbands, 6 (2.9 per cent) were widowed, 9 (4.3 per cent) were divorced and 22 (10.6 per cent) were separated. Most, but not all, of these 37 were pregnant to a man other than their husband.

Older applicants (30+) apparently had a more stable marriage than the under thirties. They were more often living with their husbands and made relatively fewer complaints of severe disharmony. Wives of semi-skilled and unskilled workers (classes IV and V) applying for abortion had a particularly high incidence of an unhappy or broken marriage compared to the upper socio-economic groups. The wives of skilled workers (class III) showed the least degree of marital disruption.

It was hypothesised that carrying an unwanted pregnancy and applying for an abortion in the context of a broken or strife-torn marriage would be a more distressing event than where the husband provided a harmonious or at least a neutral relationship. When compared with the 'no disharmony admitted' group, both the women 'parted' from their husbands and the 'disharmony' group scored as significantly more depressed and hostile, with a marked tendency to direct hostility outwards. Those still living with husband but complaining of serious conflict rated as the most depressed and hostile (Tables 5:13 and 5:14).*

It was further postulated that personality disorders would be more prominent among the 'parted' and 'disharmony' group than among those apparently living peacefully with their husbands. A gradation of character disorder (CD > 3) was noted, ranging from 'disharmony' (75.7 per cent), through the separated (63.7 per cent), divorced (62.5 per cent), the widowed (50 per cent) to the 'no disharmony' group with the least proportion (38.3 per cent). With the last named as the reference group, those 'parted' from their husbands scored as significantly more suspicious L(+), self-absorbed M(+), and uncontrolled and

190

showed a trend to more emotional instability C(−). The 'disharmony' group exhibited still more prominent emotional instability C(−) as well as the self-absorbed trait M(+). Individuals with a C(−) trait are described by Cattell as being easily perturbed, changeable, readily annoyed by people and objects and having general difficulty in coping with life. It is sometimes characterised as weak 'ego strength' and is one of the most general contributions to the personality profiles of psychiatric patients. Increased suspiciousness L(+) and lack of control Q_3(−) differentiated those who had left their husbands from those who had stayed and suffered.

These traits may have developed secondary to a long-standing marital conflict, but alternatively they may have pre-dated the marriage and contributed to its strain or ultimate breakdown.[54]

THE SINGLE APPLICANTS WHO SUBSEQUENTLY GOT MARRIED

Forty-five (27.6 per cent) of the single women's cohort were recorded as having married by October 1970, i.e. within a period of two to three years after referral. They comprised 23.2 per cent of those who aborted the index pregnancy and 34.4 per cent of those who continued to term. The younger women and members of the student and professional groups showed the greatest incidence of marriage in this period. Twenty-two continued the pregnancy to term and got married, 18 before the birth of the baby. A high proportion – 17 (77.7 per cent) – were thought to have married the putative father. Rather surprisingly 15 (65.2 per cent) of the 23 in the aborted group who married eventually, married the putative father in the period of observation. Thus 32 (19.6 per cent) of the original 163 women in the cohort appeared to have married the putative father.

Women who subsequently married scored as significantly more shy, timid, readily reacting to threat H(−) and a tendency to be more sensitive, dependent and overprotected I(+).† Cattell related the H(−) trait to difficulties in making social contacts, having feelings of inferiority and difficulties in self-expression. Apparently it was the more insecure individuals among the applicants who tended to marry soon after referral.

† Married v. not married: 16 PF, t values H(−) 2.22, $P < 0.05$; I(+) 1.78, $P < 0.1$, NS.

CONTRACEPTIVE PRACTICE AND THE ABORTION APPLICANTS

All the applicants in one sense had been inefficient contraceptors in that they had become pregnant, apparently for the most part involuntarily. Nevertheless it seemed that there was a wide spectrum of contraceptive endeavour, some had made determined efforts to avoid pregnancy whereas with many no precautions whatever had been taken. Tables 5:15 and 5:16 analyse the contraceptive practice reported by the single and ever-married women in terms of regularity of use rather than type of device or technique employed. Coitus interruptus was not categorised as contraception in these tables. Strict operational definitions of regularity could not be readily applied to the data available. However, 'regular use' implied that contraceptive measures were deliberately taken in the large majority of occasions when sexual intercourse took place, though not necessarily on every occasion. 'Irregular use' denoted the absence of consistent attempts at contraception in the recent past, though contraceptive measures had been used on occasion. A further sub-group of ever-married women who insisted that they had been obsessional and 'meticulous' in their observance of contraceptive procedures was also delineated.

Nearly three-quarters of the *single women* (74.8 per cent) applying for abortion had taken no contraceptive precautions during their relationship with the putative father. Only 9.2 per cent could be described as having used regular contraceptive measures. There was little variation in contraceptive practice with age but marked class differences were evident. Student applicants had used contraception significantly more often than the other occupation groups (Table 5:15).* Even here only 14.5 per cent regularly used contraceptive measures and 24.2 per cent used them irregularly. More than 80 per cent of the manual, clerical and distributive workers had totally neglected to take precautions against pregnancy.

The pattern of contraception in *ever-married women* was quite different from the unmarried applicants. Only 29.5 per cent had completely neglected contraception and 44.4 per cent reported regular use. Twenty-seven married women (13 per cent) claimed that they had been particularly careful in the strict observance of contraceptive precautions and could not understand why they had become pregnant. Only two single women (1.2 per cent), both students, claimed to have been so particular.

Neglect of contraception was the hallmark of the single applicants whereas contraceptive failure was the prominent feature of the ever-married group. Women with illegitimate pregnancies in the ever-married group were rather an exception. Their pattern of contraception closely resembled the unmarried group with 75.7 per cent totally neglecting to take precautions. There was little difference in contraceptive practice with age, but there was a marked class variation. Neglect of contraception was particularly high (46.9 per cent) among the wives of unskilled workers (class v). Class III wives reported the highest proportion of regular contraception (55.3 per cent) and the lowest proportion of complete neglect (18.1 per cent) (Tables 5:15 and 5:16).*

It must, however, be re-emphasised that these are findings from a group of pregnant women referred for termination and do not necessarily represent the patterns in the general population.

PSYCHOLOGICAL FACTORS IN CONTRACEPTIVE PRACTICE

Fourteen (93.3 per cent) of the 15 unmarried girls who were regular contraceptors relied on their partner's use of the sheath as the principal measure of birth control. Two substituted the 'safe period' method from time to time and another girl supplemented the sheath with vaginal suppositories. It seems likely that many of this group of 'careful' girls would have used the more effective oral contraceptives had they thought that these could be obtained. At least one girl was under the impression that she would not have been allowed 'the pill' as an unmarried woman. Embarrassment at making application to a general practitioner known to the family can also be a deterrent.

Education about effective contraception and readier access to oral contraceptives would seem to be important ways of reducing the incidence of unwanted pregnancy. Several studies have indicated a general lack of information about birth control and also the considerable difficulty in obtaining oral contraceptives experienced by many single girls who were nevertheless regularly risking a pregnancy.[55, 56]

Apart from the more conscious motivations such as the above, a number of writers discuss motivations to avoid contraception at a much less conscious level. Sandberg and Jacobs list fourteen categories associated with contraception misuse and rejection in married and unmarried individuals who profess the need to avoid an unwanted pregnancy.[57] Among these are the denial of personal responsibility for contraception or the possibility that pregnancy could occur to them. Alternatively, sex without contraception may be seen as a demonstration of her depth of commitment to her boyfriend or the pleasure may be considerably enhanced by the thrill of risk-taking. The unconscious need in some women to prove their femininity and bolster up a low self-esteem by pregnancy is commented upon as is the use of a pregnancy to express hostility to partner or family or to control a relationship.

Bakker and Dightman discuss personality factors in married women who forget to take their oral contraceptives.[58] They are characterised as immature women who have a tendency to acting out and to avoid responsibilities.

It would seem that there can be many different motivations for avoiding or discontinuing effective contraception. For instance one girl among the regular unmarried contraceptors refused her fiancé's request to use oral contraceptives rather than the sheath until he had fixed the wedding date! She became pregnant before he had been pressured into a decision whereupon he broke off the engagement. Another single girl, applying for an abortion, a Roman Catholic, regularly using the 'safe' period was quite shocked to hear of a girlfriend who had been prescribed an oral contraceptive.

It was hypothesised that personality traits might be important determinants of contraceptive practice and thus the regular contraceptors would show different personality characteristics from those who totally neglected or made irregular use of birth control measures. Forty-one *single* women who used contraception, whether irregularly or regularly, were in fact more experimenting and radical $Q_1(+)$ and more group-dependent $Q_2(-)$ on the 16 PF than the 122 single women who gave no evidence of birth control measures being taken either by themselves or their partners (Table 5:17).*

The small group of 15 single women who reported *regular* contraception were significantly more practical $M(-)$ as opposed to self-absorbed, and group-dependent $Q_2(-)$ than the no contraception group. There were also non-significant trends for the 'regulars' to be less suspicious $L(-)$, more controlled $Q_3(+)$ and more emotionally stable $C(+)$.

A cluster of traits associated with stability, control, relating satisfactorily to others and a practical, reality-oriented approach differentiated the unmarried girls whose regular contraceptive measures had failed, from those who had never taken precautions. It should be noted that superiority in intelligence was not a differentiating factor.

The group of 92 regular *ever-married* contraceptors was more apprehensive and guilt-prone O(+), and more conscientious and persevering G(+) than the rest of the ever-married women. A sub-group of 27 who claimed they had used birth control measures meticulously and could not understand why they had become pregnant scored still higher on O(+) and G(+) but also showed high scores on practicability M(−), emotional warmth A(+), and tension Q_4(+), compared to those who used no contraception (Table 5:18).* These results suggest that psychological factors are involved in the use of contraception.

In the present study the 32 *unmarried applicants with a previous pregnancy* were singularly lacking in contraceptive measures. Twenty-eight (87.5 per cent) were taking no precautions. They were mainly older women with clerical, distributive or manual occupations. A significantly higher proportion of the 37 *married women with illegitimate pregnancies* (75.7 per cent) had totally neglected contraception compared to 19.4 per cent of those with legitimate pregnancies. In some cases contraception had been discontinued after separation or divorce. All but 2 of the 37 had prior experience of pregnancy, over half had 3 or more previous pregnancies. At least 9 (24.3 per cent) had been illegitimately pregnant before. So, despite considerable experience of pregnancy and in particular of 'unwanted' pregnancy, an appreciable group of women had neglected contraception. These statistics lend some support to the idea of a group of women who find it difficult to learn from experience or organise their life to avoid an unwanted pregnancy.

Kane *et al.* quote an estimate of 15 to 20 per cent American women in their childbearing years who are poorly motivated for contraception yet consciously wish to avoid pregnancy.[59] Such women are likely to be over-represented among abortion applicants. In the Aberdeen study for example, 31.9 per cent of the single women had high sten scores of 8 to 10 on 'self-absorbed', impractical factor pole M(+), a trait probably conducive to neglect of contraception.

It would appear that an effective programme to reduce the incidence of unwanted pregnancy must include a scheme for detecting women in this category and paying particular attention to initiating and maintaining their motivation for contraception.

PETER C. OLLEY

REFERRAL FOR A PSYCHIATRIC OPINION ON ABORTION OF THE INDEX PREGNANCY

A psychiatric opinion was sought for 66 (40.5 per cent) of the single women and 53 (25.6 per cent) of the ever-married applicants – a significantly higher rate for the unmarried.† Mostly this took place after the gynaecological examination. A few women though referred to a psychiatrist did not arrive at the outpatient clinic and instead had decided to continue the pregnancy. These are listed below as 'uneventuated'. The diagnoses reported below are those of numerous consulting psychiatrists and not those of the research psychiatrist. Thus they cannot be considered as an entirely consistent assessment, but only give an overall impression of the major categories of mental disorder. It should be noted that 'no psychiatric diagnosis' was recorded for sizeable proportions of the referred women. Frequently this seemed to indicate that a formal psychiatric illness was not considered to be present, though in some instances it might be a substitute for a diagnosis of 'situational maladjustment'. Nevertheless 6 single and 8 ever-married women in this category were recommended for termination.

Neurotic reactions and personality disorders constituted the majority of the diagnoses made by the psychiatrists.

Psychiatric diagnoses

	Single	Ever-married
Neurotic or 'reactive' depression	24	17
Anxiety state	6	4
Depression with personality disorder	5	2
Anxiety with personality disorder	0	1
Personality disorder	15	6
Mentally subnormal	1	1
Paranoid state	0	1
No psychiatric diagnosis	13	16
Uneventuated	2	5
	66	53

Personality disorders formed a larger percentage of diagnoses in the case of the single women than for the ever-married. A varied collection of descriptive terms were used, many expressing the concepts of

† Referrals, single v. ever-married: $\chi^2 = 8.59$, d.f. $= 1$, $P < 0.01$.

196

instability, inadequacy or immaturity. Major mental illness formed only a small proportion of those referred to a psychiatrist for an opinion on abortion of the index pregnancy.

It was postulated that women referred for a psychiatric opinion on abortion would be more mentally disturbed and show greater personality deviations than applicants who were not so referred.

Single women sent to psychiatrists in fact scored as significantly more depressed and extropunitive, but also reported an excess of suicidal feelings that was not matched by the degree of inward directed hostility (see Table 5:19). There were no clear personality differences evident on the 16 PF, though there was a trend approaching significance to be more self-absorbed and fantasy-dominated M(+).

Ever-married women referred for a psychiatric opinion were also significantly more depressed than their colleagues who only consulted the gynaecologists, but they tended to score higher on inward-directed hostility. However they did show prominent personality traits, being significantly more aloof and reserved A(−); emotionally unstable C(−); self-absorbed and imaginative M(+); tense and driven $Q_4(+)$† (Table 5:20).

A(−) represents a detached, cool, critical characteristic whereas $Q_4(+)$ according to Cattell implies a trait of turmoil and frustrated drive that is disruptive of steady application and emotional balance. It is an important component in the cluster of factors related to anxiety. These frustrated drives may be sexual in nature but they also involve aggressiveness or escape tendencies.[30] Referral to a psychiatrist seemed closely related to a highly disturbed mental state at the time of the initial consultation. Gynaecologists seemed to have selected the more vulnerable and introverted personalities among the married women, but failed to make such a clear differentiation for the unmarried applicants.

LATER REFERRALS TO THE PSYCHIATRIC SERVICES

The Regional Psychiatric Case Register enabled checks to be made on further psychiatric referrals of women from the cohorts in the period up to October 1970.

Some of the *single women* were offered psychiatric treatment at or

† Referred to psychiatrist v. not referred, ever-married: 16 PF, t values A(−) 2.86, $P < 0.01$; C(−) 2.02, $P < 0.05$.

near the time of the abortion decision. Four of the 6 women who were given *continued psychiatric support* in relation to the index pregnancy were aborted, 3 of them on psychiatric grounds. This constituted 4.0 per cent of the total aborted in the single cohort. Unresolved grief about her mother's recent death which had antedated the index pregnancy was thought to be central to one girl's depression and she was given outpatient psychotherapy for fourteen months. Another was admitted to the psychiatric hospital in a state of severe neurotic depression before termination. She came from an unhappy home with continual parental quarrelling. This was her second pregnancy. Her son, by a different father, was looked after by her parents. There was no question of marriage. The putative father (himself married) had said 'it was her problem' and she feared being turned out of her home by her rather strict father. Her mother had a depressive illness three years before.

A third girl, considered to have an immature personality, with a previous history of depression related to educational and home problems, was supported satisfactorily as an outpatient for eight months after her termination. The fourth single woman, with a marked family history of mental illness and suicide, was given day-hospital group-psychotherapeutic treatment and outpatient support for ten months after the index pregnancy was terminated. She had become guilty and fearful that she herself was going to die. The year before the pregnancy crisis she apparently suffered an hysterical fugue.

Two single women (3.1 per cent of those who continued the pregnancy) made suicidal attempts shortly after their request for termination was refused and were treated as psychiatric inpatients. One, a student with a history of periodic bouts of depression and an unhappy home life, had a succession of unsatisfactory affairs. Her studies had suffered and she considered the putative father to be too unreliable to marry. She had been too frightened to seek advice in the earlier stages of her pregnancy. At five months she took an overdose of aspirin and was admitted for a short period to the psychiatric clinic. She was considered essentially to have a personality disorder and was supported as an outpatient until after her baby was born. The other girl, a nurse from a very puritanical home, was refused termination and became deeply depressed when her parents found out about the pregnancy. She also required inpatient psychiatric treatment after a suicidal attempt.

Few of the single women found their way to the north-east Scotland psychiatric services *after* the referral period for the index pregnancy. Prior to October 1970 only 5 single women, 3.1 per cent of the original cohort, had been referred to a psychiatrist for a further assessment after the immediate pregnancy crisis. Three of these (1.8 per cent of CS) were again illegitimately pregnant and a psychiatric opinion on termination had been requested. Of the other two girls, one, whose abortion request had been refused one month previously and now four months pregnant, had been admitted to the casualty department having threatened to throw herself under the wheels of a passing car. She was transferred to the psychiatric clinic, where it emerged that she had seen the putative father in the company of another girl and had become quite histrionic. A diagnosis was made of an acute situational maladjustment in a young pregnant woman with a personality disorder. She settled with supportive treatment, decided not to see her boyfriend again and to have her baby adopted.

The other girl had been subject to recurrent depressive episodes even before the index pregnancy and became acutely depressed shortly after an abortion was carried out on medico-psychiatric grounds. There had been two previous illegitimate pregnancies by different men. The current putative father declined marriage. After the abortion she became severely depressed and was treated with ECT as an inpatient. She made satisfactory progress in hospital and was followed up as an outpatient. Nine months later she was still seeing the putative father and having occasional moods of depression.

Three *ever-married women* (1.5 per cent) were given outpatient support after an initial psychiatric assessment at the time of the index pregnancy. Two were aborted and the other continued the pregnancy. Fourteen ever-married women were subsequently referred to the psychiatric services (6.8 per cent). One of these was sent for a psychiatric opinion about abortion of another unwanted pregnancy. The 13 other women (6.3 per cent) were referred for other psychiatric upsets not related to pregnancy. This comprised 5.2 per cent of women who had been aborted and 8.3 per cent of those who had continued the pregnancy to term. Psychiatric diagnosis was mainly that of neurotic (reactive) depression with or without personality problems.

Four had made suicidal attempts. Most of the breakdowns were closely related to marital stress, separation or divorce, poor housing or finance. A barbiturate addict suffered a puerperal depression in a later pregnancy and an amphetamine addict was also referred again. One woman became depressed after a hysterectomy carried out for a condition detected at the time of termination.

Only a tiny minority of *single* women were referred to the regional psychiatric services in the two or three years after the pregnancy crisis. Despite a considerable number of suicidal threats and feelings at the time of referral, known suicidal attempts were few in number. *Ever-married* women were referred significantly more often for further psychiatric assessment ($\chi^2 = 4.76$, d.f. = 1, $P < 0.05$), but there was no significant difference in the rates for aborted and non-aborted. In fact referrals were slightly less common in the aborted group despite their greater vulnerability as judged by their test scores.

PSYCHOLOGICAL TEST SCORES AND MAIN INDICATIONS FOR TERMINATION AS CLASSIFIED BY GYNAECOLOGISTS

As reported in Chapter 2, two of the gynaecologists in the study (IMacG and JD) retrospectively classified the indications for abortion in each woman's case, whether abortion occurred or not. This categorisation took place without knowledge of psychological test results. Often there were multiple indications but in this section, for the sake of simplicity, only the main indications have been used. These five categories are: medico-psychiatric, socio-psychiatric, social, medical, and eugenic.

When major psychiatric, medical or eugenic aspects were not involved, a main social indication was recorded by the classifying gynaecologists. Table 5:21 shows the distribution of the various main indications for the single and ever-married cohorts.

Inherent in the definitions of the various categories was a gradation of psychological disturbance at referral and a personality vulnerability ranging from the most marked deviation from the norm with the 'medico-psychiatric' group, through lesser deviations for 'socio-psychiatric' and 'social' and in the case of the 'medical' and 'eugenic' categories the absence of specific reference to personality problems. It was to be expected that the last two groups would show the least degree of psychological disturbance and personality deviation at referral.

The scores on psychological tests closely related to the presence of psychiatric symptoms clearly illustrated these trends for both single and ever-married women, particularly with the depression scores (B_1) and the intropunitive scores at referral $(In)_1$, though outward-directed hostility $(Ex)_1$ did not connect up so closely with the definitions (Tables 5:22 and 5:23). Percentages of character disordered women in the various indication categories showed similar gradations for both single and ever-married women with medico-psychiatric as the most disordered and medical group as the least.

Percentage character disordered (CD > 3)

Main indication	Single	Ever-married
Medico-psychiatric	85.7	72.2
Socio-psychiatric	59.5	51.0
Social	46.2	49.5
Medical	—	31.8

Single women assigned to the medico-psychiatric category had a 'psychopathic' type of hostility pattern with high extropunitiveness and high intropunitiveness. Ever-married women with the same main indication had a more 'neurotic' pattern with high intropunitive but unremarkable extropunitive scores.

The 16 PF scores reflected similar trends in personality pathology with medico-psychiatric groups scoring as the most deviant in such vulnerability traits as $C(-)$, $H(-)$, $I(+)$, $M(+)$, $O(+)$, and $Q_3(-)$ with lesser deviations occurring for socio-psychiatric and social groups. By contrast the medical group of ever-married women were the most stable in the cohort, being comparatively out-going $A(+)$, venturesome $H(+)$, most controlled $Q_3(+)$ and placid $Q_4(-)$, though they scored quite high on guilt-proneness $O(+)$ (Tables 5:24 and 5:25).

The gynaecological classifications are thus generally consistent with the psychological test scores and would appear to possess a fair degree of validity.

PSYCHOLOGICAL STATE AT REFERRAL IN RELATION TO DECISIONS ABOUT ABORTION

The final decision about the application for abortion was mostly made by the gynaecologist, frequently with a second opinion from a psychiatrist. In three instances in which the patient saw a psychiatrist initially, she was refused at this point, there was no referral to a gynaecologist and the pregnancy was continued.

Between 50 and 60 per cent of the total applicants were accepted for abortion by the Aberdeen gynaecologists – by no means a situation of abortion on demand! Approximately 30–40 per cent were refused termination and continued the pregnancy to term. A further group, mainly married women, changed their minds about an abortion after interviews with the research workers and the clinicians, withdrew their application and decided to continue the pregnancy. They are listed as 'Patient changed her mind' (Tables 5:26 and 5:27). Nine single and 14 ever-married women had aborted the pregnancy shortly after referral without induction by the gynaecologists. Another single girl who was refused termination, aborted over a month after referral, and 2 married women who had also been refused went into premature labour at 27 and 28 weeks respectively with resultant neo-natal deaths. All these cases were reported under the heading of 'spontaneous abortion'.

Probably most of these were genuine spontaneous abortions since only a minority had been definitely refused termination before they aborted. A self-induced abortion after refusal was however carried out by one ever-married woman who had also aborted herself on a previous occasion. One unmarried woman refused by the Aberdeen gynaecologists subsequently obtained a termination in London. It was notable that this was the only instance where the Aberdeen decision was reversed – quite a different situation to other series where a large proportion of those refused obtained an abortion elsewhere.

The eventual outcome was established for all the women in the cohorts, and Tables 5:26 and 5:27 show the different categories of outcome for the single and the ever-married women.

Making a decision to abort or recommend continuation of an unwanted pregnancy was clearly a complex process involving many diverse social, obstetric and psychological factors. The test scores at referral allowed a broad examination to be made of psychological features of women who were accepted contrasted with the features of those who were refused termination.

It was hypothesised that there would be marked psychological differences between the two groups. *Single* women who were accepted for abortion were significantly more depressed (BDI), extropunitive $(Ex)_1$ and intropunitive $(In)_1$ than those who were refused. They also registered a significant excess of suicidal thoughts on the Beck Depression

Inventory (Table 5:28). Differences in personality structure for these two groups were only slight, though the accepted group showed rather more deviant scores on factors often associated with psychological maladjustment such as aloof A($-$), suspicious L($+$), self-absorbed M($+$), and uncontrolled Q_3($-$) (Table 5:29).

Ever-married women who were recommended for abortion also displayed a significant excess of depression and inner-directed hostility but were not notably more extropunitive. Definite personality factor differences were apparent. Those accepted were significantly more guilt-prone O($+$) but had a greater degree of self-control Q_3($+$).* The more impulsive, uncontrolled, ever-married women, lacking clear self-identity, tended to be refused an abortion.

Single and ever-married women who showed a marked depressive reaction at the time of referral tended to be accepted for an abortion. A decision to abort the single women was evidently related more to the current mental state and situational factors than any personality vulnerability. Personality factors in the ever-married women however appeared much more important in determining whether abortion was or was not carried out.

DECISIONS ABOUT STERILISATION

Sterilisation was carried out for 106 (51.2 per cent) of the ever-married women and significantly more often for those who were aborted than those continuing the pregnancy to term. 61.5 per cent of those who aborted the pregnancy were also sterilised and tubal ligation in association with hysterotomy was the most favoured procedure. Post-partum sterilisation was carried out in 23 instances, i.e. 31.9 per cent of those who went to term. A progressive increase in the rate of *sterilisation* occurred with increasing *age* at referral, except for the 40–44 age group which has a particularly low rate. This increase in sterilisation with age was mainly contributed by the women who were *aborted*. *Non-aborted* women had a rate of sterilisation essentially independent of age (Table 5:30).*

There were also significant *social class* variations in sterilisation. The incidence of sterilisation was greatest in class III, followed by class I and II, class IV and class V in decreasing proportions. Class dependence of sterilisation was only a feature of the ever-married women who were aborted (Table 5:31).* Most of the ever-married women with a main *medical* indication (90.9 per cent) were sterilised, whether or not they were aborted. Comparative percentages of those with main medico-psychiatric, socio-psychiatric and social indications who were sterilised were 65.0, 59.6 and 38.0 per cent respectively. In each main indication group women who continued the pregnancy were less likely to be sterilised than those who were aborted. Only three *single women* were sterilised, all of whom had two or more previous pregnancies.

One woman had cohabited with the putative father for many years and already had two children by him. She considered that her family was large enough to bring up with their limited finances. Her relationship was a stable one and they planned to marry when his divorce was finalised. Abortion was in fact refused but post-partum sterilisation was carried out. Another unmarried woman in her late thirties was living with her two illegitimate children and was pregnant again to the youngest child's father. Apparently he was an extremely unstable and unreliable man and she had broken with him at the time of the referral. She lived on social security in cramped housing conditions and didn't wish to continue the pregnancy. She was aborted and sterilised by the gynaecologists. The third single woman in her mid-twenties was mentally subnormal and liable to be seduced by any stranger who took an interest in her. She had two young children, looked after by her parents, who were both conceived after casual encounters. Abortion as well as sterilisation was performed.

THE INFLUENCE OF THE GYNAECOLOGISTS

There was considerable variation in the proportion of applicants who were terminated by the different gynaecologists operating in the area. Tables 5:32 and 5:33 list the decisions made by the individual gynaecologists (denoted by capital letters), during the period of the study.

H is in fact a group of gynaecologists who each only assessed a few patients for abortion. The term 'other' includes the categories 'spontaneous abortion' and 'changed mind'. Three women in the cohorts were not assessed for termination by a gynaecologist. They were seen initially by a psychiatrist, were refused an abortion and were seen by the gynaecologist only for the purpose of managing the pregnancy.

Two distinct groups of gynaecologists A, B, C and E, F, G, H are apparent from the tables, aborting high and low proportions of applicants, with gynaecologist D intermediate between them. Similar rankings occurred in previous years. These main groups have been labelled 'liberal' and 'conservative' respectively, and D has been included in the conservative group for some aspects of the analysis. 'Liberal' gynaecologists aborted a significantly higher proportion of both single and ever-married applicants than the 'conservatives'; whereas the 'liberals' aborted similar proportions of unmarried and ever-married applicants, the 'conservatives' aborted a rather higher proportion of the ever-married than the single.*

However, were these apparent differences in abortion practice really due to different attitudes towards this procedure or were they due to a different clientele that was referred?

In the earlier part of the *psychological* study individual gynaecologists saw the patients specifically referred to them by the general practitioner. It was not until the last six months of this study that a random allocation system was adopted and referrals were 'pooled' (see Introduction).

There were in fact marked differences in the social class of single women who were referred to the 'liberal' and 'conservative' groups. 'Students' and 'professionals' formed a significantly higher proportion of those referred to the 'liberals', whereas 'conservatives' assessed a significantly higher proportion of clerical and distributive workers (Table 5:34). There were also differences by main indication for referral. The 14 single women with medico-psychiatric indications were seen exclusively by the 'liberal' group, whereas the 'conservatives' more frequently dealt with unmarried women with main social indications (Table 5:36).

These differences were reflected in the scores on the 16 PF, with single women referred to 'liberal' gynaecologists scoring as significantly more emotionally unstable $C(-)$, serious and over-inhibited $F(-)$, and uncontrolled $Q_3(-)$ and having trends to be timid $H(-)$, experimenting $Q_1(+)$, and tense $Q_4(+)$, traits mostly associated with a tendency to psychiatric disturbance (Table 5:38).*

On the other hand the *ever-married* women referred to the 'liberals' closely resembled those seen by the 'conservatives' on social class and main indications (Tables 5:35 and 5:37). Personality traits were also similar except that the 'conservatives' group of ever-married applicants scored as significantly more shrewd and worldly wise $N(+)$ than the 'liberals' group.* This factor has not been considered important in distinguishing the psychologically vulnerable from the psychologically stable and the implication of this difference is uncertain.

Thus there were notable differences in the 'liberal' and 'conservative' clientele of unmarried applicants but not for the ever-married applicants.

Examination of the decisions taken by the two groups of gynaecologists about women with the same main indications for abortion allowed a rough comparison of abortion attitudes. Tables 5:36 and 5:37 illustrate the abortion practice analysed by main indication. In these tables abortion comprised both that induced by the gynaecologists and 'spontaneous' abortions.

For the single women there were significant differences evident in abortion of both the social and social psychiatric groups, even when 'spontaneous' abortions and 'changed mind' groups were allowed for. 'Liberals' aborted significantly higher percentages of both social psychiatric and social groups than the 'conservatives'.* In the case of the ever-married women where the populations referred to the two types of gynaecologist were psychologically much more similar, the only significant difference was the higher abortion rate among women referred with main social indications to the 'liberal' gynaecologists. However, the 'liberals' dealt with married women presenting a main medical or psychiatric indication similarly to the 'conservatives'. The concept of 'liberal' and 'conservative' types of gynaecologist would appear to have some substance with significantly different decisions about abortion being taken for roughly comparable populations.

Though these groups came to widely different decisions on abortion their practice as regards sterilisation of the ever-married women was very similar (Table 5:39). There were no significant differences though 'conservatives' offered sterilisation rather more frequently to those they accepted for termination.

SUMMARY

The first part of the psychological study was concerned with a description of social, obstetric and psychological characteristics of the large majority of a city's abortion applicants during a fourteen-month period in 1967–8. Evaluation was carried out before and independently of the decision-making process. The group that was studied reflected the major features noted by Jean Aitken-Swan in her epidemiological study (Chapter 1), and was considered in most respects to give a representative picture of abortion practice in Aberdeen during that period. Unmarried applicants formed a population distinct from the ever-married cohort and in particular displayed a different personality structure. Both groups showed abnormal psychological characteristics compared to control groups. Neurotic personality patterns were more prevalent among the ever-married whereas more psychopathic features with 'accident prone' tendencies were prominent in the single women's cohort.

Though the majority presented in a state of depression, major mental illness both in the past and at the time of referral was quite uncommon in the cohorts.

Unmarried manual workers and older single women, younger ever-married women, the wives of unskilled workers, and those with broken or strained marriages appeared to be the most distressed sub-groups at the time of referral and also possessed the most deviating personality patterns. Ever-married women with illegitimate pregnancies, however, showed considerable personality resemblances to women in the unmarried cohort. Scores on the questionnaires also suggested that psychological factors were of importance both in the occurrence of an illegitimate conception and in the regular use of contraception among the applicants.

The validity of the main indication categories assigned by the gynaecologists checked with the expected ranking of psychological disturbance assessed by the questionnaires. Overall only about 60 per cent of the women were granted an abortion by the gynaecologist. Women who were aborted were significantly more depressed at referral and especially in the case of the ever-married had more vulnerable personality characteristics than women who continued the pregnancy.

Two groups of gynaecologists were distinguished who differed significantly in the proportion they aborted when assessing patients with similar social and psychological characteristics. The gynaecologists' attitudes to abortion were most divergent concerning women with main social indications. Their attitudes to sterilisation, however, were quite similar.

Thus the scene was set for the next stage of the research project, the follow-up and evaluation of long-term effects of abortion, continuing to term and sterilisation.

REFERENCES

1 Sim, M. (1963) 'Abortion and the psychiatrist', *Brit. med. J.*, **2**, 145.
2 British Medical Association Committee on Therapeutic Abortion (1968) 'Indications for termination of pregnancy', *Brit. med. J.*, **1**, 171–5.
3 Anderson, E. W. (1966) 'Psychiatric indications for the termination of pregnancy', *J. psychosom. Res.*, **10**, 127–34.
4 Simon, N. M., Senturia, A. G. (1966) 'Psychiatric sequelae of abortion', *Arch. gen. Psychiat.*, **15**, 378–89.
5 Ekblad, M. (1955) 'Induced abortion on psychiatric grounds', *Acta psychiat. neurol. scand.*, Suppl. 99.
6 Margolis, A. J., Davison, L. A., Hanson, K. H., Loos, S. A., Mikkelsen, M. S. W. (1971) 'Therapeutic abortion follow-up study', *Am. J. Obstet. Gynec.*, **110**, 243–9.
7 Patt, S. L., Rappaport, R. G., Barglow, P. (1969) 'Follow-up of therapeutic abortion', *Arch. gen. Psychiat.*, **20**, 408–14.
8 Simon, N. M., Senturia, A. G., Rothman, D. (1967). 'Psychiatric illness following therapeutic abortion', *Am. J. Psychiat.*, **124**, 59–65.
9 Niswander, K. R., Patterson, R. J. (1967) 'Psychologic reaction to therapeutic abortion. 1. Subjective patient response', *Obstetrics and Gynecology*, **29**, 702–6.
10 Peck, A., Marcus, H. (1966) 'Psychiatric sequelae of therapeutic interruption of pregnancy', *J. nerv. ment. Dis.*, **143**, 417–25.
11 Brody, H., Meikle, S., Gerritse, R. (1971) 'Therapeutic abortion: a prospective study 1', *Am. J. Obstet. Gynec.*, **109**, 347–53.
12 Levene, H. I., Rigney, F. J. (1970) 'Law, preventive psychiatry and therapeutic abortion', *J. nerv. ment. Dis.*, **151**, 51–9.
13 Jansson, B. (1965) 'Mental disorders after abortion', *Acta psychiat. scand.*, **41**, 87–110.
14 Höök, K. (1963) 'Refused abortion. A follow-up study of 249 women whose applications were refused by the National Board of Health in Sweden', *Acta psychiat. scand.*, Suppl. 168.
15 Clark, M., Forstner, I., Pond, D. A., Tregold, R. F. (1968) 'Sequels of unwanted pregnancy. A follow-up of patients referred for psychiatric opinion', *Lancet*, **2**, 501–3.
16 Pare, C. M. B., Raven, H. (1970) 'Follow-up of patients referred for termination of pregnancy', *Lancet*, **1**, 635–8.
17 Kenyon, F. E. (1969) 'Termination of pregnancy on psychiatric grounds. A comparative study of 61 cases', *Brit. J. med. Psychol.*, **42**, 243–54.
18 McCoy, D. R. (1968) 'The emotional reaction of women to therapeutic abortion and sterilisation', *J. Obstet. Gynaec. Brit. Cmwlth.*, **75**, 1054–7.
19 Todd, N. A. (1972) 'Follow-up of patients recommended for therapeutic abortion', *Brit. J. Psychiat.*, **120**, 645–6.
20 Ingham, C., Simms, M. (1972) 'Study of applicants for abortion at the Royal Northern Hospital, London', *J. Biosoc. Sci.*, **4**, 351–69.

21 Beck, A. T., Ward, C. H., Mendelson, M., Mock, J., Erbaugh, J. (1961) 'An inventory for measuring depression', *Arch. gen. Psychiat.*, **4**, 561–71.

22 Schwab, J., Bialow, M., Clemmons, R., Martin, P., Holzer, C. (1967) 'The Beck Depression Inventory with medical in-patients', *Acta psychiat. scand.*, **43**, 255–66.

23 Metcalfe, M., Goldman, E. (1965) 'Validation of an inventory for measuring depression', *Brit. J. Psychiat.*, **111**, 240–2.

24 Foulds, G. A. (1965) *Personality and Personal Illness*, Tavistock, London.

25 Philip, A. E. (1969) 'The development and use of the Hostility and Direction of Hostility Questionnaire', *J. psychosom. Res.*, **13**, 283–7.

26 Foulds, G. A., Hope, K. (1968) *Manual of the Symptom Sign Inventory*, University of London Press, London.

27 Foulds, G. A. (1967) 'Some differences between neurotics and character disorders', *Brit. J. soc. clin. Psychol.*, **6**, 52.

28 Philip, A. E. (1970) 'Traits, attitudes and symptoms in a group of attempted suicides', *Brit. J. Psychiat.*, **116**, 475–82.

29 Foulds, G. A. (1968) 'Neurosis and character disorder in hospital and in prison', *Brit. J. Crim.*, **8**, 46.

30 Cattell, R. B., Eber, H. W., Tatsuoka, M. M. (1970) *Handbook for the Sixteen Personality Questionnaire* (16PF), IPAT Champaign, Illinois.

31 Cattell, R. B. (1962) *Handbook Supplement for Form C of the Sixteen Personality Factor Test*, IPAT Champaign, Illinois.

32 Anastasi, A. (1961) *Psychological Testing*, Macmillan, New York.

33 Vernon, P. E. (1964) *Personality Assessment*, Methuen, London.

34 Treadway, C. R., Kane, F. J., Jarrahi-Zadeh, A., Lipton, M. A. (1969) 'A psychoendocrine study of pregnancy and puerperium', *Am. J. Psychiat.*, **125**, 1380–6.

35 Philip, A. E. (1968) 'The constancy of structure of a hostility questionnaire', *Brit. J. soc. clin. Psychol.*, **7**, 16.

36 Weir, S. (1970) 'A study of unmarried mothers and their children in Scotland', *Scottish Health Service Studies*, no. 13, Scottish Home and Health Department.

37 Mayo, P. R. (1969) 'Women with neurotic symptoms who do not seek treatment', *Brit. J. med. Psychol.*, **42**, 165–9.

38 Cattell, R. B. (1962) *Handbook Supplement for Form C of the Sixteen Personality Factor Test*, IPAT Champaign, Illinois.

39 Ekblad, M. (1955) 'Induced abortion on psychiatric grounds. A follow-up of 479 women', *Acta psychiat. neurol. scand.*, Suppl. 99.

40 Philips, A. E. (1970) 'Traits, attitudes and symptoms in a group of attempted suicides', *Brit. J. Psychiat.*, **116**, 475–82.

41 Baldwin, J. A., Innes, G., Miller, W. M., Sharp, G. A., Dorricott, N. (1965) 'A psychiatric case register in NE Scotland', *Brit. J. prev. soc. Med.*, **19**, 38–42.

42 Illsley, R. A., Gill, D. (1968) 'Changing trends in illegitimacy', *Soc. Sci. and Med.*, **2**, 415–33.

43 Aarons, Z. A. (1967) 'Therapeutic abortion and the psychiatrist', *Am. J. Psychiat.*, **124**, 745–54.

44 Patt, S. L., Rappoport, R. G., Barglow, P. (1969). 'Follow-up of therapeutic abortion', *Arch. gen. psychiat.*, **20**, 408–14.

45 Biele, A. M. (1971) 'Unwanted pregnancy: symptom of depressive practice', *Am. J. Psychiat.*, **128**, 748–54.

46 Bowlby, J. (1957) *Maternal Care and Mental Health*, WHO, HM Stationery Office.

47 Giel, R., Kidd, C. (1965) 'Some psychiatric observations on pregnancy in the unmarried student', *Brit. J. Psychiat.*, **3**, 591.

48 Nilsson, A., Kaij, L., Jacobson, L. (1967) 'Postpartum mental disorder in an unselected sample. The importance of the unplanned pregnancy', *J. psychosom. Res.*, **10**, 341–7.

49 Babikian, H. M., Goldman, A. (1971) 'A study in teen-age pregnancy', *Am. J. Psychiat.*, **128**, 755–60.

50 Vincent, C. (1961) *Unmarried Mothers*, Free Press of Glencoe, Chicago.

51 Schmideberg, M. (1951) 'Psychiatric social factors in young unmarried mothers', *Social Casework*, **32**, 3–7.

52 Suhr, V. W. (1953) 'The Cattell 16PF test as a prognosticator of accident susceptibility', Proceedings of *Iowa Acad. Sci.*, **60**, 558–61.

53 Marshall, J. W., Waxman, B. D. (1959) 'An empirical study of the relationship between certain personality dimensions and the incidence of accidental injuries', *Connecticut Health Bulletin*, **73**, 11.

54 Kreitman, N., Collins, J., Nelson, B., Troop, J. (1970) 'Neurosis and marital interaction. I. Personality and symptoms', *Brit. J. Psychiat.*, **117**, 33–46.

55 Schofield, M. (1968) *The Sexual Behaviour of Young People*, Penguin Books, London.

56 McCance, C., Hall, D. J. (1972) 'Sexual behaviour and contraceptive practice of unmarried female undergraduates at Aberdeen University', *Brit. med. J.*, **11**, 694–700.

57 Sandberg, E. C., Jacobs, R. I. (1971) 'Psychology of the misuse and rejection of contraception', *Am. J. Obstet. Gynec.*, **110**, 227–42.

58 Bakker, C. B., Dightman, C. R. (1964) 'Psychological factors in fertility control', *Fertility and Sterility*, **15**, 559–67.

59 Kane, F. J., Lachenbruch, P. A., Lokey, L., Chafetz, N., Auman, R., Pocuis, L., Lipton, M. A. (1971) 'Motivational factors affecting contraceptive use'. *Am. J. Obstet. Gynec.*, **110**, 1050–4.

APPENDIX 5:A

Significance test values

p. 178   Tables 5:1 and 5:13, single cohort v. single control: (BDI) B $\geqslant$ 10, $\chi^2 = 143.7$, d.f. = 3, $P < 0.001$; CD > 3, $\chi^2 = 20.37$, d.f. = 1, $P < 0.001$; (Ex), $t = 0.34$, NS; (In), $t = 2.63$, $P < 0.01$.

p. 179   Tables 5:2 and 5:14, single cohort v. single control: 16 PF, t values C($-$) 3.53; F($-$) 3.96; I($+$) 6.50; O($+$) 4.00; Q$_4$($+$) 8.84; B($-$) 10.48; M($+$) 5.84, all $P < 0.001$; Q$_1$($+$) 3.26, $P < 0.01$.

p. 179   Tables 5:1 and 5:13, married cohort v. married control: (BDI) B $\geqslant$ 10, $\chi^2 = 108.2$, d.f. = 3, $P < 0.001$; CD > 3, $\chi^2 = 13.1$, d.f. = 1, $P < 0.001$; (Ex), $t = 0.14$, NS; (In), $t = 1.73$, $P < 0.1$, NS.

p. 184   Tables 5:14 and 5:8, single cohort v. legitimate pregnancy cohort: 16 PF, t values M($+$) 4.09; G($-$) 3.95; Q$_3$($-$) 3.34; B($+$) 4.41; Q$_2$($-$) 3.75, all $P < 0.001$; E($+$) 2.21; H($-$) 2.31, both $P < 0.05$.

p. 185   Single cohort v. legitimate pregnancy cohort: 16 PF, t values O($+$) 2.35; F($-$) 2.44, both $P < 0.05$.

p. 186   Tables 5:2 and 5:11, single women, student v. control: 16 PF, t values C($-$) 2.50, $P < 0.02$; I($+$) 5.36, $P < 0.001$; Q$_4$($+$) 5.77, $P < 0.001$; F($-$) 2.27, $P < 0.05$; G($-$) 2.10, $P < 0.05$; M($+$) 4.54, $P < 0.001$; Q($+$) 4.29, $P < 0.001$; Q$_3$($-$) 1.64, NS; B($-$) 2.80, $P < 0.01$.

p. 187   Ever-married, illegitimate v. legitimate: (BDI) $t = 2.37$, $P < 0.02$; (Ex), $t = 2.03$, $P < 0.05$; (In), $t = 1.94$, $P < 0.1$, NS; 16 PF, t values M($+$) 2.95, $P < 0.01$; L($+$) 2.54, $P < 0.01$.
Ever-married, illegitimate v. married control: 16 PF, t values C($-$) 3.09, $P < 0.001$; Q$_4$($+$) 2.08, $P < 0.05$; M($+$) 3.55, $P < 0.001$.

p. 189   Tables 5:9 and 5:11, single women, manual v. student: (BDI) $t = 2.19$, $P < 0.05$; (In), $t = 2.04$, $P < 0.05$; CD > 3, $\chi^2 = 5.67$, d.f. = 1, $P < 0.02$; 16 PF, t values O($+$) 3.50, $P < 0.001$; F($-$) 1.79, $P < 0.1$, NS; B($+$) 5.45, $P < 0.01$; G($-$) 3.66, $P < 0.001$; Q$_3$($-$) 2.31, $P < 0.05$; Q$_1$($+$) 1.83, $P < 0.1$, NS.

p. 189   Tables 5:10 and 5:12, ever-married, class III v. class V: (BDI) $t = 2.63$, $P < 0.01$; (Ex), $t = 3.03$, $P < 0.01$; (In), $t = 1.89$, $P < 0.1$, NS; 16 PF, t values E($+$) 2.42; G($-$) 2.48; Q$_3$($-$) 2.57, all $P < 0.02$; M($+$) 2.91, $P < 0.01$; C($-$) 2.05, $P < 0.05$; Q$_4$($+$) 2.55, $P < 0.02$.

p. 190   Tables 5:13 and 5:14, 'parted' v. no 'disharmony' admitted: (BDI) $t = 3.30$, $P < 0.01$; (Ex)$_1$, $t = 3.53$, $P < 0.001$; (In)$_1$, $t = 2.56$, $P < 0.02$; CD > 3, $\chi^2 = 5.1$, d.f. = 1, $P < 0.05$; 16 PF, t values L($+$) 2.51, $P < 0.02$; M($+$) 3.10, $P < 0.01$; Q$_3$($-$) 2.00, $P < 0.05$; C($-$) 1.91, $P < 0.1$, NS.

'Disharmony' v. no 'disharmony' admitted: (BDI) $t = 4.06$, $P < 0.001$; $(Ex)_1$, $t = 4.15$, $P < 0.001$; $(In)_1$, $t = 2.65$, $P < 0.01$; CD > 3, $\chi^2 = 13.4$, d.f. $= 1$, $P < 0.001$.

p. 192   Table 5:15, contraception v. no contraception, students v. rest: $\chi^2 = 8.64$, d.f. $= 1$, $P < 0.01$.

p. 193   Tables 5:15 and 5:16, contraception, single v. ever-married: $\chi^2 = 81.5$, d.f. $= 2$, $P < 0.001$.
Table 5:16, ever-married, contraception: class V v. rest, $\chi^2 = 12.2$, d.f. $= 2$, $P < 0.01$; class III v. rest, $\chi^2 = 12.2$, d.f. $= 2$, $P < 0.01$.

p. 194   Table 5:17, single, use of contraception: regular or irregular v. nil, 16 PF, t values $Q_1(+)$ 1.98, $P < 0.05$; $Q_2(-)$ 1.99, $P < 0.05$; regular v. nil, t values $M(-)$ 2.22, $P < 0.05$; $Q_2(-)$ 2.89, $P < 0.01$.

p. 195   Table 5:18, ever-married, use of contraception: regular v. rest, 16 PF, t values $O(+)$ 2.59, $P < 0.02$; $G(+)$ 1.95, $P < 0.1$, NS; 'meticulous' v. no contraception, t values $O(+)$ 1.73; $G(+)$ 1.83; $M(-)$ 1.86; $A(+)$ 1.77; $Q_4(+)$ 1.81, all $P < 0.1$, NS.

p. 203   Table 5:29, ever-married, accepted v. refused abortion: 16 PF, t values $O(+)$ 2.67, $P < 0.01$; $Q_3(+)$ 2.38, $P < 0.02$.

p. 203   Ever-married, sterilised v. not sterilised: Tables 5:30 and 5:31

(a) aborted v. not aborted	$\chi^2 = 15.24$, d.f. $= 1$, $P < 0.001$
(b) total by age	$\chi^2 = 19.92$, d.f. $= 4$, $P < 0.001$
(c) aborted by age	$\chi^2 = 28.41$, d.f. $= 4$, $P < 0.001$
(d) not aborted, under 30 v. 30+	$\chi^2 = 0.04$, d.f. $= 1$, NS

p. 203

(e) total by class	$\chi^2 = 9.89$, d.f. $= 3$, $P < 0.02$
(f) aborted by class	$\chi^2 = 13.13$, d.f. $= 3$, $P < 0.01$
(g) not aborted, class III v. rest	$\chi^2 = 0.002$, d.f. $= 1$, NS
(h) medical indication v. rest	$\chi^2 = 13.80$, d.f. $= 1$, $P < 0.001$

p. 205   Tables 5:32 and 5:33, 'liberals' v. 'conservatives', accepted for abortion: single, $\chi^2 = 19.31$, d.f. $= 1$, $P < 0.001$; ever-married, $\chi^2 = 12.59$, d.f. $= 1$, $P < 0.001$.

p. 205   Tables 5:34, 5:36 and 5:38, 'liberals' v. 'conservatives', single women: students and professionals v. rest, $\chi^2 = 4.73$, d.f. $= 1$, $P < 0.05$; clerical and distributive v. rest, $\chi^2 = 9.23$, d.f. $= 1$, $P < 0.01$; medico-psychiatric v. rest, $\chi^2 = 9.94$, d.f. $= 1$, $P < 0.01$; 16 PF, t values $C(-)$ 3.46, $P < 0.001$; $F(-)$ 3.49, $P < 0.001$; $Q_3(-)$ 2.41, $P < 0.02$; $H(-)$ 1.69, $P < 0.1$, NS; $Q_1(+)$ 1.76, $P < 0.1$, NS; $Q_4(+)$ 1.90, $P < 0.1$, NS.

p. 205   Table 5:38, 'liberals' v. 'conservatives', ever-married: 16 PF, $N(+)$ $t = 2.31$, $P < 0.05$.

p. 206   Tables 5:36 and 5:37, 'liberals' v. 'conservatives', aborted and refused by gynaecologists: single women, socio-psychiatric, $\chi^2 = 12.05$, d.f. $= 1$, $P < 0.001$, social, $\chi^2 = 5.82$, d.f. $= 1$, $P < 0.02$; ever-married, social, $\chi^2 = 11.09$, d.f. $= 1$, $P < 0.001$.

TABLE 5:1. *Test scores for control groups*

| | Beck Depression Inventory (BDI) | | Fould's Hostility Scales | | Personal Illness (PI) and Character Disorder (CD) Scales | | | |
| | | | | | CD ≤ 3 Personal Illness score | | | Character Disorder CD > 3 |
	Score	No. of women	Extropunitive (Ex)	Intropunitive (In)	(0-1)	(2-4)	(5+)	
Control group of nursing students	0–9	70 (86.4%)	Mean 11.68	8.71	18 (22.2%)	30 (37.0%)	13 (16.0%)	20 (24.7%)
	10–16	7 (8.6%)	SD 4.17	4.05				
	17–24	4 (4.9%)						
	25+	0 (0.0%)						
	N = 81		N = 81		N = 81			
Control group of pregnant ever-married women	0–9	58 (75.3%)	Mean 11.35	8.51	18 (23.7%)	25 (32.9%)	15 (19.7%)	18 (23.7%)
	10–16	14 (18.2%)	SD 5.24	3.40				
	17–24	5 (6.5%)						
	25+	0 (0.0%)						
	N = 77		N = 77		N = 76			

TABLE 5:2. *Control groups: 16 PF scores*

| | | | | | | | | 16 PF (stens) | | | | | | | | | |
	A	B	C	E	F	G	H	I	L	M	N	O	Q₁	Q₂	Q₃	Q₄	MD
Nursing students, N = 619 Mean	5.10	7.44	5.23	5.95	5.38	4.32	4.02	5.15	5.79	5.10	5.79	5.26	5.43	4.36	3.81	5.75	3.29
SD	2.13	1.24	1.93	2.27	1.97	2.08	1.90	2.13	1.78	1.99	1.91	2.05	1.97	2.10	1.89	2.06	2.04
Ever-married women at ante-natal clinic, N = 80 Mean	4.90	5.70	5.74	6.46	4.60	5.13	4.73	5.84	6.10	4.84	5.69	5.98	5.48	5.11	4.74	6.40	4.43
SD	2.30	1.68	2.11	2.24	2.09	2.14	2.24	2.24	1.98	1.89	2.05	2.31	2.03	2.30	2.39	1.71	2.05

TABLE 5:3. *Age by class at referral: single women*

Social class	Age					Combined	Total in class group	Age (years)	
	15–19	20–24	25–29	30–34	35–39	25–39		Mean	SD
'Professional'	0	8	3	0	0	3	11	23.9	2.2
'Student'	30	30	2	0	0	2	62	20.2	2.8
Clerical and distributive	33	20	1	1	0	2	55	19.8	3.1
Manual	10	16	3	2	4	9	35	23.7	6.3
Total in age group	73	74	9	3	4	16	163	21.1	4.3

TABLE 5:4. *Age by class at referral: ever-married women*

Social class	Age							Total in class group	Age (years)	
	15–19	20–24	25–29	30–34	35–39	40–44	45+		Mean	SD
I and II	0	4	7	8	7	4	1	31	32.5	6.6
III	2	6	31	25	21	9	0	94	32.0	5.9
IV	0	9	18	11	6	6	0	50	30.7	6.2
V	1	12	11	4	4	0	0	32	27.2	5.3
Total in age group	3	31	67	48	38	19	1	207	31.1	6.3

TABLE 5:5. *Psychological test scores by age: single women*

Age	N		Beck Depression Inventory B_1	Fould's Hostility Scales	
				$(Ex)_1$	$(In)_1$
15–19	73	Mean	21.77	11.75	9.78
		SD	10.51	4.51	3.16
20–24	74	Mean	24.91	10.91	9.84
		SD	10.57	4.30	3.35
25+	16	Mean	26.75	12.88	11.56
		SD	9.05	3.72	3.08

TABLE 5:6. *16 PF scores by age: single women*

		16 PF (stens)																MD
Age		A	B	C	E	F	G	H	I	L	M	N	O	Q₁	Q₂	Q₃	Q₄	MD
15–19, N = 73	Mean	5.51	6.17	4.60	6.21	4.96	4.14	4.03	6.44	5.61	5.90	5.96	6.04	6.06	4.26	3.39	7.51	3.65
	SD	2.35	1.61	2.15	2.49	2.25	2.11	2.53	2.14	1.87	2.11	1.91	2.12	2.22	2.17	1.61	1.70	2.02
20–24, N = 74	Mean	4.77	6.35	4.62	6.23	4.62	4.65	4.19	6.31	5.72	6.27	6.14	5.68	6.05	4.91	3.85	7.31	3.74
	SD	2.31	1.47	2.15	2.20	1.92	2.37	1.85	2.07	1.94	2.08	1.82	1.97	2.03	1.86	2.01	2.03	2.05
25+, N = 16	Mean	4.81	5.13	4.63	5.38	3.81	5.44	3.13	6.19	6.31	6.88	5.75	7.25	5.81	5.44	4.06	6.56	4.38
	SD	2.21	1.73	1.93	2.40	1.81	2.69	1.83	1.91	1.83	1.41	1.95	1.79	2.30	1.97	1.78	2.15	2.29

TABLE 5:7. *Test scores by legitimacy: ever-married women*

| | | Beck Depression Inventory B_1 | Fould's Hostility Scales | |
			Extropunitive $(Ex)_1$	Intropunitive $(In)_1$
Illegitimate pregnancy $N = 36$	Mean	24.03	13.27	10.51
	SD	10.47	5.76	3.17
Legitimate pregnancy $N = 170$	Mean	19.07	11.25	9.32
	SD	11.50	5.30	3.38

TABLE 5:8. *16 PF scores by legitimacy: ever-married women*

		A	B	C	E	F	G	H	I	L	M	N	O	Q_1	Q_2	Q_3	Q_4	MD
										16 PF (stens)								
Illegitimate pregnancy, N = 36	Mean	4.58	5.28	4.44	6.28	4.14	5.56	3.97	6.53	6.56	6.33	6.03	6.03	5.72	5.19	4.08	7.17	3.83
	SD	2.31	1.30	2.01	2.24	2.11	2.64	2.23	1.57	1.59	2.43	1.74	2.13	1.97	1.27	1.94	2.08	2.32
Legitimate pregnancy, N = 169	Mean	4.86	5.40	4.52	5.57	4.14	5.45	4.56	6.40	5.59	5.25	5.67	6.53	5.76	5.49	4.34	7.20	4.65
	SD	2.28	1.68	2.10	2.44	1.90	2.09	2.26	1.99	1.89	1.89	1.89	2.14	2.07	1.93	1.86	2.11	2.13

TABLE 5:9. *Test scores by social class: single women*

Social class		'Depression' Beck Depression Inventory score B_1	Fould's Hostility Scales Extropunitive $(Ex)_1$	Intropunitive $(In)_1$	% Personally ill $CD \leqslant 3$ $PI (5+)$	% Character disorder $CD > 3$
'Professional', N = 11	Mean	24.64	10.46	9.36	18.2	81.8
	SD	11.94	4.11	3.44		
'Student', N = 62	Mean	21.40	10.79	9.40	29.3	41.4
	SD	10.54	4.38	3.13		
Clerical and distributive, N = 55	Mean	23.55	11.58	10.24	22.2	59.3
	SD	9.20	4.19	3.28		
Manual workers, N = 35	Mean	27.63	12.86	10.80	15.2	69.7
	SD	11.12	4.51	3.32		

TABLE 5:10. *Test scores by social class: ever-married women*

Social class		'Depression' Beck Depression Inventory score B_1	Fould's Hostility Scales		% Personally ill CD ≤ 3 PI (5+)	% Character Disorder CD > 3
			Extropunitive $(Ex)_1$	Intropunitive $(In)_1$		
I and II Professional and Management, $N = 31$	Mean	19.13	11.07	9.55	16.7	43.3
	SD	13.79	4.43	3.45		
III Skilled workers, $N = 94$	Mean	18.59	10.57	9.17	30.0	43.3
	SD	9.99	5.67	3.22		
IV Semi-skilled, $N = 49$	Mean	20.10	12.36	9.62	22.4	57.1
	SD	11.13	5.24	3.42		
V Unskilled, $N = 32$	Mean	24.44	14.03	10.44	25.0	57.1
	SD	12.88	5.13	3.61		

TABLE 5:11. *16 PF scores by social class: single women*

Social class		A	B	C	E	F	G	H	I	L	M	N	O	Q_1	Q_2	Q_3	Q_4	MD
														16 PF (stens)				
'Professional', N = 11	Mean	4.55	6.18	5.36	5.82	5.18	5.09	3.55	5.73	5.09	6.09	5.91	6.46	6.46	5.91	4.00	6.27	4.27
	SD	2.42	2.12	2.01	2.04	1.64	2.43	1.37	2.00	2.02	1.98	1.51	1.97	1.78	0.90	2.34	2.38	1.91
'Student', N = 62	Mean	4.95	6.97	4.58	5.95	4.78	3.73	4.13	6.68	5.74	6.32	6.05	5.34	6.57	4.40	3.40	7.34	3.45
	SD	2.39	1.40	2.08	2.45	2.04	2.28	2.25	2.15	1.96	2.16	1.83	1.93	2.12	2.00	1.65	2.07	1.85
Clerical and distributive, N = 55	Mean	5.64	5.78	4.60	6.46	4.86	4.64	4.26	6.13	5.67	6.00	6.33	6.11	5.46	4.46	3.47	7.53	3.69
	SD	2.21	1.30	2.04	2.42	2.30	2.19	2.47	2.10	1.89	1.98	1.92	2.04	2.22	2.12	1.57	1.75	2.02
Manual, N = 35	Mean	4.74	5.40	4.46	6.17	4.03	5.46	3.49	6.43	6.03	6.09	5.60	6.80	5.77	5.09	4.31	7.40	4.21
	SD	2.25	1.25	2.30	2.22	1.83	2.09	1.75	1.92	1.72	2.08	1.96	2.00	1.91	2.08	2.14	1.66	2.46

TABLE 5:12. *16 PF scores by social class: ever-married women*

Social class		A	B	C	E	F	G	H	I	L	M	N	O	Q₁	Q₂	Q₃	Q₄	MD
		\multicolumn{16}{c}{16 PF (stens)}															
I & II, N = 31	Mean	5.36	5.55	5.13	6.10	4.13	5.55	5.10	6.81	6.03	5.29	5.42	6.19	5.84	5.48	4.03	7.03	4.00
	SD	2.38	1.58	2.08	2.39	1.96	2.47	2.23	1.99	1.68	2.45	2.03	2.13	1.90	2.18	1.66	2.48	2.03
III, N = 93	Mean	4.58	5.31	4.54	5.38	3.91	5.86	4.50	6.43	5.53	5.03	5.67	6.23	5.52	5.70	4.58	6.90	4.92
	SD	2.20	1.74	2.16	2.32	1.90	2.05	2.27	1.83	1.82	1.93	1.80	2.12	2.03	1.64	1.95	2.14	2.22
IV, N = 49	Mean	4.96	5.67	4.59	5.51	4.35	5.14	4.41	6.39	5.37	5.84	5.84	6.67	5.80	5.08	4.41	7.35	4.53
	SD	2.47	1.22	1.93	2.57	1.89	2.07	2.24	2.05	1.98	1.93	1.83	2.07	2.14	1.93	1.75	1.86	2.02
V, N = 32	Mean	4.72	4.94	3.66	6.53	4.50	4.78	3.81	6.09	6.78	6.16	6.13	6.22	6.06	5.19	3.56	7.97	3.53
	SD	2.02	1.69	1.81	2.26	1.98	2.26	2.11	1.84	1.67	1.72	1.87	2.42	1.98	1.76	1.84	1.69	1.91

TABLE 5:13. *Test scores by marital state*

		Depression, Beck score, B_1	Fould's Hostility Scales	
			$(Ex)_1$	$(In)_1$
Single	Mean	23.68	11.48	9.98
	SD	10.47	4.35	3.25
	N	163	163	163
Total ever-married	Mean	19.99	11.61	9.53
	SD	11.47	5.43	3.37
	N	205	207	207
Living with husband	Mean	19.04	11.17	9.32
	SD	11.59	5.37	3.37
	N	169	170	170
No 'disharmony' admitted	Mean	17.16	10.30	8.96
	SD	11.39	5.02	3.17
	N	132	132	132
'Disharmony'	Mean	25.58	14.21	10.58
	SD	9.89	5.36	3.71
	N	37	38	38
'Parted' from husband	Mean	24.08	13.65	10.49
	SD	9.97	5.30	3.24
	N	36	37	37

TABLE 5:14. *16 PF scores at referral by marital state*

		16 PF (stens)																
		A	B	C	E	F	G	H	I	L	M	N	O	Q₁	Q₂	Q₃	Q₄	MD
Single, N = 163	Mean	5.11	6.18	4.61	6.16	4.68	4.50	3.99	6.37	5.74	6.14	6.04	5.99	6.01	4.67	3.66	7.34	3.75
	SD	2.34	1.54	2.12	2.38	2.09	2.32	2.20	2.09	1.90	2.08	1.89	2.06	2.15	2.05	1.83	1.93	2.07
Total ever-married, N = 205	Mean	4.81	5.38	4.50	5.70	4.14	5.47	4.46	6.42	5.76	5.44	5.73	6.44	5.75	5.44	4.30	7.20	4.51
	SD	2.28	1.62	2.08	2.43	1.94	2.20	2.26	1.92	1.88	2.03	1.87	2.15	2.05	1.84	1.88	2.10	2.19
Living with husband, N = 169	Mean	4.81	5.39	4.59	5.60	4.11	5.54	4.57	6.44	5.61	5.28	5.67	6.53	5.76	5.53	4.41	7.17	4.62
	SD	2.31	1.66	2.05	2.42	1.91	2.11	2.29	1.95	1.90	1.97	1.82	2.15	2.07	1.87	1.84	2.13	2.14
'Parted' from husband, N = 36	Mean	4.81	5.33	4.08	6.14	4.31	5.14	3.92	6.33	6.47	6.19	6.03	6.03	5.72	5.00	3.75	7.31	3.97
	SD	2.17	1.41	2.19	2.39	2.04	2.53	2.02	1.80	1.57	2.17	2.09	2.10	1.97	1.60	1.96	1.98	2.32
Living with husband 'Disharmony' not admitted, N = 131	Mean	4.65	5.35	4.82	5.51	4.00	5.62	4.57	6.49	5.61	5.02	5.65	6.53	5.74	5.56	4.46	7.02	4.82
	SD	2.24	1.67	2.01	2.39	1.98	2.15	2.33	2.01	1.88	1.95	1.79	2.15	2.11	1.86	1.84	2.12	2.09
'Disharmony' admitted, N = 38	Mean	5.37	5.50	3.79	5.92	4.47	5.29	4.58	6.29	5.61	6.16	5.74	6.53	5.82	5.45	4.26	7.71	3.92
	SD	2.43	1.60	1.96	2.49	1.62	1.95	2.18	1.70	1.99	1.77	1.92	2.14	1.92	1.90	1.82	2.06	2.16

TABLE 5:15. *Use of contraception by social class: single women*

Use of contraception	Social class				Total
	'Professional'	'Student'	Clerical and distributive	Manual	
Nil used	8 (72.7%)	38 (61.3%)	47 (85.5%)	29 (82.9%)	122 (74.8%)
Irregular	2 (18.2%)	15 (24.2%)	5 (9.1%)	4 (11.4%)	26 (16.0%)
Regular	1 (9.1%)	9 (14.5%)	3 (5.5%)	2 (5.7%)	15 (9.2%)
Total	11 (100.0%)	62 (100.0%)	55 (100.0%)	35 (100.0%)	163 (100.0%)

TABLE 5:16. *Use of contraception by social class: ever-married women*

Use of contraception	Social class				Total
	I and II	III	IV	V	
Nil used	11 (35.5%)	17 (18.1%)	18 (36.0%)	15 (46.9%)	61 (29.5%)
Irregular	5 (16.1%)	25 (26.6%)	13 (26.0%)	11 (34.4%)	54 (26.1%)
Regular	15 (48.4%)	52 (55.3%)	19 (38.0%)	6 (18.8%)	92 (44.4%)
Total	31	94	50	32	207

TABLE 5:17. *16 PF scores by use of contraception: single women*

Use of contraception		A	B	C	E	F	G	H	I	L	M	N	O	Q_1	Q_2	Q_3	Q_4	MD
Nil used, N = 122	Mean	5.08	6.15	4.59	6.15	4.57	4.54	3.89	6.39	5.84	6.05	5.98	6.04	5.82	4.85	3.57	7.30	3.76
	SD	2.18	1.56	2.17	2.40	2.12	2.29	2.23	2.03	1.82	1.93	1.90	2.22	2.22	2.04	1.83	2.02	2.05
Contraception used, N = 41	Mean	5.20	6.27	4.68	6.20	5.00	4.37	4.29	6.34	5.42	6.42	6.20	5.83	6.59	4.12	3.93	7.49	3.71
	SD	2.76	1.48	1.96	2.31	1.96	2.41	2.09	2.28	2.10	2.45	1.82	1.51	1.82	1.98	1.81	1.63	2.16
Regular contraception, N = 15	Mean	5.47	6.13	5.40	5.80	5.53	4.13	4.47	6.07	5.07	4.87	6.20	5.27	6.33	3.27	4.33	6.73	4.87
	SD	2.25	1.50	1.45	2.61	2.09	2.25	1.82	2.44	2.05	1.93	1.56	1.24	1.54	1.57	1.19	1.29	2.13

TABLE 5:18. *16 PF scores by use of contraception: ever-married women*

Use of contraception		A	B	C	E	F	G	H	I	L	M	N	O	Q_1	Q_2	Q_3	Q_4	MD
Regular contraception, N = 92	Mean	4.98	5.40	4.49	5.73	4.20	5.80	4.71	6.61	5.47	5.37	5.70	6.87	5.87	5.47	4.40	7.36	4.82
	SD	2.40	1.87	2.17	2.44	1.96	2.14	2.22	2.01	2.00	1.95	1.81	2.18	2.13	1.94	1.75	2.08	2.09
Other than regular (including no contraception), N = 113	Mean	4.67	5.35	4.51	5.67	4.10	5.20	4.26	6.27	6.00	5.50	5.76	6.10	5.66	5.42	4.21	7.06	4.25
	SD	2.18	1.38	2.01	2.41	1.92	2.21	2.27	1.84	1.74	2.10	1.92	2.06	2.25	1.75	1.97	2.11	2.23
No contraception, N = 60	Mean	4.57	5.38	4.48	5.77	4.17	5.12	4.32	6.32	6.17	5.87	5.83	6.22	5.60	5.60	4.25	7.17	4.07
	SD	2.16	1.36	1.91	2.45	1.93	2.18	2.41	1.65	1.72	2.19	1.71	2.07	2.07	1.31	1.99	1.96	2.28
'Meticulous' contraception, N = 27	Mean	5.48	5.00	3.96	5.59	4.11	6.04	4.11	6.82	5.56	4.96	5.19	7.07	5.52	5.19	4.30	7.96	4.96
	SD	2.27	1.38	2.10	2.15	2.20	2.08	2.06	1.70	2.18	1.82	1.36	2.14	2.25	1.89	1.80	1.64	2.01

16 PF (stens)

TABLE 5:19. *Test scores by referral for psychiatric opinion*

		Beck Depression Inventory		Fould's Hostility Scales	
		B_1	Suicide thoughts expressed in Beck	Extro-punitive $(Ex)_1$	Intro-punitive $(In)_1$
Single					
(a) Referred, $N = 66$	Mean	26.50	32 (48.5%)	12.39	10.23
	SD	10.22		4.74	3.53
(b) Not referred, $N = 97$	Mean	21.76	26 (26.8%)	10.86	9.81
	SD	10.30		4.00	3.07
t_{ab}		2.87		2.22	0.79
P_{ab}		<0.01		<0.05	NS
Ever-married					
(c) Referred, $N = 53$	Mean	23.02	15 (28.3%)	11.94	10.30
	SD	11.61		5.90	3.34
(d) Not referred, $N = 152$	Mean	18.93	25 (16.4%)	11.50	9.27
	SD	11.27		5.27	3.35
t_{cd}		2.25		0.67	1.93
P_{cd}		<0.05		NS	<0.1 NS

TABLE 5:20. *16 PF scores by referral for psychiatric opinion*

		A	B	C	E	F	G	H	I	L	M	N	O	Q_1	Q_2	Q_3	Q_4	MD
										16 PF (stens)								
Single women																		
Referred,	Mean	4.77	6.12	4.41	5.96	4.53	4.58	3.82	6.05	5.68	6.52	6.11	6.09	6.14	4.79	3.35	7.59	3.86
N = 66	SD	2.40	1.65	2.22	2.20	1.94	2.15	2.07	2.08	1.87	2.22	1.74	2.27	2.16	1.99	1.92	2.01	2.08
Not	Mean	5.34	6.22	4.75	6.26	4.77	4.46	4.11	6.60	5.72	5.89	5.99	5.92	5.93	4.59	3.88	7.18	3.68
referred,	SD	2.27	1.47	2.04	2.46	2.19	2.44	2.28	2.07	1.90	1.94	1.98	1.91	2.14	2.09	1.74	1.86	2.06
N = 97																		
Ever-married women																		
Referred,	Mean	4.04	5.15	4.00	5.98	3.90	5.90	4.08	6.37	5.48	5.98	5.85	6.50	5.56	5.64	3.96	7.85	4.18
N = 52	SD	1.86	1.75	1.96	2.41	2.08	2.09	2.08	1.78	1.77	1.92	1.90	2.37	2.14	1.82	1.91	1.96	2.18
Not	Mean	5.07	5.45	4.67	5.60	4.22	5.29	4.59	6.44	5.86	5.26	5.69	6.43	5.82	5.37	4.41	6.97	4.62
referred,	SD	2.36	1.56	2.10	2.42	1.88	2.20	2.31	1.97	1.90	2.04	1.86	2.06	2.01	1.84	1.85	2.11	2.18
N = 153																		

TABLE 5:21. *Main indications for the application*

	Type of main indication					
	Medico-psychiatric	Socio-psychiatric	Social	Medical	Eugenic	Total
Single women (CS)	14 (8.6%)	76 (46.6%)	69 (42.3%)	3 (1.8%)	1 (0.6%)	163 (100.0%)
Ever-married women (CM)	20 (9.7%)	52 (25.1%)	108 (52.2%)	22 (10.6%)	5 (2.4%)	207 (100.0%)

TABLE 5:22. *Test scores by main indication: single women*

Main indication		Beck Depression inventory, B_1	Fould's Hostility Scales		N
			$(Ex)_1$	$(In)_1$	
Medico-psychiatric	Mean	30.00	13.79	12.57	14
	SD	9.22	2.46	3.23	
Socio-psychiatric	Mean	24.93	11.15	9.76	76
	SD	10.77	4.95	2.96	
Social	Mean	20.86	11.39	9.49	69
	SD	9.89	3.90	3.35	

TABLE 5:23. *Test scores by main indication: ever-married women*

Main indication		Beck Depression inventory, B_1	Fould's Hostility Scales		N
			$(Ex)_1$	$(In)_1$	
Medico-Psychiatric	Mean	25.05	11.45	10.45	19
	SD	10.33	5.42	3.33	
Socio-psychiatric	Mean	23.86	11.81	9.94	52
	SD	10.98	5.72	3.06	
Social	Mean	19.25	12.26	9.54	108
	SD	11.17	5.35	3.40	
Medical	Mean	12.59	8.82	8.18	22
	SD	10.41	4.39	3.63	

TABLE 5:24. *16 PF scores by main indication: single women*

Main indication		16 PF (stens)																
		A	B	C	E	F	G	H	I	L	M	N	O	Q_1	Q_2	Q_3	Q_4	MD
Medico-psychiatric, $N = 14$	Mean	5.71	5.86	3.71	6.50	4.43	4.07	3.50	7.29	5.36	7.21	5.79	6.29	5.71	4.50	2.86	7.21	3.50
	SD	2.02	1.36	1.67	2.26	1.95	2.02	1.92	1.39	2.32	2.43	1.57	2.09	2.02	2.13	2.16	2.27	1.96
Socio-psychiatric, $N = 76$	Mean	4.67	6.30	4.63	6.09	4.61	4.66	3.88	6.25	5.84	5.96	5.99	5.84	6.29	4.74	3.70	7.37	3.83
	SD	2.35	1.56	1.99	2.12	2.05	2.43	1.96	1.96	1.88	1.97	1.89	2.25	2.09	2.01	1.30	2.01	2.05
Social, $N = 69$	Mean	5.49	6.17	4.86	6.09	4.80	4.36	4.26	6.26	5.61	6.00	6.13	6.06	5.86	4.58	3.80	7.29	3.79
	SD	2.31	1.56	2.27	2.61	2.22	2.25	2.49	2.32	1.83	2.03	1.98	1.88	2.18	2.11	1.46	1.78	2.12

TABLE 5:25. *16 PF scores by main indication: ever-married women*

Main indication		A	B	C	E	F	G	H	I	L	M	N	O	Q_1	Q_2	Q_3	Q_4	MD
												16 PF (stens)						
Medico-psychiatric, N = 20	Mean	3.75	4.95	4.20	5.35	3.60	5.45	3.85	6.65	5.25	5.80	5.80	7.05	6.30	5.20	4.05	7.60	4.60
	SD	2.41	1.32	2.14	2.71	1.91	2.09	1.96	1.53	1.87	1.86	2.11	2.75	2.17	1.94	1.75	2.33	2.15
Socio-psychiatric, N = 51	Mean	4.49	5.31	4.20	5.88	3.75	5.75	4.61	6.31	5.82	5.26	5.63	6.47	5.69	5.45	4.16	7.41	4.10
	SD	2.22	1.64	1.85	2.46	1.82	2.38	2.05	2.08	1.83	2.05	2.05	2.33	2.08	1.91	1.74	2.04	2.19
Social, N = 107	Mean	5.08	5.47	4.62	5.87	4.32	5.28	4.38	6.50	5.84	5.57	5.68	6.20	5.56	5.49	4.35	7.21	4.58
	SD	2.21	1.57	2.16	2.43	1.90	2.22	2.27	1.91	1.81	2.11	1.83	1.91	1.91	1.76	1.91	2.05	2.06
Medical, N = 22	Mean	5.27	5.36	4.36	4.91	4.46	5.59	5.55	6.27	5.82	4.96	6.05	6.91	6.23	5.36	4.64	6.73	4.77
	SD	2.40	1.99	1.75	2.07	2.06	1.64	2.48	1.71	2.21	1.61	1.52	2.02	2.35	2.06	2.08	2.00	2.58

TABLE 5:26. *Final decision and outcome by age: single women*

	Age			Total in decision group
	15–19	20–24	Combined 25–39	
Aborted by gynaecologist	33 (45.2%)	45 (60.8%)	11 (68.8)%	89 (54.6%)
Abortion refused by gynaecologist. Pregnancy continued to term	35 (47.9%)	23 (31.1%)	3 (18.8%)	61 (37.4%)
'Spontaneous abortion'	5 (6.8%)	4 (5.4%)	1 (6.3%)	10 (6.1%)
Patient 'changed mind' and continued pregnancy to term	0 (0.0%)	2 (2.7%)	1 (6.3%)	3 (1.8%)
	73 (100%)	74 (100%)	16 (100%)	163 (100%)
$\%\dfrac{\text{Aborted by gynaecologist}}{\text{Aborted} + \text{refused}}$	48.5	66.2	78.6	59.3

TABLE 5:27. *Final decision and outcome by age: ever-married women*

	Age							Total in decision group
	15–19	20–24	25–29	30–34	35–39	40–44	45+	
Aborted by gynaecologist	0 (0.0%)	15 (48.4%)	36 (53.7%)	31 (64.6%)	23 (60.5%)	12 (63.2%)	1 (100%)	118 (57.0%)
Abortion refused by gynaecologist. Pregnancy continued to term	3 (100%)	12 (38.7%)	22 (32.8%)	8 (16.7%)	12 (31.6%)	4 (21.1%)	0 (0.0%)	61 (29.5%)
'Spontaneous abortion'	0 (0.0%)	4 (12.9%)	5 (7.5%)	3 (6.3%)	2 (5.3%)	2 (10.5%)	0 (0.0%)	16 (7.7%)
Self-induced abortion	0 (0.0%)	0 (0.0%)	0 (0.0%)	1 (2.1%)	0 (0.0%)	0 (0.0%)	0 (0.0%)	1 (0.5%)
Patient changed her mind and continued to term	0 (0.0%)	0 (0.0%)	4 (6.0%)	5 (10.4%)	1 (2.6%)	1 (5.3%)	0 (0.0%)	11 (5.3%)
	3 (100%)	31 (100%)	67 (100%)	48 (100%)	38 (100%)	19 (100%)	1 (100%)	207 (100%)
% $\dfrac{\text{Aborted by gynaecologist}}{\text{Aborted + refused}}$	0.0	55.6	62.1	79.5	65.7	75.0	100	65.9

TABLE 5:28. *Test scores at referral by decision and marital state*

| | | Beck Depression Inventory, B_1 | Fould's Hostility Scales | |
			Extropunitive $(Ex)_1$	Intropunitive $(In)_1$
Single women				
(a) Accepted, $N = 88$	Mean	25.71	12.17	10.65
	SD	10.75	4.51	2.94
(b) Refused, $N = 63$	Mean	19.67	10.44	9.03
	SD	9.53	4.23	3.55
	t_{ab}	3.54	2.37	3.04
	P_{ab}	< 0.001	< 0.02	< 0.01
Ever-married women				
(c) Accepted, $N = 118$	Mean	22.20	12.08	9.98
	SD	11.76	5.61	3.35
(d) Refused, $N = 66$	Mean	17.20	10.80	8.89
	SD	10.67	4.93	3.42
	t_{cd}	2.84	1.53	2.07
	P_{cd}	< 0.01	NS	< 0.05

TABLE 5:29. *16 PF scores at referral by decision and marital state*

								16 PF (stens)									
	A	B	C	E	F	G	H	I	L	M	N	O	Q1	Q2	Q3	Q4	MD
Single women																	
Accepted, Mean	4.90	6.31	4.48	6.22	4.57	4.30	3.94	6.43	5.97	6.31	6.16	5.90	5.94	4.66	3.47	7.42	3.81
$N = 88$ SD	2.19	1.41	2.06	2.26	2.02	2.38	2.15	2.06	2.00	2.06	2.00	2.05	2.11	2.11	1.62	1.80	2.11
Refused, Mean	5.48	6.06	4.76	6.02	4.91	4.54	3.92	6.33	5.43	5.81	5.95	6.10	6.22	4.60	3.94	7.05	3.71
$N = 63$ SD	2.48	1.64	2.20	2.41	2.11	2.11	2.27	2.12	1.70	2.06	1.77	2.04	2.21	2.03	2.00	2.12	2.00
Ever-married women																	
Accepted, Mean	4.71	5.25	4.47	5.54	3.97	5.53	4.41	6.45	5.78	5.62	5.53	6.75	5.87	5.35	4.55	7.41	4.44
$N = 116$ SD	2.40	1.54	2.03	2.50	1.91	2.13	2.14	2.04	1.88	1.98	2.00	2.08	2.06	2.00	1.84	2.11	2.17
Refused, Mean	4.79	5.58	4.49	5.79	4.30	5.36	4.49	6.26	5.73	5.20	6.05	5.88	5.80	5.71	3.86	6.94	4.66
$N = 66$ SD	2.15	1.86	2.08	2.28	2.06	2.30	2.46	1.78	1.86	2.04	1.65	2.16	2.09	1.64	1.91	2.17	2.10

TABLE 5:30. *Sterilisation by age: ever-married women*

				Age				
	15–19	20–24	25–29	30–34	35–39	40–44	45+	Total
Aborted and sterilised								
Aborted and sterilised	0	4	20	28	22	8	1	83
Total aborted in age group	0	19	41	35	25	14	1	135
% Sterilised	—	21.1	48.8	80.0	88.0	57.1	100.0	61.5
Not aborted and sterilised								
Not aborted and sterilised	0	5	8	4	4	2	0	23
Total not aborted in age group	3	12	26	13	13	5	0	72
% Sterilised	0.0	41.7	30.8	30.8	30.8	40.0	—	31.9
Aborted + not aborted								
Total sterilised	0	9	28	32	26	10	1	106
Total in age group	3	31	67	48	38	19	1	207
% Sterilised in total age group	0.0	29.0	41.8	66.7	68.4	52.6	100.0	51.2

TABLE 5:31. *Sterilisation by social class: ever-married women*

	Social class				
	I and II	III	IV	V	Total
Aborted and sterilised	14	46	17	6	83
Total aborted in class group	25	60	32	18	135
% Sterilised	56.0	76.7	53.1	33.3	61.5
Not aborted and sterilised	1	12	6	4	23
Total not aborted in class group	6	34	18	14	72
% Sterilised	16.7	35.3	33.3	28.6	31.9
Total sterilised	15	58	23	10	106
Total in class group	31	94	50	32	207
% Sterilised in class group	48.4	61.7	46.0	31.3	51.2

TABLE 5:32. *Decision and outcome by gynaecologist: single women*

Gynaecologist	Accepted for abortion	Refused abortion	Other	Total	% $\dfrac{\text{Accepted}}{\text{Accepted} + \text{refused}}$
A	28 (62.2%)	11 (24.4%)	6 (13.3%)	45 (100%)	71.8
B	19 (79.2%)	3 (12.5%)	2 (8.3%)	24 (100%)	86.4
C	17 (77.3)%	5 (22.7%)	0 (0.0%)	22 (100%)	77.3
Total for 'liberals'	64 (70.3%)	19 (20.9%)	8 (8.8%)	91 (100%)	77.1
D	10 (52.6%)	9 (47.4%)	0 (0.0%)	19 (100%)	52.6
E	2 (25.0%)	6 (75.0%)	0 (0.0%)	8 (100%)	25.0
F	3 (21.4%)	10 (71.4%)	1 (7.1%)	14 (100%)	23.1
G	8 (38.1%)	13 (61.9%)	0 (0.0%)	21 (100%)	38.1
H	1 (12.5%)	4 (50.0%)	3 (37.5%)	8 (100%)	20.0
Total for 'conservatives'	24 (34.3%)	42 (60.0%)	4 (5.7%)	70 (100%)	36.4

TABLE 5:33. *Decision and outcome by gynaecologist: ever-married women*

Gynaecologist	Accepted for abortion	Refused abortion	Other	Total	% $\dfrac{\text{Accepted}}{\text{Accepted}+\text{refused}}$
A	33 (68.8%)	9 (18.8%)	6 (12.5%)	48 (100%)	78.6
B	19 (76.0%)	5 (20.0%)	1 (4.0%)	25 (100%)	79.2
C	28 (63.6%)	10 (22.7%)	6 (13.6%)	44 (100%)	73.7
Total for 'liberals'	80 (68.4%)	24 (20.5%)	13 (11.1%)	117 (100%)	76.9
D	16 (61.5%)	9 (34.6%)	1 (3.8%)	26 (100%)	64.0
E	4 (40.0%)	4 (40.0%)	2 (20.0%)	10 (100%)	50.0
F	9 (34.6%)	13 (50.0%)	4 (15.4%)	26 (100%)	40.9
G	7 (36.8%)	9 (47.4%)	3 (15.8%)	19 (100%)	43.8
H	2 (25.0%)	4 (50.0%)	2 (25.0%)	8 (100%)	33.3
Total for 'conservatives'	38 (42.7%)	39 (43.8%)	12 (13.5%)	89 (100%)	49.4

TABLE 5:34. *Type of gynaecologist by social class of applicant: single women*

| | Type of gynaecologist | |
Social class	'Liberal'	'Conservative'
'Professionals'	7 (7.7%)	3 (4.3%)
'Students'	41 (45.1%)	21 (30.0%)
Clerical and distributive	21 (23.1%)	33 (47.1%)
Manual	22 (24.2%)	13 (18.6%)
Total	91 (100%)	70 (100%)

TABLE 5:35. *Type of gynaecologist by social class of applicant: ever-married women*

| | Type of gynaecologist | |
Social class	'Liberal'	'Conservative'
I and II	20 (17.1%)	11 (12.4%)
III	50 (42.7%)	43 (48.3%)
IV	28 (23.9%)	22 (24.7%)
V	19 (16.2%)	13 (14.6%)
Total	117 (100%)	89 (100%)

TABLE 5:36. *Final outcome by main indication and type of gynaecologist: single women*

| | Type of gynaecologist | | | | | |
| | 'Liberal' | | 'Conservative' | | Grand total | |
Main indication	Total	% Aborted	Total	% Aborted	Total	% Aborted
Medico-psychiatric	14	100	0	0.0	14	100
Socio-psychiatric	43	83.7	31	54.8	74	71.6
Social	33	60.6	36	25.0	69	42.0
Medical and eugenic	2	100	2	50.0	4	75.0

TABLE 5:37. *Final outcome by main indication and type of gynaecologist: ever-married women*

| | Type of gynaecologist | | | | | |
| | 'Liberal' | | 'Conservative' | | Grand Total | |
Main indication	Total	% Aborted	Total	% Aborted	Total	% Aborted
Medico-psychiatric	12	100	8	75.0	20	90.0
Socio-psychiatric	34	79.4	18	77.8	52	78.9
Social	58	70.7	49	42.9	107	57.9
Medical and eugenic	13	46.2	14	50.0	27	48.1
Total	117	73.5	89	53.9	206	65.0

TABLE 5:38. *16 PF scores of applicants by type of gynaecologist*

	A	B	C	E	F	G	H	I	L	M	N	O	Q_1	Q_2	Q_3	Q_4	MD
								16 PF (stens)									
(CS) Single																	
Liberal gynaecologists, N = 91 Mean	4.96	6.23	4.13	6.14	4.19	4.34	3.74	6.51	5.91	6.24	6.14	5.99	6.27	4.71	3.37	7.59	3.64
SD	2.36	1.56	1.91	2.50	2.01	2.43	2.23	1.90	2.00	2.12	1.89	2.08	2.02	2.07	1.66	1.87	2.02
Conservative gynaecologists, N = 70 Mean	5.31	6.11	5.26	6.13	5.31	4.73	4.33	6.20	5.43	6.01	5.90	6.09	5.67	4.61	4.06	7.01	3.90
SD	2.29	1.52	2.21	2.15	2.03	2.16	2.12	2.32	1.70	2.02	1.88	1.98	2.27	2.02	1.96	1.95	2.13
(CM) Ever-married																	
Liberal gynaecologists, N = 117 Mean	4.88	5.33	4.43	5.69	4.10	5.33	4.42	6.42	5.92	5.53	5.48	6.54	5.72	5.53	4.36	7.33	4.44
SD	2.36	1.55	2.20	2.48	1.88	2.16	2.26	2.01	1.77	2.08	1.91	2.10	2.09	1.82	1.85	2.01	2.15
Conservative gynaecologists, N = 89 Mean	4.71	5.44	4.60	5.71	4.20	5.61	4.52	6.43	5.55	5.31	6.08	6.31	5.79	5.31	4.21	7.01	4.59
SD	2.17	1.71	1.91	2.35	2.02	2.21	2.26	1.79	1.99	1.96	1.76	2.20	2.00	1.85	1.91	2.21	2.23

TABLE 5:39. *Sterilisation offered by abortion decision and gynaecologist: ever-married women*

Gynaecologist	Accepted for abortion and offered sterilisation	Refused abortion and offered sterilisation	'Other', offered sterilisation	Total offered sterilisation
A	20 (60.6%)†	5 (55.6%)	1 (16.7%)	26 (54.2%)
B	11 (57.9%)	2 (40.0%)	0 (0.0%)	13 (52.0%)
C	18 (64.3%)	1 (10.0%)	4 (80.0%)	23 (52.3%)
Total for 'liberals'	49 (61.3%)	8 (33.3%)	5 (38.5%)	62 (53.0%)
D	13 (81.3%)	2 (22.2%)	0 (0.0%)	15 (57.7%)
E	4 (100%)	0 (0.0%)	0 (0.0%)	4 (40.0%)
F	6 (66.7%)	7 (53.8%)	0 (0.0%)	13 (50.0%)
G	5 (71.4%)	4 (44.4%)	0 (0.0%)	9 (47.4%)
H	1 (50.0%)	3 (75.0%)	0 (0.0%)	4 (50.0%)
Total for 'conservatives'	29 (76.3%)	16 (41.0%)	0 (0.0%)	45 (50.6%)

† Figures on parentheses are % of decision group that were offered sterilisation.

6 LONG-TERM PSYCHIATRIC FOLLOW-UP

Colin McCance, Peter C. Olley and Vivien Edward

INTRODUCTION

Emotional disturbance in the first few weeks following childbirth or abortion is a well-known phenomenon. In the present British social climate where more liberal abortion laws have recently been introduced and any medical practitioner is liable to be asked by a patient to recommend an abortion, it is clearly of paramount importance to know something about the psychological aftermath and the personal, demographic and other factors which may influence it. Furthermore, the immediate psychological response is perhaps less important to anticipate than the delayed and long-lasting sequelae. The close collaboration which has been fostered for a number of years between the obstetricians, sociologists and psychiatrists in Aberdeen provides a favourable opportunity to study this problem in depth and at length. This chapter describes a part of this work.

METHOD

The cohort of 370 women upon whom this study was undertaken comprised 90 per cent of all referrals for abortion to the Gynaecology Department for the fourteen months, 1 July 1967 – 31 August 1968, which was described in detail in Chapter 5.

About fifteen months after initial referral for consideration of abortion, follow-up was initiated by a letter inviting each patient to attend the Maternity Hospital for interview with a doctor. Patients were allocated alternately to PCO or CM. Each woman had been warned at the time of her original attendance that a follow-up contact would be sought and she had been asked to indicate her best address for this purpose. The follow-up appointment letter was couched in noncommittal terms which did not disclose the reason for the original attendance in case the letter was opened by somebody in whom the patient had not confided. 150 (40.5 per cent) attended at the first appointment. Those who did not were sent a second letter with another appointment time. Thirty-two (8.6 per cent) attended the second appointment. In the early stages of the follow-up work a psychiatric social worker then visited the addresses of those who had still failed to attend after the second letter, but she found only 12 patients (3.2 per cent) and was unable to continue the research collaboration owing to pressure of service commitments.

Thirteen months after the follow-up work had started, a married female psychiatrist (VE) joined the team on a part-time basis and was able to find and interview a further 91 (24.6 per cent) in their homes. In some cases it was necessary to obtain new addresses through the help of local executive councils and general practitioners. The time which elapsed between original contact and the psychiatric follow-up thus varied between 13 and 43 months, but for 83 per cent it was between 13 and 24 months (Table 6:1). Each patient who had moved to a known address outside the region was asked to supply information about her present condition, circumstances and feelings through a postal inquiry and to complete the Fould's and Beck scales. Satisfactory replies were obtained from 18 (4.9 per cent). Follow-up data was thus obtained on 303 women, 81.9 per cent of the original 370.

FOLLOW-UP INTERVIEW

The objectives were broadly threefold. Firstly, to direct a semi-structured inquiry into various areas of special interest and to make an on-the-spot rating of what emerged. Secondly, to allow the patient an opportunity for spontaneous unstructured dialogue with the psychiatrist. Thirdly, to obtain the completion of the Beck Depression scale and Fould's Hostility Scale which each patient had previously done at her first referral.

In almost all cases the interview was opened by some simple inquiries about menstrual, urinary and sexual function at a straightforward physical level. This information was obtained on behalf of a collaborator in the Obstetrics Department. Attention then passed to assessing various feelings and attitudes and rating certain aspects of social and psychological function. As the various topics were discussed, digressions would often occur and problems would sometimes emerge which were allowed full ventilation as they did so. In some cases, the patient was asked to do the Beck and Fould's questionnaires after the clinical interview but occasionally it was more convenient for her to do the questionnaires first. In this event, no perusal of the answers was made before the interview, as this might have biassed the clinical assessment.

In asking the women to come back for follow-up it was felt proper to indicate to them that the interview with the doctor could be expected to last about half an hour. This was therefore the usual duration but if an individual seemed anxious for a longer discussion of her problems it was usually possible to extend the interview for a further fifteen minutes or even half an hour. Occasionally a second appointment was arranged.

In the cases who failed to attend hospital and who were therefore visited at home, the interview situation was obviously less standardised. The commonest reason for non-attendance was the inability to leave a young family. Some interviews were thus hampered by the presence of children or other people in the home, leading to divided attention and some inhibitions in discussion of intimate details. On the other hand, a more objective assessment could be made of the way in which the woman was coping with her domestic duties and the care of her children. Sometimes a further dimension could be added by the husband's impressions of his wife's state.

Finally, in those cases who were only able to supply a written account of their feelings, it was impressive how full and how revealing many of these were: so much so as to suggest that this method might have been a valuable adjunct to the interview in all cases.

RELIABILITY

The clinical assessment of patients in psychiatry or indeed in medicine as a whole is not amenable to absolute measurement though some phenomena can be more accurately gauged than others. Such things as patients' moods, feelings, attitudes and the quality of their relationships and social function are all areas where there is ample room for differences of opinion amongst observers. An attempt was thus made to assess the reliability between the three observers of the ratings made at follow-up interviews and between the individual observer's ratings on different occasions (which we term within-observer reliability).

Twenty-two married women who had requested abortion some fifteen to thirty months previously but after July 1968 and who were therefore not included in the main research cohort were asked to attend for an interview. It was explained to each of them that their interview would be recorded on video tape for research purposes. CM did eight interviews, PCO six and VE eight, each interview being rated at the time by the person conducting it as in the main follow-up study. About a month after the recording, each video tape was played back and the interview rated by all three psychiatrists. Details of the measurement of reliability may be found in Appendix 6:A to this chapter. Briefly, however, it was found that for 16 items in the 22 patients, where a subjective judgement is concerned there was total agreement on 260 occasions (80.2 per cent), agreement between 2 out of 3 observers on 60 occasions (18.5 per cent) and total disagreement only 4 times (1.1 per cent). For the 16 items which were regarded as having a reliability which warranted their application to the main cohort, there were $16 \times 22 = 352$ pairs of observations. Of these 28 concerned only a matter of fact and 25 were recorded differently by the observer on the two occasions. The rate of agreement was therefore $\dfrac{(352 - 28 - 25)}{(352 - 28)} = 92.3\%$.

STATISTICS OF THE FOLLOW-UP

From the original group of 370 women applying for termination 303 (81.9 per cent) were eventually contacted and re-tested. 117 single and 186 ever-married women, forming 71.8 per cent and 89.9 per cent of their respective cohorts, were re-assessed and are termed the 'follow-up groups'. Sixty-seven women comprising 46 single and 21 ever-married could not be found and are called the 'missed' groups.

The single and ever-married cohorts in fact formed two distinct populations with regard to age, legitimacy of pregnancy, parity and social class distributions and were accordingly analysed separately in the follow-up study. Marital status grouping *at referral* was preserved for the purpose of the analysis. Thus, women who were single at referral but had married in the interim period were still included in the single group for general follow-up assessment.

Fourteen single and 4 ever-married women (12 and 2.2 per cent respectively of the follow-up groups) could not be interviewed personally at follow-up but were contacted by post. Students and women with psychiatric indications were over-represented in this postal group. The postal replies to questions other than the entirely structured type in the Beck Depression Inventory and Fould's Hostility Scales were remarkably detailed and expressive as though many welcomed the opportunity to write about their experiences. Likewise most of the interviewed women were quite ready to discuss their present and past situation. A few mentioned spontaneously how glad they were to have this opportunity of discussing their experiences.

Significantly more single than ever-married women eluded follow-up and similar significant differences obtained when the aborted and non-aborted groups were considered separately (Tables 6:2 and 6:3). Missed groups contained a marginally higher proportion of women who continued the pregnancy to term.

The 'missed' groups were lost to the follow-up broadly in three ways (see Table 6:4). 'No trace' women had left the address they gave at referral, without leaving a forwarding address. Attempts to locate their new place of residence had been unsuccessful. Another group whose present address was known did not reply to letters requesting a follow-up interview, though it was reasonably certain that the messages had been conveyed to them. The smallest group comprised those who had explicitly refused a follow-up assessment. It is possibly worthy of note that non-aborted women were over-represented in the 'no reply' and 'refused' follow-up groups, whereas those vanishing without trace had very similar proportions of aborted women to their respective follow-up groups.

At this point some of the distinctive features of this study's follow-up are worth re-emphasising.

(i) The completeness of information obtained from records about the eventual outcome, i.e. whether aborted or delivered at term, even where the woman herself was not contacted again.

(ii) The fact that only one woman who was refused an abortion by the Aberdeen clinicians obtained a legal abortion elsewhere.

Apart from a few possible cases of self-induced abortion the large majority seemed to abide by the Aberdeen decision. This may be due to the remoteness of Aberdeen from other major centres where abortion could be obtained, or possibly the idea that refusal in a comparatively liberal centre such as Aberdeen at that time made acceptance for termination elsewhere unlikely.

The lower rate of follow-up for the *single* women was mainly accounted for by the omission of 'students'.† They were followed up significantly less frequently (61.3 per cent) than the non-students (78.2 per cent). This was however the only major difference between the 'missed' and follow-up groups. Basic characteristics such as age, number of previous pregnancies, main indications for the abortion and percentage aborted were very similar in these groups. 'Students' lost to the study also had similar characteristics on these variables and virtually identical scores on mental state tests at referral to the students who were followed up.

It would seem that difficulties in follow-up of students had little connection with whether abortion had been carried out or not, but were probably more closely related to other factors such as high geographical and job mobility. More 'students' had their homes and centres of interest outside north-east Scotland than the non-student group.

To what extent were the follow-up groups representative of the original cohorts?

Comparison of the social, obstetric and psychological characteristics measured at the time of referral enabled such an estimate to be made.

Psychologically it was those women who scored as more suspicious and difficult to get on with L($+$) who tended to be missed from the follow-up study, and in fact Cattell also associated this trait with reluctance to give test information.‡

Aborted single women *missed* from the follow-up displayed a cluster of self-reliant qualities, being especially tough-minded I($-$), experimenting and independent minded $Q_1(+)$ and self-sufficient $Q_2(+)$, compared to *aborted single* women who were followed up.* They also scored as rather less depressed and intropunitive at referral than the latter whereas the converse obtained for single women who continued the pregnancy. Though these mental state differences were not significant at the 5% level, the mean values nevertheless gave the best available estimate of the psychological state at referral. Thus if there were a bias in the follow-up sampling from the original cohort this would tend to exaggerate the psychological vulnerability of the aborted women and underestimate that of the non-aborted group (Tables 6:5 and 6:6).

Similarly the 'follow-up' and 'missed' groups of *ever-married* women showed close resemblances on most of the basic social and obstetric

† 'Students' are all those in full-time education including schoolgirls.
‡ Significance test values are given in Appendix 6:B at the end of this chapter. An *
in the text in the remainder of this chapter denotes the existence of such a test value.

variables. The only significant difference between the groups concerned parity. Women with more than one previous pregnancy were more likely to be included in the follow-up.* This could be understood as a function of the practical difficulties of moving away with a family of small children.

The only major personality difference was on the expedient–conscientious dimension. Ever-married women missed from the follow-up scored as significantly more conscientious and persevering G(+).* This trait also involves concern about rules and moral standards and the difference might be interpreted as avoidance of follow-up by a group of women whose dread of social disapproval had led them to conceal the abortion application from relatives. Though only small numbers were involved in the missed group, the scores on the personality and mental state tests indicated that the aborted women who were *not* followed up were, if anything, rather less vulnerable and less psychiatrically disturbed at referral than those who were included in the follow-up. The converse held for those who were continuing the pregnancy. As in the case of the single women, the most likely bias from the sampling would be to exaggerate the disturbance in the aborted group and underestimate that of the non-aborted (Tables 6:7 and 6:8).

CONCLUSION

The composition of the follow-up groups measured at the time of referral closely resembled those of the original cohorts on most relevant variables. An overall estimate of an urban community's experience with abortion application and the later sequelae of various modes of management could therefore be derived with a fair degree of confidence from study of these follow-up groups. In a few respects the latter were distorted samples of the cohorts and so in these areas conclusions had perforce to be tentative. Generally results from the ever-married group were likely to be more representative and accurate than those from the single women's group because of the former's higher rate of follow-up. Even so the single women's follow-up group apart from its low proportion of students remained a fair approximation to the original referral cohort.

Particular caution must be exercised in interpreting results applying to 'students', to ever-married women of upper social class, of low parity or with main medical indications for abortion. Further studies concentrating especially on these sub-groups would help to fill in some of the gaps in the present project.

COLIN MCCANCE, PETER C. OLLEY AND VIVIEN EDWARD

CRITERIA FOR EVALUATING SOCIAL AND PSYCHOLOGICAL DYSFUNCTION AT FOLLOW-UP

Several different indices were used to assess the outcome state at follow-up.

(*a*) The *psychiatrists'* rating of the presence of depression, anxiety or other psychiatric disturbance at interview.

(*b*) *Self report by the patient* of:

(i) Her attitudes and feelings about the 'treatment' she had undergone, e.g. abortion, continuing to term, sterilisation, adoption of her baby.

(ii) The state of her relationship with significant people in her life, e.g. husband, putative father (PF), mother, new baby.

(iii) Her past and present ability to cope with any other children, job situation, and any history of psychiatric treatment.

(*c*) *Scores on psychological tests completed at follow-up.* The Beck Depression Inventory (BDI) and Fould's Hostility Scales gave measures of the current mental state and could be contrasted with scores at referral. Groups were compared by mean scores or proportions of 'impaired' individuals.

In addition to a clinical evaluation of psychiatric impairment, an operational definition of depression derived from the Beck Depression Inventory was used in the study. Previous projects using this test had suggested useful gradings of depression: 0–9, depression absent; 10–16, mild depression; 17–24, moderate depression; 25+, severe depression (see Chapter 5). Thus, depression was operationally defined to exist with a score of 10 or more on the BDI.

(*d*) A less operationally defined *global assessment* attempting to take into account the welter of variables in each individual case. The results of this overall assessment are presented in Chapter 7.

COMPARISON OF THE CHARACTERISTICS OF ABORTED AND NON-ABORTED FOLLOW-UP GROUPS AT THE TIME OF REFERRAL

A major objective of the follow-up study for both single and ever-married cohorts was a comparison of the late effects of abortion with the late effects of continuing the index pregnancy to term. In a strictly controlled scientific study women would have been assigned at random to the abortion or pregnancy continuation groups. Medical ethics precluded such an arrangement in the context of the research study. Gynaecologists and psychiatrists made the selection for abortion on clinical criteria, and not surprisingly social and psychological character-istics of the abortion group at the time of referral differed considerably from those who continued the pregnancy.

1 Psychological test scores at referral

Both the single and the ever-married women who were aborted were significantly more depressed (BDI) and intropunitive (In) than those who continued the pregnancy (Tables 6:9 |and 6:10).*

There were no significant 16 PF personality trait differences for unmarried women, though aborted single women scored as rather more aloof A($-$) and tense $Q_4(+)$ (see Table 6:5). Among the ever-married women in the follow-up it was the guilt-prone and the apprehensive O($+$) who were selected for abortion, but also to some extent those scoring as shrewd, astute and worldly N($+$) – as opposed to naive, forthright and unpretentious (Table 6:7).* Probably the shrewd and sophisticated woman was able to manipulate the situation and present her case for abortion in a more convincing manner than the naive, unpolished applicant.

2 Psychiatric treatment in the year prior to referral (Table 6:11)

On this measure, ever-married women in the follow-up had received psychiatric treatment significantly more often than the unmarried group ($\chi^2 = 8.67$, d.f. $= 1$, $P < 0.01$). Regardless of marital status, aborted women reported twice the incidence of treatment (mainly from general practitioners) than those who continued the pregnancy. This was however not an effect significant at the 5% level.

3   Other social indices

Self-reports of the quality of interpersonal and sexual relationships with husband or putative father and the ability to cope with existing children all indicate that the aborted groups prior to the index pregnancy had a marginally less satisfactory level of adjustment, but the difference was not significant at the 5% level.

The balance of evidence indicates that it tended to be the more vulnerable and maladjusted women who were selected for abortion and the more stable who continued the pregnancy. In assessing progress between the time of referral and the follow-up it must therefore be borne in mind that the aborted group were at a disadvantage from the start.

THE CHARACTERISTICS OF ABORTED AND NON-ABORTED GROUPS AT FOLLOW-UP

1   Psychological test scores at follow-up

The Beck Depression Inventory (BDI) and Fould's Hostility Scales (Ex) and (In) were completed at follow-up as well as at referral. The incidence of depression in *single women* did not differ significantly between aborted and non-aborted groups, being 20.0 and 22.2 per cent respectively. Moderate and severe depressions were infrequent in both groups (Table 6:9). Two aborted women failed to complete the BDI at follow-up, and one of these was judged clinically to be mentally disturbed. The levels of outward and inward directed hostility were equivalent in both groups (Table 6:10).*

In *ever-married women* a pattern emerged similar to that of the unmarried group. 23.8 per cent of the aborted and 25.4 per cent of the non-aborted were rated as depressed and hostility scores at follow-up were also not significantly different. One aborted woman failed to complete the Beck test. Ever-married women registered a significantly greater depth of depression than single women at follow-up, however.* A total of 10 ever-married (5 aborted and 5 non-aborted) scored as severely depressed compared to only one unmarried applicant. This was consistent with the greater degree of neuroticism noted among the ever-married women at the time of referral.

The most significant finding was that all four groups showed dramatic reductions in depression and hostility between the time of referral and follow-up. *As measured by the psychological questionnaires highly disturbed and depressed groups at referral had been transformed into groups with essentially normal scores approximately eighteen months later.* The aborted groups of both single and ever-married women were the ones that showed the greatest improvement. They had rated as significantly more depressed at the time of referral than the women who continued the pregnancy. At follow-up they registered similar levels of depression and hostility.*

2 Clinical assessment of mental state at follow-up (Table 6:12)

Unmarried aborted women were assessed as less depressed than their non-aborted colleagues. One in nine of the aborted group rated as depressed as compared with one in four of those continuing the pregnancy – an effect which approached the 5% level of significance. Most of the affected women were only mildly depressed. Eleven (15.3%) of the aborted and 12 (26.7 per cent) of the non-aborted were considered to be 'disturbed', i.e. depressed and/or anxious.

Differences in the mental state of the *ever-married* aborted and non-aborted groups at follow-up were minimal. Thirty-seven (30.1 per cent) of the aborted and 19 (30.2 per cent) of the non-aborted were rated as 'disturbed'. Approximately one in four were considered to be depressed, mostly to a mild degree, with a slight excess of depression in women who had gone to term. As in the case of the single women, severe depressions were infrequent late sequelae, only occurring in about 2 per cent of cases.

Depression *after abortion* was more common among ever-married than single women whereas there were equivalent reactions after going to term in these groups.*

3 Attitudes to the outcome of the index pregnancy (Table 6:13)

The women were asked to describe specifically how they felt about the outcome of the pregnancy as the solution to the particular set of problems they had faced at the time of referral. They were asked to distinguish these feelings from any general regrets at having become pregnant at that time.

Aborted women were generally more satisfied with the result than those who carried the pregnancy to term. At the time of the follow-up approximately one in five of the aborted *single women* regretted the abortion compared with two in five of the non-aborted group who regretted having their baby. There was a significantly greater proportion both of total regrets and of severe regrets among those who were not aborted. The excess of regrets at continuing the pregnancy was less clear cut among the *ever-married* women at the follow-up. One in three regretted going to term compared with one in five regretting the abortion. The proportion with severe regrets in the non-aborted group was also greater, but again, not significantly so.*

Inquiry was also made at the time of follow-up about attitudes experienced three months after the abortion. A larger proportion of single women retrospectively reported regrets soon after the abortion (36.1%) than did married women (25.2%). In the interim period to the time of follow-up there appeared to have been a significant improvement for the aborted single women but little change for the ever-married group.*

These results, however, must be regarded with reservation as this item did not rate highly in the reliability study and the reports are liable to considerable retrospective distortion. However, whether or not these attitudes were actually held at the three-month stage, by approximately eighteen months the single women saw themselves as having shaken off a substantial proportion of their previous regrets at having had an abortion.

SINGLE WOMEN WHO CONTINUED THE PREGNANCY TO TERM

The role of *adoption* in the solution of problems posed by an unwanted pregnancy appears to be changing. There are reports of a shortage of babies for adoption and an increasing tendency for unmarried mothers to look after their children, and certainly many of the abortion applicants were reluctant to consider adoption as an alternative to abortion.

In the present study 16 single women, 35.6 per cent of those continuing their pregnancy, had their babies adopted. At follow-up they were asked about their attitude to the adoption. Six (37.5 per cent) were glad, 9 (56.3 per cent) had mixed feelings and regrets and one (6.3 per cent) had severe regrets. Thus 10 (62.5 per cent) had some regrets at the adoption arrangement. Of the 16 who had their babies adopted, 9 had regrets about having to continue the pregnancy and of those 7 had *severe* regrets.

One woman who had married the putative father was glad she had the baby adopted, but strongly regretted having continued the pregnancy. Yet another who had broken with the putative father and married another man was glad both that she had continued the pregnancy to term and had her baby adopted. Two-thirds of the 'professional' women who continued the pregnancy had their baby adopted compared to approximately one in three in the other occupational groups.

From the woman's standpoint therefore adoption had not been a very satisfactory solution to their problems. There were fewer and less severe regrets at having continued the pregnancy among those who had kept their baby, whether they had or had not remained unmarried (Table 6:14).

The 29 single applicants at follow-up *who kept their babies* were asked about their attitude to their child. Twenty-six reported 'normal maternal' feelings, but 2 (6.9 per cent) felt they hadn't developed these. One woman's baby died the day after delivery. She expressed considerable regrets that she hadn't been granted an abortion.

EVER-MARRIED WOMEN WHO CONTINUED THE PREGNANCY TO TERM

Sixty-three women in the follow-up group continued the index pregnancy to term, two of them (3.2 per cent) delivering still-born babies. One of these women, nominally a Roman Catholic, was divorced and illegitimately pregnant. At follow-up she expressed severe regrets at having continued the pregnancy. The other woman, also a Roman Catholic, had a legitimate conception, was on good terms with her husband, and was glad that she went to term despite her child's death.

Two other women (3.2 per cent) had their babies adopted. Both had severe regrets about having done this and also having continued the pregnancy. One was divorced and with an illegitimate pregnancy and the other, legitimately pregnant, was separated from her husband at referral and had obtained a divorce by the time of the follow-up. Fifty-four women (85.7 per cent) of the non-aborted group described 'normal feelings' that they had for their baby. The remaining 5 (7.9 per cent) described 'less than normal feelings' for their child amounting to a degree of rejection. All 5 had regrets about having continued the pregnancy. One with a history of criminal abortions had produced an illegitimate premature infant which survived. There may also have been an attempt at self-induction in this instance. Another woman also with an illegitimate pregnancy was separated from her husband and a third with a medical psychiatric indication was in severe conflict with her husband. In the other two instances relationships with the husbands were quite satisfactory but the financial and housing situations were made more difficult by the arrival of the new baby.

THE EFFECTS OF STERILISATION

In evaluating the long-term sequelae of aborting or of continuing an 'unwanted' pregnancy to term, an additional major variable – sterilisation, had to be taken into account for the ever-married women. Seventy-six (61.8 per cent) of the aborted group in the follow-up had been sterilised and 23 (36.5 per cent) of those who delivered had been sterilised post-partum. The great majority of the sterilised group (over 80 per cent) were glad that this procedure had been carried out. There was no significant difference in the incidence of regrets between those sterilised with abortion, and the group with post-partum sterilisation, though the former expressed rather deeper regrets (Table 6:15).

Depression scores following abortion were apparently independent of sterilisation, but if the index pregnancy had been continued a sterilisation was associated with a lesser degree of depression at follow-up (Table 6:16).

At follow-up the ever-married women were asked to describe the quality of the general (as opposed to sexual) relationship with their husband both currently and in the period shortly before the index pregnancy.

Tables 6:17 and 6:18 list the findings of this inquiry for women who were aborted and also for those who continued the pregnancy. The variable sterilised/not sterilised refers always to the state at follow-up, whereas the relationship category refers to the state of the marriage, firstly before the index pregnancy, and secondly at follow-up. Those classified as having a 'broken relationship' comprised those 'parted' from their husband by death, divorce or separation.

A definite overall improvement in relationship with husband *after abortion* of the index pregnancy was evident for both sterilised and non-sterilised groups, though a number of women whose marriage was initially under strain and who had not been sterilised had broken with their spouse by the time of follow-up. By contrast, little change in the quality of the marital relationship seemed to have occurred for ever-married women who *continued the pregnancy*, whether or not they were sterilised.

The groups who were sterilised had significantly better marital relationships prior to the index pregnancy than those who were not sterilised, an effect particularly marked in the non-aborted group. Sterilisation was apparently contra-indicated in most situations where there was a broken or insecure marriage. The possibility of a remarriage or occasionally of a reconciliation may have weighed heavily in these decisions. At follow-up the sterilised groups still maintained relationships with their husbands that were generally more satisfactory than those of the non-sterilised groups.*

The ever-married women were also asked at follow-up to comment on their sexual adjustment both at the present and prior to the index pregnancy. Their sexual partner was not necessarily the legal husband. 'Not applicable' was a category used where the women were unable to rate an isolated sexual encounter which resulted in the index pregnancy or where they claimed sexual relationships had been discontinued.

Sexual adjustment was significantly improved in those who were *aborted*. Improvement however occurred mainly in *aborted* women who were also *sterilised*. In fact the non-sterilised group as a whole reported a deterioration in the degree of sexual adjustment by the time of follow-up, mainly due to women breaking with their previous partner and becoming sexually abstinent. Before the index pregnancy the two groups apparently had similar levels of sexual adjustment, but by the follow-up they had diverged considerably, with the sterilised aborted group reporting a significantly better sexual relationship than the non-sterilised, aborted women.*

Women who were *not aborted* showed overall only a marginal increase in the proportion who reported a satisfactory sexual relationship at follow-up. The limited amount of improvement that did occur took place among those with post-partum *sterilisation*. An appreciable proportion of the ever-married women with 'lukewarm' sexual relationships who continued the pregnancy but were not sterilised reported even greater difficulties or were sexually abstinent at the time of follow-up. Once more, the sterilised group was chosen from women with much superior sexual adjustment prior to the index pregnancy. They retained this advantage over the non-sterilised women who had gone to term when assessed at follow-up (Tables 6:19 and 6:20).*

The proportion of ever-married women reporting a satisfactory general relationship with their husband exceeded the proportion who claimed a satisfactory sexual adjustment. Women with post-partum sterilisation already enjoyed good general marital relationships before the pregnancy. The quality of this was maintained, but the sterilisation was associated with an increase in the proportion reporting sexual satisfaction from 65.2 per cent to 78.3 per cent.

Thus to most women who applied for termination sterilisation had been a benign and welcome event and was associated with an improvement in general marital and sexual relationships.

DEPRESSION ASSOCIATED WITH UNFAVOURABLE ATTITUDES TO THE PREGNANCY OUTCOME

A state of depression at follow-up may be reactive to events associated with the index pregnancy or may be related to other problems, e.g. poor housing, inadequate finances or a turbulent relationship with husband or boyfriend. It is therefore relevant to inquire which women were assessed as depressed on the Beck Depression Inventory at follow-up, and also regretted the abortion, having their baby or a subsequent sterilisation. A score of 10 or more was the operational definition of depression.

Four single women (5.7 per cent) of the aborted group were depressed and also regretted the abortion, whereas 6 single women (13.3 per cent) were depressed and regretted going to term. Nine (7.4 per cent) of the aborted ever-married women were both depressed and had misgivings about the abortion compared to 10 (15.9 per cent) of those who continued the pregnancy.

A greater incidence of depression associated with regrets at the outcome of the pregnancy was thus encountered in women who were not aborted – whether single or ever-married, though these effects were not significant at the 5% level.

FURTHER ANALYSIS OF OUTCOME STATES

To what extent are unfavourable sequelae associated with key variables other than the fact of abortion, sterilisation or continuing the pregnancy to term? The influence of a number of these basic variables is discussed below.

1 Age and social class

Tables 6:21 to 6:26 illustrate the *age* and *social class* composition of the follow-up groups and analyse long-term sequelae in terms of these variables.

The notable feature of the unmarried group was the regular gradation with social class of regrets about abortion or continuing the pregnancy, the highest incidence being among the professional group and the lowest reported by the manual workers. This finding might be connected with differing attitudes to illegitimate pregnancy in the various social classes.

For each individual class group the proportion of regrets at abortion was less than the proportion among those continuing to term. The professional group registered the highest incidence of depression on the Beck Depression Inventory and the students the lowest incidence at follow-up. With the exception of the clerical and distributive workers, aborted women were marginally more depressed than non-aborted. It should be noted however that numbers involved were small and these effects were not significant at the 5% level (Table 6:23).

The lowest proportion of regrets at abortion in the unmarried group occurred among women in the 20–24 age category, with teenagers reporting the highest incidence of regrets.* On the other hand chagrin at continuing the pregnancy steadily increased with increasing age at referral (Table 6:22).

With the ever-married the process of continuing the pregnancy and rearing the child would seem to have been most traumatic for the class v women – the wives of unskilled workers. They reported a higher incidence of regrets at going to term than all the other social class groups, though no regrets at all at having had an abortion. However class v registered a higher incidence of depression for both non-aborted and aborted groups, again underlining the fact that many depressed women at follow-up do not specifically regret the abortion but are probably responding to other stresses.*

Younger married women tended to regret an abortion less and having their baby more than the over thirties, but whatever the 'treatment' were generally more depressed at follow-up than the latter (Tables 6:25 and 6:26).

2 State of marriage

A state of depression on the Beck Depression Inventory at follow-up was particularly associated in the case of ever-married women with those who at the time of referral were '*parted*' from their husband or who though still living with him had complained of severe '*disharmony*', whether or not they had been aborted. In this context 'parted' included those divorced, separated or widowed. Women living with their husbands who did not complain of severe marital strain at the time of referral (the 'harmony' group) were significantly less depressed at follow-up than either of the above groups.*

Women living with their husbands at the time of referral also registered a higher incidence of regrets about their abortion than those 'parted' from husband. Few of the latter group in fact made any complaints about termination* (Table 6:27).

CHANGES IN MARITAL STATUS BY THE TIME OF FOLLOW-UP

A number of women in the follow-up groups were known to have changed their marital status in the period between referral and reassessment.

Thirty-three (28.2 per cent) of the *single women's* follow-up group had married by the time they were contacted again. This sub-group comprised 17 (23.6 per cent) of those aborted and 16 (35.6 per cent) of those not aborted. Ten (13.9 per cent) of the aborted single women appeared to have married the putative father of the index pregnancy compared with 15 (33.3 per cent) of those who continued the pregnancy to term. In the case of abortion applicants who were unmarried at the time of referral, subsequent marriage is clearly another important variable that must be taken into account when assessing outcome at the time of the follow-up.

Tables 6:28 to 6:32 describe the attitudes to abortion or continuing the pregnancy to term, Beck Depression Inventory (BDI) scores and sexual adjustment as reported at follow-up by those who had married since referral, and separately by those who had remained unmarried.

The category 'not applicable' used in Tables 6:31 and 6:32 describing sexual adjustment, refers to a situation prior to the index pregnancy where a regular sexual relationship had not taken place and the index pregnancy was allegedly the result of a casual encounter which could not be rated on the scale of satisfaction. However, 'not applicable' when applied to the follow-up period signified total lack of a sexual relationship. For women who were single at referral, regrets about having an abortion differed little whether they had subsequently married or not. About 80 per cent were glad they had been aborted. A majority of those who continued the pregnancy were glad they went to term, but there was a slightly higher incidence of regrets among those who remained unmarried. Of the women who married, there was a greater degree of depression among those who were aborted than those who continued the pregnancy whereas the converse obtained for those who did not marry. Unmarried women who aborted showed a marginally lower incidence of depression than the women who had married by the time of follow-up. For those who continued to term, not surprisingly, there was a greater incidence of depression among the unmarried company compared with the married.

As regards the quality of sexual adjustment reported by the different groups at follow-up, those who had married had considerably improved their level of sexual satisfaction, whether or not they had been aborted. At follow-up about a half of the unmarried group claimed they were not having sex and there seemed to be little difference in this whether the index pregnancy had resulted in abortion or in having a full-term child. The recent pregnancy seemed to have acted as a deterrent. Some girls reported how their parents were now more restrictive and others who were now bringing up a young child how their changed situation had hindered their social life. Many however had themselves avoided further relationships with men. Forty-four per cent of the unmarried women who had been aborted and were continuing to have sex reported a good adjustment compared to 68 per cent of those who had gone to term and had remained unmarried.

Nineteen (10.2 per cent) of women classified as *ever-married* at the time of referral and included in the follow-up group had altered their marital state. This total was made up of 11 (8.9 per cent) of those aborted and 8 (12.7 per cent) of those who had continued the pregnancy and had been reassessed. Six (31.6 per cent) of those who changed status had illegitimate index pregnancies compared with 15 per cent of those who remained in the same marital state. Mostly the change was a separation or a divorce from the husband, but 4 women resumed cohabitation with formerly estranged husbands. Two of these had apparently effected a satisfactory reconciliation but the other 2 continued to have strained relationships.

Changes in marital status at follow-up

	At referral	At follow-up		Total
Aborted				
	Living with husband	Separated	4	6
		Divorced	1	
		Widowed	1	
	Separated	Divorced	2	5
		Living with husband again	3	
				11
Not aborted				
	Living with husband	Separated	1	2
		Divorced	1	
	Separated	Divorced	5	6
		Living with husband again	1	
				8

3 Outcome for ever-married women with illegitimate index pregnancies

Thirty-one ever-married women with illegitimate index pregnancies were included in the follow-up study. Eighteen (85.7 per cent) of the 21 women who were aborted, had broken with the putative father by this time. The break-up or the impending break-up seemed to have been an important factor in the decision to abort. Four (40 per cent) of the 10 who continued the pregnancy had discontinued their relationship with the father of their child. Of the remaining 6 women, 2 had married the putative father and 4 maintained close relations with him.

There seemed to be no major differences in outcome between those with illegitimate and legitimate pregnancies. The illegitimate group were marginally more depressed and had rather more regrets at continuing the pregnancy, but reported a slightly reduced incidence of regrets at having had an abortion (Tables 6:33 and 6:34).

Aborted women with illegitimate pregnancies were sterilised much less frequently than the legitimate group.*

4 Main indications for abortion

Principal indications for abortion had been earlier assigned to each applicant by two of the gynaecologists (see Chapter 2). A number of trends were evident when the follow-up groups were analysed in terms of the main indication and the outcome state. The highest incidences of depression on the Beck Inventory at follow-up for both the single and the ever-married groups occurred in those who had presented at referral with a main medico-psychiatric indication. With the exception of the very small medical group of single women there was a steady decrease in the proportion depressed from the medico-psychiatric through socio-psychiatric and social to the lowest in the medical group in the case of the ever-married women. A similar ranking of depression scores had been noted in these indication groups at referral. Thus those groups who were most depressed at referral were likely to remain most depressed at follow-up. With respect to the aborted women, those with main medico-psychiatric, or socio-psychiatric indications tended to be more depressed at follow-up than those with social or medical indications. The dichotomy between depression and regrets was further illustrated in that single women with psychiatric indications had a significantly lower level of regrets than the social group but a higher level of depression on the Beck Inventory at the time of reassessment (Table 6:35).*

5 The type of termination and its relation to the outcome

Unfavourable sequelae of termination may occur more frequently with some types of procedure than with others. For instance, saline termination involving a miniature labour may be considered far more distressing than a D & C. On the other hand a spontaneous abortion may be regarded as an 'Act of God' with no personal responsibility involved. Tables 6:36 and 6:37 list the sequelae for different types of termination.

Single women who had saline or suction terminations reported the greatest incidence of regrets experienced three months after the operation, though differences were not significant at the 5% level. By the time of follow-up, approximately eighteen months after termination, differences in regrets were less remarkable, though only women with saline or suction operations were observed to be clinically depressed or anxious. Unmarried women with D & C or spontaneous abortions rated as the least distressed or regretful at follow-up.

The type of abortion employed is however a dependent variable being closely related to the stage of pregnancy. Women with delayed referral would tend to be given saline or a hysterotomy, whereas D & C or suction would be employed at a shorter period of gestation. The results were not conclusive but suggested that saline and suction terminations may be initially more stressful than other modes of abortion.

In the case of the *ever-married* women, the greatest incidence of both early and late regrets occurred after hysterotomy, the most frequently used method of termination.* There was little change in the reported frequency of regrets between the immediate post-operative period and the time of the follow-up. Hysterotomy patients were significantly more clinically depressed or anxious at follow-up than the rest of the ever-married group (see Table 6:37).*

Women receiving hysterotomy also tended to be older women with a completed family and were mostly sterilised at the same time. The type of operation was thus only one of several important factors relating to the outcome. As for single women, 'spontaneous' abortion was associated with remarkably few psychiatric sequelae.

When corrections were made for women who had aborted 'spontaneously' no new patterns emerged different from the outcome figures for aborted and non-aborted groups referred to above.

Single women aborted by the gynaecologists experienced significantly greater satisfaction at the time of follow-up than single women who continued the pregnancy to term. Fifty-three (80.3 per cent) out of 66 aborted by the gynaecologists were glad at this mode of treatment as were 82 (76.7 per cent) of the ever-married group. As before the difference in satisfaction was not significantly greater than ever-married women who went to term.

Depression on the Beck Inventory at follow-up* ($B_2 \geqslant 10$) was registered by 21.9 per cent of the single women and 27.4 per cent of the ever-married women aborted by the gynaecologists. Thus, as before there were no significant differences in the levels of depression between aborted and non-aborted groups at the time of the follow-up.

THE OUTCOME AND THE GYNAECOLOGIST

It is clear from Chapter 5 that there were groups of gynaecologists who aborted significantly different proportions of applicants referred to them even where there were comparable psychological and social characteristics. Those aborting a large proportion of applicants were labelled as 'liberal' gynaecologists and those aborting a small percentage as 'conservative' gynaecologists.

Though this individual pattern was evident for a number of years prior to and following the study, it should not be assumed that this is a permanently 'fixed' attitude on the gynaecologist's part. In the light of further experience 'liberals' may begin to abort a smaller percentage or 'conservatives' a larger percentage. Again attitudes may change towards single women but not towards ever-married, and vice versa.

It seems likely that there are women who would be aborted by a 'liberal' and refused abortion by a 'conservative' gynaecologist, though there will be many where a consensus would occur. Unfortunately the extent of the first group, where differing decisions would be made, is unknown in the present study. Comparisons between the outcome for the 'liberal' and 'conservative' groups will therefore tend to blur the essential differences in practice as there will be a proportion who would be accepted for abortion or refused abortion by each type of gynaecologist.

At the time of follow-up, there were no conclusive differences in mental state or regrets at treatment evident between those women dealt with by the two groups of 'liberal' and 'conservative' gynaecologists (Tables 6:38 and 6:39, 6:40 and 6:41). Overall, the 'liberals' group expressed marginally fewer regrets but scored as being rather more frequently depressed at follow-up. It should be remembered that at referral the unmarried group seen by the 'liberals' were more distressed and vulnerable than those seen by the 'conservatives', though the ever-married groups were of equivalent psychological status.

The most marked differences in abortion practice between the gynaecologists occurred for women who had a main social indication for abortion (see Chapter 5). When the outcomes for ever-married women with this indication were compared it was found that 17.3 per cent of the 52 women in the 'liberals' group had regrets and 31.1 per cent of the 45 in the 'conservative' group. Attitudes to abortion were equivalent, with the proportion of regrets being 21.1 per cent and 20 per cent respectively. However, 40 per cent of the 'conservatives' who continued the pregnancy regretted this compared with only 7.1 per cent of the 'liberals'.

The total incidence of depression was however virtually identical in the two groups, though the 'liberal' group were more frequently depressed if aborted (26.3 per cent cf. 10 per cent) and less depressed (14.3 per cent cf. 40 per cent) if they continued the pregnancy compared to the 'conservatives' group of patients.

These trends suggest that the conservative's practice of frequently refusing abortion to those with social indications resulted in a more regretful though not a more depressed group of patients at follow-up. It must be re-emphasised however that none of these differences were significant at the 5% level.

THE RELATIONSHIP BETWEEN REFERRAL AND FOLLOW-UP CHARACTERISTICS

What were the psychological characteristics at *referral* in those women who were depressed at *follow-up* or had regrets about the decision at this stage?

Table 6:42 compares 16 PF scores in women who were 'depressed' on the Beck Depression Inventory with those who did not score as depressed at follow-up.

For the *single women* there were no significant differences between these two groups on the 16 PF factors though there were more deviating scores with the 'depressed' women on a number of factors including: $G(+)$ conscientious, $H(-)$ timid, $L(+)$ suspicious, $M(+)$ self-absorbed, $Q_3(-)$ uncontrolled.

On the other hand, ever-married women who scored as depressed on the Beck Depression Inventory at follow-up, showed *significant* differences on several factors of the 16 PF completed at the time of referral, compared with those not depressed.

The 'depressed' group ($B_2 \geqslant 10$) were significantly more: $C(-)$ emotionally unstable ($t = 3.05$, $P < 0.01$); $L(+)$ suspicious ($t = 2.71$, $P < 0.01$); $Q_1(+)$ experimenting, radical ($t = 2.08$, $P < 0.05$); $Q_4(+)$ tense ($t = 2.43$, $P < 0.02$). Thus, later depression in the ever-married was related to the presence of neurotic personality traits evident at the time of referral. By contrast women with regrets at treatment displayed more stable personality traits.

A state of depression at follow-up seemed to be more closely related to the type of treatment in the non-aborted groups than in those who had been aborted. Thus in the aborted groups of single and ever-married women only 28.6 per cent and 34.5 per cent respectively of those who were depressed regretted having an abortion whereas 60 per cent and 56.3 per cent of their depressed non-aborted groups regretted going to term. Many women with regrets about abortion or going to term nevertheless did not register as depressed on the BDI. Thus only 28.6 per cent and 38.4 per cent respectively of the single and ever-married aborted groups who had regrets about abortion were also depressed. The equivalent figures for the non-aborted groups were similar, viz. 40.9 per cent and 31.6 per cent.

Women who were depressed at follow-up and women who expressed regrets about the treatment were drawn from largely different populations.

SUMMARY

A number of major conclusions emerged from the first part of the follow-up study.

(i) Few severe depressive reactions were evident in aborted women at the time of follow-up though moderate degrees of depression were not uncommon.

(ii) These depressive states appeared to be frequently related to current marital or other external stresses or personality factors rather than the fact of abortion. Depression among those who had continued the pregnancy was more often associated with regrets at going to term.

(iii) At follow-up, the aborted women were no more depressed than women who had continued the pregnancy, despite the fact that the former group were significantly more depressed at referral and displayed more vulnerable personality traits.

Both aborted and non-aborted groups had improved psychologically since the time of referral, but the aborted group showed the greatest change.

(iv) Regrets about continuing with the pregnancy were more common than regrets about abortion in both single and ever-married groups, but especially so in the former.

(v) Few regrets occurred concerning abortion in women with major psychiatric problems, though they tended to be the most depressed groups both at referral and follow-up.

(vi) Sterilisation combined with abortion appeared to be particularly beneficial for ever-married applicants and these procedures were associated with improved relationships with husband and improved sexual adjustment.

(viii) Adoption for single women appeared to be generally unsatisfactory as far as the woman was concerned.

Thus in the context of Aberdeen at this particular period the practice of abortion to solve the problems of the women with an unwanted pregnancy was not specifically associated with a high degree of later social and psychological difficulties. On balance the outcome was apparently more beneficial to the women concerned than the outcome for those who continued the pregnancy.

APPENDIX 6:A

Analysis of reliability

It was possible to study 29 items which were open to disagreement on rating judgements (items 1, 2, 5, 6, 9, 10, 13–16, 18–21, 24, 25, 27–34, 39–43).

The sub-group of 22 married women were not suitable for the study of 5 further items which were nonetheless open to disagreement on rating judgements (items 22, 26, 23, 7 and 8). This lack of data on reliability of these items must therefore temper the conclusions drawn from them in the results as a whole.

Returning to the 29 items which it was possible to study, 14 could have included matters of fact as opposed to a subjective judgement of the rater, e.g. the item 'feelings about having had abortion' would have been considered a matter of fact if there had been no abortion – i.e. rated as 'not applicable', but otherwise it would have been a judgement permitting the possibility of a different rating.

For each item, the number of times that there was complete agreement between all three observers, between 2 out of 3, or worse was set out. Any item which did not show total agreement in a proportion of at least 72 per cent of the subjective judgements was not considered reliable enough to warrant serious study in the results of the main cohort. These items were 1, 2, 14, 15, 16, 20, 27, 28, 29, 31, 32, 33, 39, and for simplicity, have not been shown below in the tabulation.

Between-observer reliability

Item	All 3 agreeing	2 agreeing	None agreeing	Matters of fact
5	19	3	0	0
6	18	4	0	0
9	14 (18.1)†	3 (3.9)	0	5
10	14 (19.2)	2 (2.8)	0	6
13	16	6	0	0
18	16	6	0	0
19	17	5	0	0
21	13 (17.9)	3 (4.1)	0	6
24	13 (17.9)	3 (4.1)	0	6
25	15 (19.4)	2 (2.6)	0	5
30	19	3	0	0
34	17	5	0	0
40	18	3	1	0
41	18	4	0	0
42	16	4	2	0
43	17	4	1	0
Total	260	60	4	28
Total scaled†	283.5	64.5	4	28
Mean scaled	17.7	4.0	0.2	

† Items where matters of fact are involved for some of the patients have been scaled up to give a result as if there were 22 patients.

Rating scheme for psychiatric and social assessment at follow-up

Name   Identifying number – Patient

                                                          Psychiatrist

Age   Marital status at follow-up

Domestic duties:	None	0	One year up to
	Managed easily	1	index pregnancy Now
	Managed with difficulty	2	
	Cannot cope	3	☐ 1 ☐ 2

Outside job: None 0   Full-time 1
               Part-time 2   ☐ 3   ☐ 4

Relationship   N/a   0   Good 1
with husband   Strained 2   Broken 3   ☐ 5   ☐ 6

Relationship   N/a   0   Good 1
with putative Strained 2   Broken 3   ☐ 7   ☐ 8
father:

Relationship   N/a   0   Good 1
with mother: Strained 2   Broken 3   ☐ 9   ☐ 10

Frequency of   Living with mother 1
seeing mother: Based with mother but
away for spells, e.g.
university term, weekly
digs, etc.   2
Home of own but sees
mother:
  (*a*) at least once a week 3
  (*b*) at least once a
    month   4
  (*c*) at least once a year 5
  (*d*) less than once a
    year   6   ☐ 11   ☐ 12
Mother dead   7

Ability of patient   N/a   0
to cope with her   Good   1
other children: Indifferent 2   ☐ 13   ☐ 14
Bad   3

Evidence of   N/a   0
emotional   None   1
disturbance in   Slight   2   ☐ 15   ☐ 16
other children: Severe   3

Number of
children alive at
home at time of   ☐ 17
abortion request:

Sexual relationships: Abstinence socially   0
appropriate
Intercourse at mutually
satisfactory frequency
with orgasm usually   1
Intercourse not greatly
enjoyed but practised
regularly   2
Intercourse disliked,
avoided if possible   3   ☐ 18   ☐ 19

       3 months after
       request for abortion   Now

Feelings about abortion*   ☐ 20   ☐ 21

Feelings about going to term*   ☐ 22

Feelings about adoption*   ☐ 23

Feelings about sterilisation*   ☐ 24   ☐ 25

```
   ⎧ Not applicable                                  0
   ⎪ No regrets, the right decision, glad            1
 * ⎨ Some regrets, second thoughts, mixed feelings   2
   ⎩ Serious regrets, the wrong decision             3
```

Feelings for baby,   Not applicable   0
  if caring for it: Normal love and care   1
                   Less than normal love
                    and care   2   [ ] 26

	The year preceding index pregnancy	At time of request for abortion	3 months after request for abortion	Now
Mental state:				
Depression absent 0 mild 1 severe 2	[ ] 27	[ ] 28	[ ] 29	[ ] 30
Anxiety absent 0 mild 1 severe 2	[ ] 31	[ ] 32	[ ] 33	[ ] 34
Other absent 0 mild 1 severe 2	[ ] 35	[ ] 36	[ ] 37	[ ] 38
(specify)				

	Longer ago than the year preceding index pregnancy	The year preceding index pregnancy	At time of request for abortion	3 months after request for abortion	Now
Psychiatric treatment:					
None 0					
Treatment for 'nerves' from GP 1	[ ] 39	[ ] 40	[ ] 41	[ ] 42	[ ] 43
'Seen and advised' type psychiatric consultation 2					
Course of psychiatric treatment, predominantly:					
(a) out-patient 3					
(b) day-patient 4					
(c) in-patient 5					

Has there been or is there now another   No 1
pregnancy since abortion was requested?   Uncertain 1   [ ] 44
                                    Yes 2

Are you hoping for another pregnancy   No 0
  in the future?   Uncertain 1   [ ] 45
                                    Yes 2

APPENDIX 6:B
Significance test values

p. 250   16 PF, L(+) $t = 2.52$, $P < 0.02$.

p. 250   16 PF, t values I($-$) 2.19, $P < 0.05$; $Q_1(+)$ 2.19, $P < 0.05$; $Q_2(+)$ 2.25, $P < 0.05$.

p. 251   Follow-up v. missed, previous pregnancies (0–1) v. 2+ : $\chi^2 = 5.38$, d.f. = 1, $P < 0.05$.

p. 251   G(+) $t = 2.11$, $P < 0.05$.

p. 253   Suffix 1 denotes referral and suffix 2 denotes follow-up.
Aborted v. non-aborted, single women: (BDI) $t = 3.73$, $P < 0.001$; (Ex)$_1$, $t = 1.46$, NS; (In)$_1$, $t = 2.84$, $P < 0.01$; ever-married women: (BDI) $t = 2.28$, $P < 0.05$; (Ex)$_1$, $t = 1.39$, NS; (In)$_1$, $t = 2.64$, $P < 0.01$.

p. 253   Aborted v. non-aborted, single women: 16 PF, t values A($-$) 1.85; $Q_4(+)$ 1.74, both $P < 0.1$, NS; ever-married: O(+) 2.47, $P < 0.02$; N(+) 1.94, $P < 0.1$, NS.

p. 254   Aborted v. non-aborted: single women: (BDI) $B_2 \geqslant$ 10, $\chi^2 = 0.003$, d.f. = 1, NS (χ^2 was used because of the non-normality of B_2 distribution); (Ex)$_2$, $t = 0.21$, NS; (In)$_2$, $t = 1.11$, NS; ever-married women: (BDI) $B_2 \geqslant$ 10, $\chi^2 = 0.004$, d.f. = 1, NS; (Ex)$_2$, $t = 0.04$, NS; (In)$_2$, $t = 0.72$, NS.

p. 254   Total ever-married and total sample: (BDI) $B_2 \geqslant$ 17, $\chi^2 = 4.56$, d.f. = 1, $P < 0.05$.

p. 255   Changes in test scores: single women

	Aborted	
$B_1 \rightarrow B_2$, B < 10 v. B $\geqslant$ 10	$\chi^2 = 77.6$, d.f. = 1, $P < 0.001$	
(Ex)$_1 \rightarrow$(Ex)$_2$	$t = 4.03$,	$P < 0.001$
(In)$_1 \rightarrow$(In)$_2$	$t = 6.39$,	$P < 0.001$

	Not aborted	
$B_1 \rightarrow B_2$, B < 10 v. B $\geqslant$ 10	$\chi^2 = 27.8$, d.f. = 1, $P < 0.001$	
(Ex)$_1 \rightarrow$(Ex)$_2$	$t = 2.21$,	$P < 0.05$
(In)$_1 \rightarrow$(In)$_2$	$t = 3.77$,	$P < 0.001$

Ever-married women:

	Aborted	
$B_1 \rightarrow B_2$, B < 10 v. B $\geqslant$ 10	$\chi^2 = 79.03$, d.f. = 1, $P < 0.001$	
(Ex)$_1 \rightarrow$(Ex)$_2$	$t = 3.52$,	$P < 0.001$
(In)$_1 \rightarrow$(In)$_2$	$t = 6.20$,	$P < 0.001$

$\begin{array}{lll} & & \text{Not aborted} \\ \text{B}_1 \rightarrow \text{B}_2, \text{B} < \text{10 v. B} \geqslant \text{10} & & \chi^2 = 26.7, \text{d.f.} = 1, P < 0.001 \\ (\text{Ex})_1 \rightarrow (\text{Ex})_2 & & t = 1.34, \text{NS} \\ (\text{In})_1 \rightarrow (\text{In})_2 & & t = 3.27, \qquad P < 0.01 \end{array}$

p. 255 Presence of clinical depression:
Aborted v. non-aborted, single $\chi^2 = 3.70$, d.f. = 1, $P < 0.1$, NS
ever-married $\chi^2 = 0.03$, d.f. = 1, NS
Aborted, single v. ever-married $\chi^2 = 3.82$, d.f. = 1, $P < 0.1$, NS

p. 256 Aborted v. not-aborted:
Regrets, single women $\chi^2 = 6.02$, d.f. = 1, $P < 0.02$
ever-married $\chi^2 = 3.45$, d.f. = 1, $P < 0.1$, NS
Severe regrets,
single women $\chi^2 = 4.48$, d.f. = 1, $P < 0.05$
ever-married $\chi^2 = 0.44$, d.f. = 1, NS

p. 256 Aborted, regrets at three months, single v. ever-married: $\chi^2 = 2.11$, d.f. = 1, NS.
Reduction in regrets, three months to follow-up, single: $\chi^2 = 4.19$, d.f. = 1, $P < 0.05$; ever-married: $\chi^2 = 0.37$, d.f. = 1, NS.

p. 259 Relationship with husband, good v. not good:
Aborted, totals, before index pregnancy v. follow-up: $\chi^2 = 5.98$, d.f. = 1, $P < 0.02$;
sterilised v. non-sterilised, before index pregnancy: $\chi^2 = 6.85$, d.f. = 1, $P < 0.01$.
Not aborted, sterilised v. non-sterilised, before index pregnancy: $\chi^2 = 16.54$, d.f. = 1, $P < 0.001$.

p. 259 Aborted, sexual adjustment, good v. not good: total group before v. follow-up, $\chi^2 = 4.19$, d.f. = 1, $P < 0.05$; sterilised v. non-sterilised, before: $\chi^2 = 0.003$, d.f. = 1, NS; at follow-up, $\chi^2 = 12.05$, d.f. = 1, $P < 0.001$.

p. 260 Non-aborted, sexual adjustment, good v. not good: sterilised v. non-sterilised, before, $\chi^2 = 5.08$, d.f. = 1, $P < 0.05$; at follow-up, $\chi^2 = 10.47$, d.f. = 1, $P < 0.01$.

p. 261 Regrets at treatment, 20–24 v. rest: $\chi^2 = 4.99$, d.f. = 1, $P < 0.05$.

p. 261 Total depression (BDI), class v v. rest: $\chi^2 = 13.85$, d.f. = 1, $P < 0.001$.

p. 262 Depression at follow-up: harmony v. disharmony, $\chi^2 = 12.83$, d.f. = 1, $P < 0.001$; harmony v. parted, $\chi^2 = 15.76$, d.f. = 1, $P < 0.001$.
Aborted, regrets, living with husband v. parted, $\chi^2 = 2.98$, d.f. = 1, $P < 0.10$, NS.

p. 264 Legitimate v. illegitimate: (BDI) $B_2 \geqslant 10$, $\chi^2 = 1.96$, d.f. $= 1$, NS.
Sterilisation in aborted groups: $\chi^2 = 13.6$, d.f. $= 1$, $P < 0.001$.

p. 265 Total regrets, medico-psychiatric and socio-psychiatric v. rest: $\chi^2 = 5.82$, d.f. $= 1$, $P < 0.02$.
Regrets at abortion, medico-psychiatric and socio-psychiatric v. rest: $\chi^2 = 3.74$, d.f. $= 1$, $P < 0.1$, NS.

p. 266 Regrets at follow-up, hysterotomy v. rest: $\chi^2 = 4.4$, d.f. $= 1$, $P < 0.05$.

p. 266 Hysterotomy v. rest, clinical state: $\chi^2 = 5.5$, d.f. $= 1$, $P < 0.02$.

p. 266 Regrets at abortion v. regrets at going to term: single women, $\chi^2 = 5.56$, d.f. $= 1$, $P < 0.02$; ever-married, $\chi^2 = 2.10$, d.f. $= 1$, NS.

TABLE 6:1. *Time elapsing between referral interview and follow-up*

Time in months	No. of patients		% of all	
13	3 ⎤		⎡ 1.0	
14	16 ⎟		⎜ 5.3	
15	64 ⎬ 175	57.8 ⎨	21.1	
16	55 ⎟		⎜ 18.2	
17	37 ⎦		⎣ 12.2	
18–23	68		22.4	
24–29	29		9.6	
30–35	21		6.9	
36+	10		3.3	
	303		100	

TABLE 6:2. *Follow-up and missed groups by marital status and abortion status*

		Marital status at referral		
		Single		Ever-married
Follow-up group	Aborted	72		123
	Not aborted	45		63
	Total followed up	117	Total followed up	186
	% Aborted	61.5		66.1
Missed group	Aborted	27		12
	Not aborted	19		9
	Total	46	Total	21
	% Aborted	58.7		58.1

TABLE 6:3. *Percentage follow-up by marital status and abortion status*

	Single	Ever-married
% Follow-up for aborted group	72.7	91.1
% Follow-up for not aborted group	70.3	87.5
% Follow-up for total group	71.8	89.9

TABLE 6:4. *Categories of response in missed groups*

	Single		Ever-married	
	No.	% Aborted	No.	% Aborted
No trace	33	63.6	9	66.7
No reply	11	45.5	6	66.7
Refused follow-up	2	50.0	6	33.3
Total	46		21	

TABLE 6:5. *16 PF scores at referral for follow-up and missed groups: single women*

16 PF (stens)

		A	B	C	E	F	G	H	I	L	M	N	O	Q_1	Q_2	Q_3	Q_4	MD
									Follow-up group									
Aborted, N = 72	Mean	4.81	6.26	4.44	6.17	4.53	4.57	4.03	6.64	5.63	6.18	6.18	6.00	5.71	4.42	3.47	7.63	3.75
	SD	2.29	1.32	2.05	2.36	2.05	2.43	2.16	1.92	1.99	2.12	1.97	2.05	1.89	2.07	1.58	1.63	2.11
Not aborted, N = 45	Mean	5.64	6.16	4.73	5.93	4.80	4.78	3.96	6.20	5.31	5.89	5.73	6.00	6.02	4.67	4.00	7.00	3.62
	SD	2.48	1.79	2.23	2.53	2.07	2.19	2.18	2.12	1.68	1.98	1.79	2.12	2.20	2.09	2.02	2.20	2.06
Total, N = 117	Mean	5.13	6.22	4.56	6.08	4.63	4.65	4.00	6.47	5.50	6.07	6.01	6.00	5.83	4.51	3.68	7.39	3.70
	SD	2.40	1.52	2.12	2.43	2.06	2.34	2.17	2.01	1.88	2.07	1.92	2.08	2.02	2.08	1.78	1.89	2.09
									Missed group									
Aborted, N = 27	Mean	5.19	6.11	4.63	6.56	4.78	4.15	4.19	5.63	6.48	6.63	5.82	5.78	6.70	5.44	3.41	7.00	4.00
	SD	2.07	1.79	2.06	2.17	2.10	2.32	2.16	2.26	1.97	1.89	1.89	2.23	2.26	1.83	1.91	2.11	2.28
Not aborted, N = 19	Mean	4.90	6.00	4.95	6.11	4.79	4.05	3.68	6.84	6.11	5.90	6.53	6.21	6.16	4.53	3.95	7.58	3.68
	SD	2.29	1.26	2.16	2.29	2.26	2.09	2.43	2.08	1.55	2.27	1.60	1.67	2.54	1.90	1.96	1.82	1.59
Total, N = 46	Mean	5.07	6.07	4.76	6.37	4.78	4.11	3.98	6.13	6.33	6.33	6.11	5.96	6.48	5.07	3.63	7.24	3.87
	SD	2.17	1.59	2.11	2.23	2.17	2.23	2.29	2.27	1.82	2.09	1.81	2.03	2.39	1.92	1.95	2.01	2.03

TABLE 6:6. *Psychological test scores at referral for follow-up and missed groups: single women*

		Beck (B)$_1$	Fould's Extropunitive (Ex)$_1$	Fould's Intropunitive (In)$_1$	N
		Follow-up group			
Aborted	Mean	26.92	12.07	10.72	72
	SD	10.30	4.48	2.93	
Not aborted	Mean	19.60	10.87	8.96	45
	SD	10.11	3.98	3.70	
		Missed group			
Aborted	Mean	23.41	11.82	9.74	27
	SD	10.59	4.51	3.07	
Not aborted	Mean	21.47	10.21	9.95	19
	SD	8.58	4.48	3.15	

TABLE 6:7. *16 PF scores at referral for follow-up and missed groups: ever-married women*

		A	B	C	E	F	G	H	I	L	M	N	O	Q_1	Q_2	Q_3	Q_4	MD
										16 PF (stens)								
								Follow-up group										
Aborted, N = 123	Mean	4.74	5.33	4.50	5.75	3.98	5.48	4.36	6.45	5.84	5.45	5.56	6.68	5.88	5.34	4.46	7.21	4.56
	SD	2.42	1.48	2.01	2.50	1.87	2.17	2.23	1.98	1.85	2.08	1.92	2.02	2.06	1.98	1.85	2.06	2.23
Not aborted, N = 63	Mean	4.98	5.57	4.44	5.83	4.46	5.16	4.84	6.37	5.71	5.22	6.11	5.87	5.62	5.60	4.16	7.13	4.34
	SD	2.13	1.89	2.27	2.09	2.05	2.22	2.35	1.74	1.99	1.93	1.66	2.24	2.16	1.69	1.96	2.08	2.12
Total, N = 186	Mean	4.82	5.41	4.48	5.78	4.14	5.37	4.52	6.42	5.80	5.37	5.75	6.41	5.79	5.43	4.36	7.18	4.49
	SD	2.33	1.64	2.11	2.37	1.94	2.19	2.28	1.90	1.90	2.03	1.86	2.13	2.10	1.89	1.90	2.07	2.20
								Missed group										
Aborted, N = 12	Mean	5.09	4.46	4.82	5.09	4.82	6.91	4.55	6.46	5.27	6.09	6.00	6.36	5.55	5.73	4.46	7.09	4.64
	SD	1.51	1.50	2.04	2.58	1.64	1.83	1.67	2.27	1.60	1.89	2.34	2.39	1.23	1.36	1.50	2.81	2.23
Not aborted, N = 9	Mean	4.22	5.78	4.56	4.78	3.33	5.89	3.00	6.44	5.67	6.00	5.11	7.33	5.22	5.33	2.89	7.67	4.67
	SD	2.10	0.79	1.57	3.05	1.83	2.03	2.00	1.83	1.70	2.05	1.37	1.89	1.81	1.05	1.29	1.70	1.89
Total, N = 21	Mean	4.70	5.05	4.70	4.95	4.15	6.45	3.85	6.45	5.45	6.05	5.60	6.80	5.40	5.55	3.75	7.35	4.65
	SD	1.85	1.40	1.85	2.80	1.88	1.99	1.98	2.09	1.66	1.96	2.01	2.23	1.53	1.24	1.61	2.39	2.08

TABLE 6:8. *Psychological test scores at referral for follow-up and missed groups: ever-married women*

		Beck (B₁)	Fould's Extropunitive (Ex)₁	Fould's Intropunitive (In)₁	N
		Beck (B_1)	Fould's Extropunitive $(Ex)_1$	Fould's Intropunitive $(In)_1$	N
		Follow-up group			
Aborted	Mean	21.22	12.15	10.08	123
	SD	11.50	5.62	3.25	
Not aborted	Mean	17.18	10.95	8.71	63
	SD	11.20	5.34	3.45	
		Missed group			
Aborted	Mean	22.82	10.42	7.67	12
	SD	13.56	5.05	3.39	
Not aborted	Mean	18.22	10.56	10.22	9
	SD	6.82	6.11	2.59	

TABLE 6:9. *BDI scores at referral (B_1) and follow-up (B_2) by outcome*

Beck score	Aborted B_1	Aborted B_2	Not aborted B_1	Not aborted B_2
	Single women			
0–9 'Depression absent'	4 (5.5%)	56 (80%)	9 (20%)	35 (77.8%)
10–16 'Mild depression'	7 (9.7%)	10 (14.3%)	8 (17.8%)	9 (20%)
17–24 'Moderate depression'	17 (23.6%)	3 (4.3%)	14 (31.1%)	1 (2.2%)
25+ 'Severe depression'	44 (61.1%)	1 (1.4%)	14 (31.1%)	0 (0.0%)
Total	72 (100%)	70 (100%)	45 (100%)	45 (100%)
	Ever-married women			
0–9 'Depression absent'	23 (18.7%)	93 (76.2%)	17 (27.0%)	47 (74.6%)
10–16 'Mild depression'	21 (17.1%)	14 (11.5%)	14 (22.2%)	8 (12.7%)
17–24 'Moderate depression'	30 (24.4%)	10 (8.2%)	15 (23.8%)	3 (4.8%)
25+ 'Severe depression'	49 (39.8%)	5 (4.1%)	17 (27.0%)	5 (7.9%)
Total	123 (100%)	122 (100%)	63 (100%)	63 (100%)

TABLE 6:10. *Scores on Fould's Hostility Scales at referral and follow-up by outcome*

		Aborted	N	Not aborted	N
		Single women			
(Ex)$_1$	Mean	12.07	72	10.87	45
	SD	4.48		3.98	
(Ex)$_2$	Mean	9.13	70	8.96	45
	SD	4.15		4.10	
(In)$_1$	Mean	10.72	72	8.96	45
	SD	2.93		3.70	
(In)$_2$	Mean	7.04	70	6.29	45
	SD	3.84		2.90	
		Ever-married women			
(Ex)$_1$	Mean	12.15	123	10.95	63
	SD	5.62		5.34	
(Ex)$_2$	Mean	9.65	123	9.66	62
	SD	5.46		5.34	
(In)$_1$	Mean	10.08	123	8.71	63
	SD	3.25		3.45	
(In)$_2$	Mean	7.12	123	6.68	62
	SD	4.15		3.43	

TABLE 6:11. *Psychiatric treatment reported by patient at follow-up*

	Treatment in year before index pregnancy		Treatment at follow-up	
	Aborted ($N = 72$)	Not aborted ($N = 45$)	Aborted ($N = 72$)	Not aborted ($N = 45$)
Single women				
Treatment by GP for 'nerves'	6	1	3	3
Seen and advised by psychiatrist	0	1	0	0
Psychiatric outpatient	0	0	1	0
Psychiatric day-patient	0	0	0	0
Psychiatric inpatient	0	0	0	0
Total treated	6	2	4	3
	Aborted ($N = 123$)	Not aborted ($N = 63$)	Aborted ($N = 123$)	Not aborted ($N = 63$)
Ever-married women				
Treatment by GP for 'nerves'	24	6	16	3
Seen and advised by psychiatrist	2	1	2	0
Psychiatric outpatient	2	1	1	0
Psychiatric day-patient	0	0	0	0
Psychiatric inpatient	1	0	0	0
Total treated	29	8	19	3

TABLE 6:12. *Clinical assessment and mental state at follow-up*

	Aborted		Not aborted	
	Depression	Anxiety	Depression	Anxiety
Single women				
Nil	64 (88.9%)	69 (95.8%)	33 (73.3%)	41 (91.1%)
Mild	7 (9.7%)	3 (4.2%)	11 (24.4%)	4 (8.9%)
Severe	1 (1.4%)	0	1 (2.2%)	0
	72 (100%)	72 (100%)	45 (100%)	45 (100%)
Ever-married women				
Nil	94 (76.4%)	108 (87.8%)	45 (71.4%)	55 (87.3%)
Mild	26 (21.1%)	15 (12.2%)	17 (27.0%)	8 (12.7%)
Severe	3 (2.4%)	0	1 (1.6%)	0
	123 (100%)	123 (100%)	63 (100%)	63 (100%)

TABLE 6:13. *Attitude to the outcome of the index pregnancy*

	Single	Ever-married
At follow-up:		
Attitude to the abortion:		
Glad had abortion	58 (80.6%)	97 (78.9%)
Mixed feelings, mild regrets	10 (13.9%)	19 (15.4%)
Severe regrets	4 (5.6%)	7 (5.7%)
	72 (100%)	123 (100%)
Attitude to continuing the pregnancy to term:		
Glad went to term	26 (57.8%)	41 (65.1%)
Mixed feelings, mild regrets	10 (22.2%)	16 (25.4%)
Severe regrets	9 (20.0%)	6 (9.5%)
	45 (100%)	63 (100%)
Attitude to abortion three months after the event as reported at follow-up:		
Glad had abortion	46 (63.9%)	92 (74.8%)
Mixed feelings, mild regrets	14 (19.4%)	19 (15.4%)
Severe regrets	12 (16.7%)	12 (9.8%)
	72 (100%)	123 (100%)

TABLE 6:14. *Attitude to continuing pregnancy by adoption and marriage*

Regrets at having continued the index pregnancy	Baby adopted	Baby not adopted	Baby not adopted, unmarried at follow-up
Nil	7 (43.8%)	19 (65.5%)	9 (64.3%)
Mild	2 (12.5%)	8 (27.6%)	4 (28.6%)
Severe	7 (43.8%)	2 (6.9%)	1 (7.1%)
	16 (100%)	29 (100%)	14 (100%)

TABLE 6:15. *Attitudes to sterilisation at follow-up*

	Aborted	Not aborted
Glad at sterilisation	62 (81.6%)	19 (82.6%)
Mixed feelings at sterilisation	8 (10.5%)	4 (17.4%)
Severe regrets at sterilisation	6 (7.9%)	0
Total	76 (100%)	23 (100%)

TABLE 6:16. *BDI scores at follow-up by sterilisation: ever-married women*

B_2	Sterilised	Not sterilised
	Aborted	
0–9	58 (76.3%)	35 (76.1%)
10–16	10 (13.2%)	4 (8.7%)
17–24	5 (6.6%)	5 (10.9%)
25+	3 (3.9%)	2 (4.3%)
Total	76 (100%)	46 (100%)
	Not aborted	
0–9	20 (87.0%)	27 (67.5%)
10–16	1 (4.3%)	7 (17.5%)
17–24	2 (8.7%)	1 (2.5%)
25+	0 (0%)	5 (12.5%)
Total	23 (100%)	40 (100%)

TABLE 6:17. *Relationship with husband as rated by the women at follow-up: ever-married aborted*

State of relationship	Before index pregnancy			At follow-up		
	Not sterilised	Sterilised	Total	Not sterilised	Sterilised	Total
Good	14 (30.4%)	43 (56.6%)	57 (46.7%)	22 (47.8%)	55 (72.4%)	77 (63.1%)
Strained	19 (41.3%)	28 (36.8%)	47 (38.5%)	6 (13%)	15 (19.7%)	21 (17.2%)
Broken	13 (28.3%)	5 (6.6%)	18 (14.8%)	18 (39.1%)	6 (7.9%)	24 (19.7%)
Total	46 (100%)	76 (100%)	122 (100%)	46 (100%)	76 (100%)	122 (100%)

TABLE 6:18. *Relationship with husband as rated by the women at follow-up: ever-married not aborted*

State of relationship	Before index pregnancy			At follow-up		
	Not sterilised	Sterilised	Total	Not sterilised	Sterilised	Total
Good	14 (35.0%)	21 (91.3%)	35 (55.6%)	15 (37.5%)	21 (91.3%)	36 (57.1%)
Strained	13 (32.5%)	2 (8.7%)	15 (23.8%)	11 (27.5%)	1 (4.3%)	12 (19.0%)
Broken	13 (32.5%)	0	13 (20.6%)	14 (35.0%)	1 (4.3%)	15 (23.8%)
Total	40 (100%)	23 (100%)	63 (100%)	40 (100%)	23 (100%)	63 (100%)

TABLE 6:19. *Sexual adjustment as rated by ever-married aborted women at follow-up*

Sexual adjustment	Before index pregnancy			At follow-up		
	Not sterilised	Sterilised	Total	Not sterilised	Sterilised	Total
Good	18 (38.3%)	30 (39.5%)	48 (39%)	15 (31.9%)	50 (65.8%)	65 (52.8%)
Lukewarm	13 (27.7%)	29 (38.2%)	42 (34.1%)	10 (21.3%)	16 (21.1%)	26 (21.1%)
Poor	12 (25.5%)	16 (21.1%)	28 (22.8%)	9 (19.1%)	8 (10.5%)	17 (13.8%)
Not applicable	4 (8.5%)	1 (1.3%)	5 (4.1%)	13 (27.7%)	2 (2.6%)	15 (12.2%)
	47 (100%)	76 (100%)	123 (100%)	47 (100%)	76 (100%)	123 (100%)

TABLE 6:20. *Sexual adjustment as rated by non-aborted ever-married women at follow-up*

Sexual adjustment	Before index pregnancy			At follow-up		
	Not sterilised	Sterilised	Total	Not sterilised	Sterilised	Total
Good	13 (32.5%)	15 (65.2%)	23 (44.4%)	13 (32.5)	18 (78.3%)	31 (49.2%)
Lukewarm	18 (45.0%)	7 (30.4%)	25 (39.7%)	13 (32.5%)	4 (17.4%)	17 (27.0%)
Poor	5 (12.5%)	1 (4.3%)	6 (9.5%)	8 (20.0%)	0 (0.0%)	8 (12.7%)
Not applicable	4 (10.0%)	0	4 (6.3%)	6 (15.0%)	1 (4.3%)	7 (11.1%)
Total	40 (100%)	23 (100%)	63 (100%)	40 (100%)	23 (100%)	63 (100%)

TABLE 6:21. *Social class by age: single women*

Social class	Aborted				Not aborted				Grand total			
	15–19	20–24	25+	Total	15–19	20–24	25+	Total	15–19	20–24	25+	Total
Professional	0	0	3	3	0	6	0	6	0	6	3	9
Student	12	13	0	25	7	6	0	13	19	19	0	38
Clerical and distributive	11	12	0	23	15	3	1	19	26	15	1	42
Manual	7	8	6	21	2	2	3	7	9	10	9	28
Totals	30	33	9	72	24	17	4	45	54	50	13	117

TABLE 6:22. *Regrets about 'treatment' by class and age: single women*

Social class	Aborted				Not aborted				Grand total			
	15–19	20–24	25+	Total	15–19	20–24	25+	Total	15–19	20–24	25+	Total
Professional	0	0	1 (50)	1 (33.3)	0	4 (66.7)	0	4 (66.7)	0	4 (66.7)	1 (33.3)	5 (55.6)
Student	5 (41.7)	0	0	5 (20)	2 (28.6)	4 (66.7)	0	6 (46.2)	7 (36.8)	4 (21.2)	0	11 (28.9)
Clerical and distributive	3 (27.3)	1 (8.3)	0	4 (17.4)	6 (40)	0	1 (100)	7 (36.8)	9 (34.6)	1 (6.7)	1 (100)	11 (26.2)
Manual	1 (14.3)	1 (12.5)	1 (16.7)	3 (14.3)	1 (50)	0	1 (33.3)	2 (28.6)	2 (22.2)	1 (10.0)	2 (22.2)	5 (17.9)
Totals	9 (30)	2 (5.9)	2 (25)	13 (18.1)	9 (37.5)	8 (47.1)	2 (50)	19 (42.2)	18 (33.3)	10 (20)	4 (30.8)	32 (27.4)

Figures in brackets denote respective % of age–class group.

TABLE 6:23. *Depression on the Beck Inventory ($B_2 \geqslant 10$) by class and age: single women*

Social class	Aborted				Not aborted				Grand total			
	15–19	20–24	25+	Total	15–19	20–24	25+	Total	15–19	20–24	25+	Total
Professional	0 (0.0)	0 (0.0)	2 (100)	2 (66.7)	0	3 (50)	0	3 (50)	0	3 (50)	2 (66.7)	5 (55.6)
Student	3 (25.0)	1 (9.1)	0	4 (16)	0	1 (16.7)	0	1 (7.7)	3 (15.8)	2 (10.5)	0	5 (13.2)
Clerical and distributive	1 (9.1)	2 (16.7)	0	3 (13)	6 (40)	0	0	6 (31.6)	7 (26.9)	2 (13.3)	0	9 (21.4)
Manual	2 (28.6)	3 (37.5)	0	5 (23.8)	0	0	0	0	2 (22.2)	3 (30)	0	5 (17.9)
Total	6 (20.0)	6 (17.6)	2 (25)	14 (19.4)	6 (25)	4 (23.5)	0	10 (22.2)	12 (22.2)	10 (20)	2 (15.4)	24 (20.5)

Figures in brackets denote respective % of age–class group.

288

TABLE 6:24. *Social class by age: ever-married women*

Social class	Aborted			Not aborted			Grand total		
	Under 30	30+	Total	Under 30	30+	Total	Under 30	30+	Total
I and II	8	14	22	1	4	5	9	18	27
III	16	40	56	18	11	29	34	51	85
IV	17	11	28	6	9	15	23	20	43
V	13	4	17	10	4	14	23	8	31
Totals	54	69	123	35	28	63	89	97	186

TABLE 6:25. *Regrets about the 'treatment' by class and age: ever-married women*

Social class	Aborted			Not aborted			Grand total		
	Under 30	30+	Total	Under 30	30+	Total	Under 30	30+	Total
I and II	1 (12.5)	1 (7.1)	2 (9.1)	0	0	0	1 (11.1)	1 (5.6)	2 (7.4)
III	4 (25.0)	12 (30.0)	16 (28.6)	7 (38.9)	4 (36.4)	11 (37.9)	11 (32.4)	16 (31.4)	27 (31.8)
IV	4 (23.5)	4 (36.4)	8 (28.6)	2 (33.3)	3 (33.3)	5 (33.3)	6 (26.1)	7 (35.0)	13 (30.2)
V	0	0	0	5 (50.0)	1 (25.0)	6 (42.9)	5 (21.7)	1 (12.5)	6 (19.4)
Totals	9 (16.7)	17 (24.6)	26 (21.1)	14 (40.0)	8 (28.6)	22 (34.9)	23 (25.8)	25 (25.8)	48 (25.8)

Figures in brackets denote % of respective age–class group.

TABLE 6:26. *Depression on the Beck Inventory ($B_2 \geq 10$) by class and age: ever-married women*

Social class	Aborted			Not aborted			Grand total		
	Under 30	30+	Total	Under 30	30+	Total	Under 30	30+	Total
I and II	1 (12.5)	4 (28.6)	5 (22.7)	0	0	0	1 (11.1)	4 (22.2)	5 (18.5)
III	6 (37.5)	6 (15.0)	12 (21.4)	4 (22.2)	0	4 (13.8)	10 (29.4)	6 (11.8)	16 (18.8)
IV	3 (17.6)	3 (27.3)	6 (21.4)	1 (16.7)	1 (11.1)	2 (13.3)	4 (17.4)	4 (20.0)	8 (18.6)
V	6 (42.6)	0	6 (35.3)	6 (60.0)	4 (100)	10 (71.4)	12 (52.2)	4 (50.0)	16 (51.6)
Total	16 (29.6)	13 (18.8)	29 (23.6)	11 (31.4)	5 (17.9)	16 (25.4)	27 (30.3)	18 (18.6)	45 (24.2)

Figures in brackets denote % of respective age–class group.

TABLE 6:27. *Attitude to 'treatment' and presence of depression on the BDI by marital status: ever-married women*

	Aborted			Not aborted			Total		
	N	% Regrets	% De-pressed B_2	N	% Regrets	% De-pressed B_2	N	% Regrets	% De-pressed B_2
'Harmony'	80	23.8	15.2	42	31.0	14.3	122	26.2	14.9
'Disharmony'	22	27.3	50.0	11	45.5	36.4	33	33.3	45.5
'Parted' from husband	21	4.8	28.6	10	40.0	60.0	31	16.1	38.7

TABLE 6:28. *Attitude to the abortion as determined at the time of follow-up by marital status*

Aborted	Unmarried at referral and follow-up	Unmarried at referral but married at follow-up
Glad had abortion	44 (80.0%)	14 (82.4%)
Mixed feelings	8 (14.5%)	2 (11.8%)
Severe regrets	3 (5.5%)	1 (5.9%)
Total	55 (100%)	17 (100%)

TABLE 6:29. *Attitude to continuing the pregnancy to term as determined at the time of follow-up by marital status*

Not aborted	Unmarried at referral and follow-up	Unmarried at referral but married at follow-up
Glad went to term	16 (55.2%)	10 (62.5%)
Mixed feelings	6 (20.7%)	4 (25.0%)
Severe regrets	7 (24.1%)	2 (12.5%)
Total	29 (100%)	16 (100%)

TABLE 6:30. *Beck Depression Inventory scores at follow-up* (B_2) *for single women by marital status at follow-up*

B_2		Aborted		Not aborted	
		Unmarried	Married	Unmarried	Married
0–9	'Depression absent'	43 (81.1%)	13 (76.5%)	19 (65.5%)	16 (100.0%)
10–16	'Mild depression'	6 (11.3%)	4 (23.5%)	9 (31.0%)	0 (0.0%)
17–24	'Moderate depression'	3 (5.7%)	0 (0.0%)	1 (3.4%)	0 (0.0%)
25+	'Severe depression'	1 (1.9%)	0 (0.0%)	0 (0.0%)	0 (0.0%)
Total		53 (100%)	17 (100%)	29 (100%)	16 (100%)

TABLE 6:31. *Sexual adjustment as rated at follow-up by single aborted women*

Sexual adjustment in aborted group	Before index pregnancy			At follow-up		
	Unmarried	Married	Total	Unmarried	Married	Total
Good	19 (35.2%)	4 (23.5%)	23 (32.4%)	12 (22.2%)	14 (82.4%)	26 (36.6%)
Lukewarm	17 (31.5%)	3 (17.6%)	20 (28.2%)	4 (7.4%)	2 (11.8%)	6 (8.5%)
Poor	5 (9.3%)	3 (17.6%)	8 (11.3%)	11 (20.4%)	1 (5.9%)	12 (16.9%)
Not applicable	13 (24.1%)	7 (41.2%)	20 (28.2%)	27 (50.0%)	0 (0.0%)	27 (38.0%)
Total	54 (100%)	17 (100%)	71 (100%)	54 (100%)	17 (100%)	71 (100%)

TABLE 6:32. *Sexual adjustment as rated at follow-up by single women who were not aborted*

Sexual adjustment in 'not aborted' group	Before index pregnancy			At follow-up		
	Unmarried	Married	Total	Unmarried	Married	Total
Good	13 (44.8%)	8 (50.0%)	21 (46.7%)	9 (31.0%)	14 (87.5%)	23 (51.1%)
Lukewarm	7 (24.1%)	1 (6.3%)	8 (17.8%)	0 (0.0%)	2 (12.5%)	2 (4.4%)
Poor	3 (10.3%)	0 (0.0%)	3 (6.7%)	4 (13.8%)	0 (0.0%)	4 (8.9%)
Not applicable	6 (20.7%)	7 (43.8%)	13 (28.9%)	16 (55.2%)	0 (0.0%)	16 (35.6%)
Total	29 (100%)	16 (100%)	45 (100%)	29 (100%)	16 (100%)	45 (100%)

TABLE 6:33. *Outcome by legitimacy of index pregnancy: aborted ever-married women*

Index of outcome	Illegitimate ($N = 21$)	Legitimate ($N = 102$)
% of aborted group in follow-up	17.1	82.9
Beck Depression $B_2 \geqslant 10$	6 (28.6)	23 (22.5)
Clinical depression or anxiety	6 (28.6)	31 (30.4)
Regrets about abortion	3 (14.3)	23 (22.5)
Number sterilised	5 (23.8)	71 (69.6)
Regrets about sterilisation	3	11
% of those sterilised with regrets	60.0	15.5

Figures in parentheses refer to % of respective group, i.e. illegitimate or legitimate.

TABLE 6:34. *Comparison of outcome for non-aborted ever-married women with illegitimate and legitimate pregnancies*

Index of outcome	Illegitimate ($N = 10$)	Legitimate ($N = 53$)
% of not aborted group in follow-up	15.9	84.1
Beck Depression $B_2 \geqslant 10$	5 (50.0)	11 (20.8)
Clinical depression or anxiety	3 (30.0)	16 (30.2)
Regrets about continuing the pregnancy	4 (40.0)	18 (34.0)
Number sterilised	0 (0.0)	23 (43.4)
Regrets about sterilisation	0	4
% of those sterilised with regrets	0	17.4

Figures in parentheses refer to % of the respective pregnancy group, i.e. illegitimate or legitimate. 'Aborted' includes spontaneous and self-induced types as well as those performed by a gynaecologist.

TABLE 6:35. *Attitude to treatment and presence of depression on the BDI at follow-up by main indication*

	Aborted			Not aborted			Total		
	N	% Regrets	% Depressed B_2	N	% Regrets	% Depressed B_2	N	% Regrets	% Depressed B_2
				Single women					
Medico-psychiatric	11	18.2	†50.0	0	0.0	0.0	11	18.2	†50.0
Socio-psychiatric	38	10.5	†18.9	16	37.5	18.8	54	17.0	†18.9
Social	20	35.0	5.0	28	46.4	25.0	48	41.7	16.7
Medical and eugenic	3	33.3	33.3	1	0.0	0.0	4	25.0	25.0
				Ever-married women					
Medico-psychiatric	17	11.8	23.5	2	50.0	100.0	19	15.8	31.6
Socio-psychiatric	34	26.5	32.4	10	50.0	20.0	44	31.8	29.5
Social	59	20.3	†20.7	39	30.8	25.6	98	24.5	†22.7
Medical and eugenic	13	23.1	15.4	12	33.3	16.7	25	28.0	16.0

Depression defined as Beck score $B_2 \geqslant 10$.
† Denotes one woman in the section had not completed the BDI.

TABLE 6:36. *Outcome at follow-up by type of termination: single women*

	D & C	Suction	Saline	Hysterotomy	'Spontaneous'	Total
Number terminated	15	11	31	9	6	72
Beck score $B_2 \geqslant 10$	3 (20.0)	3 (27.3)	8 (25.8)	1 (11.1)	0	15 (20.8)
Clinical depression or anxiety	0	3 (27.3)	8 (25.8)	0	0	11 (15.3)
Regrets at the abortion						
3 months after abortion	2 (13.4)	5 (45.5)	15 (48.4)	3 (33.3)	1 (16.7)	26 (36.1)
At follow-up	1 (6.7)	3 (27.3)	7 (22.6)	2 (22.2)	1 (16.7)	14 (19.4)

Figures in brackets denote % of termination type.

TABLE 6:37. *Outcome at follow-up by type of termination: ever-married women*

	D & C	Suction	Saline	Hystero-tomy	'Spontaneous' or 'criminal'	Total
Number terminated	15	17	5	70	16	123
Beck score $B_2 \geqslant$ 10	5	3	2	19	0	29
	(33.3)	(17.6)	(40.0)	(27.1)	(0.0)	(23.6)
Clinical depression	2	6	1	26	2	37
or anxiety	(13.3)	(35.3)	(20.0)	(37.1)	(12.5)	(30.1)
Regrets at the abortion						
3 months after	3	5	1	22	0	31
abortion	(20.0)	(29.4)	(20.0)	(31.4)		(25.2)
At follow-up	2	3	0	20	1	26
	(13.3)	(17.6)	(0.0)	(28.6)	(6.3)	(21.1)

Figures in brackets denote % of termination type.

TABLE 6:38. *Beck score at follow-up by type of gynaecologist: single women*

	Aborted		Not aborted		Total aborted and not aborted	
	'Liberal'	'Conservative'	'Liberal'	'Conservative'	'Liberal'	'Conservative'
0–9 'Depression absent'	36 (73.5%)	20 (92.3%)	11 (78.6%)	23 (79.3%)	47 (74.6%)	43 (86.0%)
10–16 'Mild depression'	9 (18.4%)	1 (7.7%)	3 (21.4%)	5 (17.2%)	12 (19.0%)	6 (12.0%)
17–24 'Moderate depression'	3 (6.1%)	0	0	1 (3.4%)	3 (4.8%)	1 (2.0%)
25+ 'Severe depression'	1 (2.0%)	0	0	0	1 (1.6%)	0
	49 (100%)	21 (100%)	14 (100%)	29 (100%)	63 (100%)	50 (100%)

TABLE 6:39. *Beck score at follow-up by type of gynaecologist: ever-married women*

	Aborted		Not aborted		Total aborted and not aborted	
	'Liberal'	'Conservative'	'Liberal'	'Conservative'	'Liberal'	'Conservative'
0–9 'Depression absent'	57 (72.2%)	36 (83.7%)	21 (80.8%)	25 (69.4%)	78 (74.3%)	61 (77.2%)
10–16 'Mild depression'	10 (12.7%)	4 (9.3%)	0	8 (22.2%)	10 (9.5%)	12 (15.2%)
17–24 'Moderate depression'	9 (11.4%)	1 (2.3%)	3 (11.5%)	0	12 (11.4%)	1 (1.3%)
25+ 'Severe depression'	3 (3.8%)	2 (4.7%)	2 (7.7%)	3 (8.3%)	5 (4.8%)	5 (6.3%)
	79 (100%)	43 (100%)	26 (100%)	36 (100%)	105 (100%)	79 (100%)

TABLE 6:40. *Attitude to outcome by type of gynaecologist: single women*

Attitude to outcome	Aborted		Not aborted		Total aborted and not aborted	
	'Liberal'	'Conservative'	'Liberal'	'Conservative'	'Liberal'	'Conservative'
Glad	40 (80.0%)	18 (85.7%)	8 (57.1%)	17 (58.6%)	48 (75.0%)	35 (70%)
Mild regrets	8 (16.0%)	2 (9.5%)	2 (14.3%)	7 (24.1%)	10 (15.6%)	9 (18.0%)
Severe regrets	2 (4.0%)	1 (4.8%)	4 (28.6%)	5 (17.2%)	6 (9.4%)	6 (12.0%)
Total	50 (100%)	21 (100%)	14 (100%)	29 (100%)	64 (100%)	50 (100%)

TABLE 6:41. *Attitude to outcome by type of gynaecologist: ever-married women*

Attitude to outcome	Aborted		Not aborted		Total aborted and not aborted	
	'Liberal'	'Conservative'	'Liberal'	'Conservative'	'Liberal'	'Conservative'
Glad	63 (78.8%)	34 (79.1%)	18 (69.2%)	23 (63.9%)	81 (76.4%)	57 (72.2%)
Mild regrets	14 (17.5%)	5 (11.6%)	7 (26.9%)	8 (22.2%)	21 (19.8%)	13 (16.5%)
Severe regrets	3 (3.8%)	4 (9.3%)	1 (3.8%)	5 (13.9%)	4 (3.8%)	9 (11.4%)
Total	80 (100%)	43 (100%)	26 (100%)	36 (100%)	106 (100%)	79 (100%)

TABLE 6:42. *16 PF scores of non-depressed and depressed patients at follow-up as assessed by the Beck Depression Inventory*

								16 PF (stens)									
	A	B	C	E	F	G	H	I	L	M	N	O	Q_1	Q_2	Q_3	Q_4	MD
Single women																	
'Depression absent' $B_2 < 10$ N = 91 Mean	5.25	6.23	4.69	6.24	4.67	4.45	4.18	6.43	5.41	5.93	6.14	5.85	5.87	4.47	3.79	7.36	3.69
SD	2.38	1.49	2.12	2.43	1.98	2.36	2.16	2.03	1.92	2.09	1.90	2.10	2.01	2.01	1.87	1.88	2.12
'Depressed' $B_2 \geqslant 10$ N = 24 Mean	4.63	6.29	4.08	5.75	4.46	5.25	3.42	6.63	6.17	6.67	5.58	6.50	5.75	4.83	3.13	7.54	3.65
SD	2.48	1.64	2.14	2.20	2.33	2.17	2.10	2.00	1.34	1.95	1.89	1.94	2.24	2.25	1.20	1.98	1.99
Ever-married women																	
'Depression absent' $B_2 < 10$ N = 140 Mean	4.83	5.53	4.75	5.74	4.10	5.45	4.62	6.49	5.58	5.25	5.76	6.42	5.61	5.51	4.41	6.98	4.77
SD	2.34	1.64	2.15	2.43	2.00	2.24	2.34	1.88	1.89	2.08	1.76	2.11	2.11	1.91	1.87	2.16	2.15
'Depressed' $B_2 \geqslant 10$ N = 44 Mean	4.86	5.05	3.66	5.84	4.27	5.14	4.18	6.21	6.46	5.71	5.61	6.36	6.36	5.14	4.14	7.84	3.62
SD	2.26	1.60	1.73	2.16	1.78	2.03	2.06	1.97	1.79	1.80	2.10	2.23	1.98	1.82	1.96	1.60	2.10

7 OVERALL CLINICAL PSYCHIATRIC ASSESSMENT

Colin McCance, Peter C. Olley and Vivien Edward

INTRODUCTION

An unwanted pregnancy inevitably presents a dilemma. For a married woman, especially if she is already extended in her roles as wife and mother, an extra child which she had not intended to have, will increase the demands upon her and further tax her psychological, physical and material resources, possibly to her own serious detriment and to that of her family. For a single woman, an illegitimate child is likely to narrow her options, may ruin her career prospects, force her into an undesirable marriage or force her to face a burden of disapprobation or even alienation from her relatives.

Yet an abortion may also be a damaging experience, physically and mentally. Which is the better of the two evils? The following clinical study of the long-term psychological and social effects of unwanted pregnancy aborted and not aborted is offered to complement the data analysis presented in the previous chapter.

The imperfections of this method and the problems of categorising complex human situations according to whether certain procedures, undertaken mainly between one and two-and-a-half years previously, have been beneficial, adverse or non-contributory, will be all too obvious. The women studied were widely different in age, parity and marital status, not to mention intelligence, personality and social circumstances. Some of their pregnancies were legitimate and others not and they had been subjected to a number of different procedures, some early and some far later in pregnancy. Furthermore, they had encountered a variety of general practitioners, gynaecologists, and in some cases psychiatrists, some harrassed and perhaps impatient, some disapproving, some sympathetic and consoling. No prospective matching or random allocation to treatment and control groups was considered either ethical or possible.

Whether or not an abortion had been done could not be concealed from the psychiatrists who saw the women at follow-up so that the judgement of each was unavoidably tainted with this knowledge as well as with personal prejudices, however genuine the attempt to be objective. By presenting a number of cases in some detail, however, it is hoped that even if the reader disagrees with the conclusions, he may at least be able to draw some of his own.

The clinical classification which follows has been orientated particularly to examine the 'effectiveness' or otherwise of abortion and sterilisation as the two main forms of active medical intervention. The case material has been set out to illustrate how a variety of personal situations has been categorised and should be read with reference to Table 7:1 and the summary classifications which follow.

Classification of case material according to the contribution of the factor-complex abortion yes/no – sterilisation yes/no, to the psychological state of each woman at follow-up

OVERALL VIEW OF CATEGORIES AND LAY-OUT

A Ever-married women who had an abortion and sterilisation.
- A1 Five examples of a *beneficial* contribution (30 cases in all).
- A2 Four examples of an *adverse* contribution (9 cases in all).
- A3 A *conflicting* contribution.
  - A3(a) Two examples where abortion made a beneficial contribution but sterilisation made an adverse one (6 cases in all).
  - A3(b) One example where abortion had made an adverse contribution but sterilisation was beneficial (3 cases in all).
  - A3(c) Two examples where abortion and sterilisation had led to ambivalent feelings and a mixed picture (4 cases in all).
- A4 A relatively *unimportant* contribution.
  - A4(a) Three examples where personality problems, adverse circumstances or other factors were largely responsible for an unsatisfactory psychological state but where there were no regrets about abortion and sterilisation (8 cases in all).
  - A4(c) Two examples where adequate personality resources and tolerable circumstances were largely responsible for a satisfactory psychological state and where there were no regrets about abortion and sterilisation (10 cases in all).
  - A4(d) One example where adequate personality resources and tolerable circumstances were largely responsible for a satisfactory psychological state, but where there were some regrets about abortion and sterilisation (3 cases in all).

B Single women who had an abortion and sterilisation.
(The question of sterilisation so seldom arises in this group that it is usually irrelevant but is included for consistency.)
B1 A *beneficial* contribution (one case which is not described).
B3 A *conflicting* contribution.
  B3(*b*) One example where abortion had made a (mildly) adverse contribution to the psychological state at follow-up but sterilisation was beneficial (the only case in this category).

C Ever-married women who had an abortion but not a sterilisation.
C1 Six examples of a *beneficial* contribution (19 cases in all).
C2 There was no case where the contribution was purely *adverse*.
C3 A *conflicting* contribution.
  C3(*a*) Two examples where abortion made a beneficial contribution but lack of sterilisation was regretted or made an adverse contribution (11 cases in all).
  C3(*b*) One example where abortion had made an adverse contribution but where retained fertility was beneficial (2 cases in all).
  C3(*c*) One example where abortion and no sterilisation had led to ambivalent feelings and a mixed picture (2 cases in all).
C4 A relatively *unimportant* contribution.
  C4(*a*) Two examples where personality problems, adverse circumstances or other factors were largely responsible for an unsatisfactory psychological state but where abortion and retained fertility were not regretted (5 cases).

D. Single women who had an abortion but no sterilisation.
D1 Four examples of a *beneficial* contribution (40 cases in all).
D2 Two examples of an *adverse* contribution (5 cases in all).
D3 A *conflicting* contribution.
  D3(*c*) Three examples where there were ambivalent feelings towards the abortion (6 cases in all).
D4 A relatively *unimportant* contribution.
  D4(*a*) One example where personality problems, adverse circumstances or other factors were largely responsible for an unsatisfactory psychological state at follow-up, but where there were no regrets about abortion (3 cases in all).
  D4(*b*) One example where personality problems, adverse circumstances or other factors were largely responsible for an unsatisfactory psychological state and where abortion was regretted (3 cases in all).
  D4(*c*) Two examples where adequate personality resources and tolerable circumstances were largely responsible for a satisfactory psychological state and where there were no regrets about abortion (2 cases in all).
  D4(*d*) One example where adequate personality resources and tolerable circumstances were largely responsible for a

satisfactory psychological state but where there were some regrets about abortion (3 cases in all).

D5 Three examples where abortion had been the source of much distress to the woman for a period, but where, by the time of follow-up, she had readjusted herself and her psychological state was found to be satisfactory or good (7 cases in all).

E Ever-married women who were sterilised but not aborted.

E1 One example of a *beneficial* contribution (4 cases in all).

E2 There were no cases where the contribution was purely *adverse*.

E3 A *conflicting* contribution.

E3(*a*) One example where continuing to term made a beneficial contribution but sterilisation was regretted (2 cases in all).

E3(*b*) Two cases where continuing to term made an adverse contribution or was regretted but sterilisation was beneficial (5 cases in all).

E3(*c*) One example where continuing to term and sterilisation had led to ambivalent feelings, and a mixed picture (4 cases in all).

E4 A relatively *unimportant* contribution.

E4(*c*) One example where adequate personality resources were largely responsible for a satisfactory psychological state and where there were no regrets about sterilisation and continuing the pregnancy to term (6 cases in all).

G Ever-married women neither sterilised nor aborted.

G1 Two examples of a *beneficial* contribution (12 cases in all).

G2 Five examples of an *adverse* contribution (10 cases in all).

G3 A *conflicting* contribution.

G3(*a*) One example where going to term was beneficial but lack of sterilisation was regretted or made an adverse contribution (2 cases in all).

G3(*c*) One example where going to term and not having a sterilisation had led to ambivalent feelings and a mixed picture (4 cases in all).

G4 A relatively *unimportant* contribution.

G4(*a*) One example where personality problems, adverse circumstances or other factors were largely responsible for an unsatisfactory psychological state but where there were no regrets about continuing the pregnancy to term, and not having a sterilisation (3 cases in all).

G4(*c*) Two examples where adequate personality resources and tolerable circumstances were largely responsible for a satisfactory psychological state and where there were no regrets about continuing the pregnancy to term and not having a sterilisation (9 cases in all).

H   Single women who had neither abortion nor sterilisation.
  Hɪ   Five examples of a *beneficial* contribution (10 cases in all).
  H2   Four examples of an *adverse* contribution (15 cases in all).
  H3   A *conflicting* contribution.
          H3(c)   One example where continuing the pregnancy to term
                  (without sterilisation) had led to ambivalent feelings and a
                  mixed picture (3 cases in all).
  H4   A relatively *unimportant* contribution.
          H4(a)   One example where personality problems, adverse circum-
                  stances or other factors were largely responsible for an
                  unsatisfactory psychological state but where there were no
                  regrets about continuing the pregnancy to term (and not
                  having a sterilisation) (2 cases in all).
          H4(c)   Two examples where adequate personality resources and
                  tolerable circumstances were largely responsible for a
                  satisfactory psychological state and where there were no
                  regrets about going to term (5 cases in all).
          H4(d)   One example where adequate personality resources and
                  tolerable circumstances were largely responsible for a
                  satisfactory psychological state but where there were some
                  regrets about going to term (4 cases in all).
  H5   One example where continuing the pregnancy to term had been a
       source of much distress for a period but where, by the time of
       follow-up, a readjustment had taken place and the psychological
       state was found to be satisfactory or good (5 cases in all).

CASE REPORTS†

A   Ever-married women who had an abortion and sterilisation

The two operations are quite frequently combined in married women
when the family is complete. Seventy-six of the women in the series
had both operations representing 25 per cent of the total cohort and
41 per cent of the ever-married women in the series. Three-fifths of the
ever-married women who had abortions also had sterilisations. In
assessing the consequences of abortion in this group of women, therefore, it is necessary to try to distinguish the separate or combined contributions of each operation to the overall outcome. In 30 of the 76
cases the overall contribution was judged beneficial.

† Throughtout the case reports, those judged to be or to have been severely upset
  by the outcome of their request for abortion are distinguished with an asterisk.
  They represent examples of the cases enumerated in parentheses in Table 7:1.

AI BENEFICIAL CONTRIBUTION

Case 171. A woman of 34 in whom a fear of pregnancy had been 'haunting her life'. She described her feelings on becoming pregnant for the fourth time with the phrase, 'The bottom was knocked out of my world.' Termination of the fifth pregnancy and tubal ligation gave her 'a new lease of life'. Sexual relationships with her husband had vastly improved. She was getting on far better with him generally and was coping much better with the children.

Case 157. A 31-year-old woman with two children who was having difficulty coping with her second baby, had lost all interest in sex and whose relationship with her husband had become strained. She hadn't been able to take the pill, a sheath did not afford her sufficient peace of mind and although the coil had allayed her fears of pregnancy, it had failed to prevent it. Following hysterotomy and tubal ligation her interest in sex returned, her relationship with her husband became good and she got on top of the domestic situation.

Case 53. A 33-year-old woman with four children living in two rooms. Her mild depression and considerable anxiety faded following hysterotomy and tubal ligation. She had some doubts about the morality of abortion but no regrets. She felt that the practical advantages outweighed any moral considerations. Sexual relationships with her husband had become more relaxed and satisfying after the sterilisation.

Case 75. A woman of 35 with two children who reported that she was 'feeling great'. She was enthusiastic that her abortion and sterilisation were absolutely right for her. Her enjoyment of sexual relationships with her husband had greatly improved.

Case 108. A woman in her early thirties with three children. She was coping well with them and doing a part-time job. She was very depressed at the time of crisis but at follow-up her mood was normal and there was much improvement in her sexual relationships since the sterilisation. She had occasionally wondered whether she could have managed the baby after all, but on balance this was seen as a beneficial procedure complex.

In contrast to the foregoing, there were 9 cases where the overall contribution of abortion and sterilisation to the person's long-term psychological and social condition was judged to be adverse. Four examples of this category follow.

A2 ADVERSE CONTRIBUTION

Case 15. The patient in her early forties had two children at the time of referral. The relationship with her husband was basically good though her interest in sex was rather luke-warm. At follow-up, though the sexual side of things had improved there had clearly been a lot of guilty unhappy soul-searching over the abortion and sterilisation which had not yet been resolved.

Case 184. A woman in her late thirties, married for the second time. She had been a regular attender at psychiatric outpatients and had inpatient treatment for depression. At follow-up she bitterly regretted both abortion and sterilisation. She felt she had denied her second husband the chance of having more than one child. (She herself had already had five children, one to her present husband and two extra-maritally.) She had lost interest in sex and felt there was 'no point in it' when she couldn't become pregnant.

Case 189. The patient in her early thirties was mildly depressed at follow-up, clearly due to the recent death of her mother. At the time of the patient's abortion the mother had been very ill: had this not been the case, the patient would have struggled through her fourth pregnancy, obtaining her mother's help with her three children instead of asking for an abortion. She felt considerable guilt over having had an abortion and since her mother had left her some money she took the view that 'the child was sacrificed unnecessarily'.

Case 195. The patient, aged 32, was depressed, due to her having had a hysterectomy for uterine pathology since when she had experienced no sexual response at intercourse. She regretted that she had had an abortion and sterilisation.

In some instances the effects of the abortion and the sterilisation seem to conflict with each other, the one having a beneficial, the other an adverse contribution. These are labelled 'conflicting' and a few examples are set out below in three sub-categories.

A3 CONFLICTING CONTRIBUTION

A3(*a*) *Case 276.* A divorced woman of 29 with three children. A basically stable person who had no regrets about the abortion but regretted sterilisation as she was wanting to remarry.

Case 102. The patient, in her early thirties, was living at home with her eight children. Her alcoholic husband used to drop in to see her occasionally. She sought an abortion on the grounds that she couldn't cope with another child at that juncture, having already got three children under 4. At follow-up she was glad she had had the abortion since pregnancy at that time was an inconvenience, but she regarded the sterilisation as 'a terrible mistake'. She never felt well unless she was pregnant and she now found that she hadn't enough to do. She wanted the operation 'reversed'.

A3(*b*) *Case 40*. A grand multipara in her late thirties who was perfectly happy about the sterilisation but there had been nearly two months delay between first going to the doctor and having the termination and by then she felt pressed by the doctors to have it and obliged to agree. At follow-up she said, 'I needed a lot of convincing. I wasn't so keen if cutting was involved. I just had to accept the fact that it had to be done. I would have been happier if it had been done earlier. Had I felt any movements I would have changed my mind.'

A3(*c*) *Case 384*. A married woman in her late twenties who had a hysterotomy and tubal ligation. When seen at follow-up she had four children under 6. One was enuretic and encopretic and was refusing to go to school. There had recently been quite a serious accident to one of the children in the home through lack of supervision. The woman's husband was inclined to gamble, drink excessively, and strike her when drunk. Since the abortion, he had been more co-operative at home. The woman, though clearly extended in the home and barely able to cope with the children, was doing a part-time job in the evenings. Since the sterilisation she had not enjoyed sex so much with her husband; she was, however, having an affair with another man. She regretted the abortion, but was not depressed in any morbid sense. (Comment – this woman shows a curious mixture of wanting to reproduce but being unable to cope with being a mother. From the point of view of her family and the wider society, an abortion and sterilisation would seem to have been a very well justified procedure, yet from her own point of view there is doubt; she has accepted the abortion as a fait accompli, as she does with all her troubles, but she really regrets it and conveys the impression that sex lacks something now that it is not aimed at procreation. There is the added problem that her husband, always jealous (and with good reason), has become worse since the sterilisation.)

Case 270. A stolid, down-to-earth woman of 27 working full-time and coping with three of her four children, the fourth being fostered. Since the sterilisation her husband has expressed regret that his sexual activity was not directed towards procreation. (Comment – this case is included as a mixed result since the husband seems not to have resolved his neurotic need to keep on fathering children, although he cannot support them. This case could be seen as the male equivalent to the preceding case.)

Sometimes the effect of abortion and sterilisation seems to be almost irrelevant or of little importance compared with the impact of social circumstances, adverse or favourable as the case may be, and the overriding influence of the woman's personality, to the picture at follow-up. These cases have been categorised separately from those where abortion and sterilisation appear to have made a fairly clear contribution. Some examples of these cases are set out below.

A4   RELATIVELY UNIMPORTANT CONTRIBUTION

A4(*a*) *Case 89.* A woman in her late thirties who had left her husband and six children and was living with a man in England. The sexual side of the relationship was highly unsatisfactory. She reported mild depression but no regrets about abortion and sterilisation.

Case 107. A neurotic woman in her late forties with two children grown up and married. She was more easily tired after her hysterotomy and sterilisation and still afraid of pregnancy. Sexual relationships with her husband were avoided if possible. (Comment – this woman's fear of pregnancy reflects a neurotic problem with the physical side of sex. Tubal ligation, predictably, has not influenced the situation greatly.)

Case 262. A lustreless, worrying woman of 32 with asthma. At referral she had three children with whom she was coping indifferently. At follow-up she was worried that she might become an alcoholic: she had begun to enjoy a drink at weekends and tended to drink avidly once she started, for this was the only time she felt relaxed. She was very glad of an opportunity to talk about her problems. She wondered if she would die of asthma.

(Comment: The 8 cases in this sub-section all had personality deficiencies. There is the probability that things would have been even worse without abortion and sterilisation but since they appeared to be much the same as before, they were not placed in category 1.)

A4(c) *Case 94.* A 38-year-old married woman with four children whose normal good function had been quite unaffected by the abortion and sterilisation.

Case 247. Patient aged 36, separated from her husband. At follow-up she had broken off her relationship with the putative father and had taken up with a new boyfriend with whom she was having a satisfactory relationship. She had three children although she actually only wanted two and was satisfied with the abortion and sterilisation.

A4(d) *Case 243.* A woman aged 37, who had been mildly depressed since her mother's death four years previously. The hysterotomy and sterilisation had contributed nothing one way or another to her mood. Her husband had wanted a third child and was opposed to the abortion but this had in no way disturbed their happy relationship and the procedure was accepted by both. (Comment – this case exemplifies the situation where most of the regrets are experienced by the husband.)

B Single women who had an abortion and sterilisation

Sterilisation is, of course, seldom carried out on single women. In this series, for example, only 2 single women had had this operation. Nevertheless, both for the sake of completeness and because they are untypical of other single women who are referred for abortion, one example will be given.

B3(b) *Case 47.* The patient was 38 years old and living with her sister on social security. She had two illegitimate children at the time of referral. At follow-up she had no current male friend and therefore no sexual relationships but she had no regrets about the sterilisation. Even though she was not coping very well with the two children she sometimes wished she had not had the abortion, but was in general quite happy and managing her domestic chores easily.

C Ever-married women who had an abortion but not a sterilisation

There were 47 women in this category, 25 per cent of ever-married women and 16 per cent of the total cohort. Once again we have set out some examples of cases where the contribution of abortion to the woman's state at follow-up was judged (1) beneficial, (2) adverse, (3) conflicting and (4) unimportant.

CI BENEFICIAL CONTRIBUTION

Case 112. A divorced woman in her early thirties, cohabiting. She had four children at the time of referral, with whom she was coping only with difficulty. Abortion by suction curettage was followed by an immediate resolution of her anxiety and depression. At follow-up she was cheerful, and relationships with her consort were good both sexually and at a social level. She was on the pill. She was now coping better with the four children.

Case 173. A woman in her early twenties, separated from her husband with two children already when her request for abortion was refused. She was living with her parents and felt that they would not have continued to have her had they known about her pregnancy. She was able to procure an abortion on herself and when seen at follow-up was very happy with the outcome. She was awaiting divorce and had been allocated a council flat.

Case 110. A woman in her late twenties. The pregnancy which was aborted to her 'marvellous relief' was an illegitimate conception, from a casual relationship. At the time of follow-up she had become divorced from her first husband and had remarried four months previously. She was now pregnant to her second husband with whom she got on well, and was very pleased.

Case 1. A divorced woman in her early thirties with no children. The pregnancy was illegitimate and the putative father only seen on the one occasion of intercourse. She was depressed to find herself pregnant but quite returned to her normal spirits following abortion. She was a person who tended to avoid deep inter-personal relationships. Her mother was the person to whom she was closest but she had never told her about the abortion.

Case 54. A woman in her late twenties, separated from her husband with three children. Following abortion the putative father, a married man, continued to visit almost every evening, yet her general practitioner would not prescribe the pill for her until her divorce was finalised. At follow-up she was probably pregnant again. She had no regrets about the abortion and would see another as the best solution of her present situation but feared that she would not be given one. In this event, she saw adoption as the best solution. (This case could perhaps have been classified in the group where abortion was regarded as beneficial but lack of sterilisation as adverse. It was felt, however, that the problem had arisen more from a failure of the general practitioner to take a realistic view and prescribe an effective contraceptive and that had she married again, she might have wanted a further child.)

Case 163. A woman of 22 with one child, mildly depressed at the time of referral. At follow-up she was pregnant again, but the environment was more favourable and she was about to move into a new house. She was quite glad about the new pregnancy, and also glad that she had not had to continue with the previous one.

C2 ADVERSE CONTRIBUTION

There were no cases in this category.

C3 CONFLICTING CONTRIBUTION

C3(*a*) *Case 67.* A happily married woman in her early thirties with two children. She had no regrets about the abortion. Indeed before the follow-up interview she had had a second abortion and on this occasion a sterilisation, since when the sexual side of her marriage had become more relaxed. She regretted that she had not had a sterilisation at the time of her first abortion.

Case 312. The patient, in her late twenties, was separated from her husband and the index pregnancy was conceived extra-maritally. She had two children, both in care. At follow-up she had returned to her husband but the general relationship was strained, unsatisfactory sexually and she had not taken her children back. (Comment – this woman seems to be incapable of caring for her two children adequately, either whilst separated from her husband, or whilst living with him. It seems probably that a sterilisation would have been well justified.)

C3(*b*) *Case 282.* A patient of 23, happily married with one child when abortion was requested. The pregnancy was sufficiently far advanced to require a saline induction. The patient saw that the foetus was a little boy and felt very depressed and 'empty' after the abortion, since when she has been very slow to reach orgasm and sex hasn't meant the same to her. At follow-up she seemed to be normal in mood, a reasonably normal personality and had recovered from her post-abortion depression now that she was pregnant again.

C3(*c*) *Case 124.* A 38-year-old widow whose pregnancy was illegitimate. At follow-up she seemed a stable, un-neurotic woman who expressed her feelings well. For the sake of her two sons, her mother and her mother-in-law (of whom she was very fond) she was glad she had had an abortion, but for herself she wished she had had the baby, or better still, twins – she was so fond of children.

C4   RELATIVELY UNIMPORTANT CONTRIBUTION

C4(*a*) *Case 58.* A divorced woman in her late twenties, clinically rather anxious, introspective and unhappy. She already had three children and the abortion didn't appear to be contributing to the overall picture. She was glad she had had it at the time of follow-up though she had had serious doubts at first.

Case 186. A woman in her early thirties who was pretty depressed at follow-up. She had become pregnant to another man and then her husband had died, never knowing about the fact that she had had an abortion. She didn't regret the abortion but felt guilty about the awful thing she had done to her husband in becoming pregnant.

D   Single women who had an abortion but no sterilisation

Seventy of the 117 single women (60 per cent) in the series fell into this category. Whilst the age range is narrower in this group than in the ever-married, and most of them were pregnant for the first time, there is still a great variety of circumstances and responses to the operation. A majority of the patients in this category were judged to have benefited from the abortion and relatively few seemed to have suffered an adverse reaction.

D1 BENEFICIAL CONTRIBUTION

Case 104. A girl of 20 who at follow-up had married the putative father but was glad she had had an abortion. Had she married at once and continued the pregnancy, she felt that she would not have been able to get three Highers and set up house, as she now had done. She intended to go to the university when she had completed her family.

Case 105. A girl of 22 who was a student at the time of her referral. At follow-up the relationship with the putative father, about whom she knew very little, was finished and she was working as a schoolteacher. She was glad she had had the abortion.

Case 199. A woman in her early twenties who at follow-up had broken with the putative father and was happily married to another man. The abortion had been discussed with her mother, and with her husband before she married him, and all three accepted it as a good solution to the predicament.

Case 119. A woman of 25 who already had one illegitimate son at referral. She had been prescribed the pill but hadn't taken it and discovered that the conception was to a married man. At follow-up she had broken with the putative father and had subsequently become engaged to somebody else, but this too had been broken off. She was not very interested in sex herself, but this seemed to be the only level at which she could relate to men. She was looking after her son and felt that it had been right to have the abortion.

D2 ADVERSE CONTRIBUTION

*Case 14. The patient, in her early twenties, had broken her relationship with the putative father, but it had been a serious affair. At follow-up she was engaged to another man but she had not told him about her abortion: in fact she had been unable to unburden herself to anybody and still felt quite bad about it, wondering if she should have had the baby. These doubts, however, were less intense than the guilt feelings she had immediately following her abortion by saline induction. The experience of illegitimate pregnancy and abortion had left her apprehensive about having sexual intercourse and mildly depressed but her general function socially and at work was unimpaired.

Case 298. The patient, aged 16, was persuaded by her parents that she was too young to have a baby. At follow-up she was enjoying sexual intercourse three times a week with the putative father and their wedding was three weeks hence. She had been very upset by the abortion at the time and was still upset that it had been carried out, but she was in no sense depressed. There was strong evidence of a neurotic personality; she had fears of going out so that her fiancé had always to come and see her at home.

D3 CONFLICTING CONTRIBUTION

D3(c) *Case 51.* A single girl in her early twenties with two illegitimate children. At follow-up interview she had broken all contact with the putative father, though she was going out with other boys. She was on the pill but not having sexual relationships. Concerning the abortion she felt it was wrong of her and was sorry about it but nonetheless glad that she had had it done.

Case 295. A teenage girl whose parents separated when she was a child. She never trusts people as everyone seems to let her down. She made a suicidal gesture when rejected by the putative father. At follow-up interview she was going with a coloured boy. She felt that the abortion was the best decision because she couldn't have kept the baby but she regrets it as she would have liked a baby. (Comment – the patient appears to be a disturbed and deprived personality. It seems possible that she wanted a baby to satisfy her own neurotic need for somebody who would be dependent on her and would not let her down.)

Case 101. A 25-year-old girl who had been fairly severely depressed at the time of referral. At follow-up there was no evidence of depression, she was functioning normally in the social setting and shortly to marry the putative father. She was glad in a way that she had had the abortion; the relationship with the putative father benefited, but nonetheless she would really rather have got married then and had the baby.

D4 RELATIVELY UNIMPORTANT CONTRIBUTION

D4(a) *Case 36.* The patient, in her early twenties, had broken with the putative father when seen at follow-up, and accepted the abortion after early guilt feelings, but had recently discovered that she was pregnant again to another man and so the wheel had come round full circle: she was in a state of anxiety and indecision as to what to do.

D4(*b*) *Case 22.* The patient, in her late teens, had a saline induction because she had denied being pregnant until gestation had progressed beyond the 13th week. When seen at follow-up she had broken with the putative father and cooled off a subsequent boyfriend with whom she had had sexual intercourse but had found it 'not worth the worry'. She was not close to anyone, did not like to be tied down and felt that her mother didn't quite trust her (small wonder). She was mildly depressed and had regrets about the abortion.

D4(*c*) *Case 30.* A patient in her early twenties who married the putative father and had a spontaneous abortion. At follow-up she was perfectly normal in mood and social function.

Case 267. A patient in her early twenties who, following the abortion, became pregnant again to the putative father and married him. At follow-up she was functioning normally both socially and sexually and had no regrets about either the abortion or the subsequent pregnancy and marriage.

D4(*d*) *Case 6.* A teenager who had some late doubts about abortion but they in no way upset her overall well-being. At follow-up the relationship with the putative father had improved socially and she was getting more out of the sexual side. She was working full-time, was cheerful but had some mild regrets.

D5 SEVERELY ADVERSE, BUT TRANSIENT, CONTRIBUTION

This additional sub-category seemed to be required to describe the experiences of certain single women who suffered marked feelings of guilt or depression for a limited period after the operation. None of the ever-married women were affected in quite this way. There were 7 aborted single women whom it seems appropriate to assign to this sub-category, and another 5 single women who were judged to have had a seriously adverse reaction to the decision not to abort but were no longer in distress at the time of follow-up. An example of this latter group will be given later.

Case 159. A girl in her early twenties who was not seen at follow-up but gave a clear account in writing. She was working full-time, living in London and had broken with the putative father. She had found the saline induction very upsetting at the time and felt very guilty and depressed afterwards. Notwithstanding this experience she had had another abortion in London since, and had again felt depressed thereafter, but at the time of writing she felt no depression over either abortion.

Case 137. A girl of 20 who had found the saline induction 'hell'. Furthermore her mother had accused her of 'murdering my first grandchild' prior to her entering hospital for it. The putative father broke off their engagement a month before she was seen at follow-up, but despite these traumatic experiences she was not depressed and did not regret the abortion.

Case 324. A single girl aged 21, pregnant following two isolated occasions of intercourse which were not enjoyed, with a casual acquaintance who meant nothing to her. There was strong pressure from her mother to have an abortion and this was carried out, despite doubts in the minds of both the girl herself and the psychiatrist whom she saw before the operation. Immediately following the abortion, she was very upset, felt that she had committed a murder and declined physically, losing some weight. She was able to unburden herself to a psychiatrist on two or three occasions with benefit, but declined the suggestion that she should continue treatment. Three-and-a-half months later, however, she had not been able to go back to work, she was frightened, constantly needing reassurance and had lost weight. She attended psychiatric day hospital for $4\frac{1}{2}$ months, her treatment being largely through group psychotherapy. There was a marked improvement after she gained the moral courage to tell her father her guilty secret about the abortion and discovered that he accepted the news calmly. She was able to leave treatment to full employment, having acquired a good deal more maturity through her experience than she had before becoming pregnant.

E Ever-married women who were sterilised but not aborted

Twenty-three of the 186 married women were given a post-partum sterilisation but were not accepted for abortion. A few examples are set out below. This combination was an unqualified success in less than half. Only occasionally were there any regrets about sterilisation but there were several women for whom refusal of abortion proved to be far from a happy decision.

E1 BENEFICIAL CONTRIBUTION

Case 215. A woman of 38 with two children at time of referral. She continued to term and gave birth to twins with whom she was highly delighted. Sexual relations with her husband had improved since her sterilisation.

E3 CONFLICTING CONTRIBUTION

E3(*a*) *Case 347.* The patient, aged 37, had three children when referred and her husband was a severe diabetic. At follow-up she was pleased with the baby and claimed that it was her doctor rather than herself who wanted her to have an abortion. She had mixed feelings about the sterilisation. (Comment – in retrospect, would it not have been more logical to sterilise the husband?)

E3(*b*) *Case 106.* A patient in her late twenties who had three children at the time of her referral and a shaky marriage. When seen at follow-up she was depressed (Beck score 21), the marriage had broken up completely ('My husband has never been the same since the fourth child'), she was poorly housed, short of money, the first two of her children – aged 8 and 6 – were 'beyond her' and the oldest was attending a psychiatrist for stealing.

Case 256. A patient in her early thirties, happily married. At the time of referral, she already had four children of her own and was looking after a fifth, which she and her husband had adopted. When seen at follow-up she was coping adequately with her domestic duties and working part-time as a cleaner. Fear of pregnancy had been removed by post-partum sterilisation which had led to improved sexual enjoyment, but she wished she had had an abortion and felt angry with the doctor who refused her, especially as her husband had asked for a vasectomy before she became pregnant and had been refused.

E3(*c*) *Case 44.* A happily married woman in her early thirties with three children at the time of her request for abortion. The request was turned down and at follow-up she said, 'I would never part with her now but I would still ask for an abortion if I could go back a year.'

E4 RELATIVELY UNIMPORTANT CONTRIBUTION

E4(c) *Case 206.* A well-adjusted woman in her early forties with an excellent husband and at follow-up seven children. She was happy with the seventh child but thinks she should have been aborted. She was relieved to find that the sterilisation did not detract from her sexual feelings. She added spontaneously at the end of the interview, 'It's fine to talk to somebody about it.'

F   There was only one case of a single woman being sterilised but not aborted and it is not reported here.

G   Ever-married women neither sterilised nor aborted

Forty (22 per cent) of the ever-married women were 'refused'.

G1 BENEFICIAL CONTRIBUTION

Case 80. A woman of 35 with five children at the time of referral, whose request for abortion had been made in order to please her husband. He, it seemed, felt badly about the size of their family, largely because his sister 'kept getting on to him' about it. The patient herself, however, had wanted to continue the pregnancy. At follow-up she reported that she was glad to have had another baby: she had not been finding enough to do since the five children she already had were growing up. She was, however, displeased that the baby had been delivered by Caesarean section: she somehow felt cheated of giving birth: 'Just an operation, that's all.' She would cheerfully accept a seventh baby, 'If you are meant to have another you will.' She and her husband attempted to practise coitus interruptus.

Case 288. At the time of referral the patient was in her early twenties, separated from her husband and pregnant to another man. She already had three children. The pregnancy continued to term and at follow-up she and her husband were reunited in a new house with the four children and appeared to have a good relationship.

G2 ADVERSE CONTRIBUTION

Case 109. A mildly depressed, anxious and rather angry patient in her early thirties. At follow-up she was on the pill but worried by the non-appearance of withdrawal bleeding, had lost interest in sex and was not coping with the three children.

Case 317. A girl of 18. At the time of follow-up she was working and her mother, who was possessive and interfering, was looking after the baby during the day. The patient was 'fed up' with her husband, dissatisfied with her marriage and wanted to be free and single again. The sexual side of the marriage was almost non-existent and she was continually worried lest she became pregnant again. She felt that she was not a good mother. She was depressed and regretted going to term. She wasn't really fond of the baby and felt that it 'trapped her in her marriage'.

Case 336. A woman in her early thirties whose request for abortion was refused. She had no children at the time of referral but her marriage was very unsatisfactory: there was very little mutual trust and consideration. The fact that the pregnancy had been conceived extra-maritally was concealed from her husband and, at follow-up, sex with him was 'a torture'. She was still having satisfactory intercourse weekly, however, with the putative father. The patient wished she could have had the baby adopted and said 'at times I feel like punching it'. (Comment – this patient was very immature and a disastrous mother. Here were the ingredients for a 'battered baby'.)

Case 114. A woman in her early thirties who at follow-up appeared mildly depressed and anxious. She was separated from her husband and her request for abortion having been turned down, her third child had been fostered and she wished she had not had to give birth to it at all. She was barely coping with the two children which he had in her care and was at the time eight months pregnant (her second illegitimate pregnancy) with no intention of marrying the putative father. She intended to get this fourth child fostered as well as the third.

Case 241. A divorced woman of 26 who at the time of referral had three children, only two of whom she was looking after herself. At follow-up she had broken with the putative father who had turned out to be married, and was having difficulty with her son who was rejecting her in favour of his grandparents. She was unhappy about having gone to term and very severely regretted having had the baby adopted. She was sad behind a façade, disinterested in sex, worried and having nightmares.

G3 CONFLICTING CONTRIBUTION

G3(*a*) *Case 310.* The patient, in her late thirties, was glad at follow-up that she had not had an abortion, but was finding four a handful and was constantly dreading another pregnancy, to the extent that all enjoyment had gone from her sexual relationships with her husband which had previously been very good.

G3(*c*) *Case 111.* A 28-year-old woman, separated from her husband with three children at the time of referral, when she was severely depressed and felt suicidal. The conception was not with her husband. At follow-up she was divorced and living with the putative father with whom relationships were strained. She was glad to have had the baby but was coping badly with the children, being mildly depressed and anxious, overtired and suffering from headaches. The sexual relationships with the putative father were satisfactory and she wanted another baby. (Comment – this is another example of a woman who wants to bear children in spite of the fact that she can't cope with them – see cases 102 and 384.)

G4 RELATIVELY UNIMPORTANT CONTRIBUTION

G4(*a*) *Case 191.* A woman in her late thirties whose husband drank excessively to the detriment of the marital relationship, and the patient's peace of mind. At follow-up she had accepted the third child and things seemed to be neither better nor worse than they had been at the time of request for abortion.

G4(*c*) *Case 136.* A woman in her late twenties who, prior to becoming pregnant and at the time of referral, had been a psychiatric patient with an episodic obsessional state, at times associated with psychotic depression. At referral there were considerable marital difficulties, hire purchase debts and the patient was housebound in a high flat. At follow-up, the financial difficulties had been cleared up, she was working in the evenings, feeling fine and taking part in a normal social and sexual life with her husband. She had a new house and was delighted with the baby. (Comment – this case illustrates the irrelevance of the abortion decision in the face of what was probably an endogenous mood swing together with beneficial changes in her environment.)

Case 316. A woman of 28 with four children when referred. She had had no difficulties and was neither depressed nor anxious when the abortion was requested, but she and her husband simply felt that their family was large enough, that the pregnancy had not been wanted and that abortion was the logical solution. At follow-up she had taken the fifth child in her stride and her sexual relationships with her husband had improved since going on the pill.

H Single women who had neither abortion nor sterilisation

Forty-four (38 per cent) of the single women applicants had their requests for abortion turned down.

H1 BENEFICIAL CONTRIBUTION

Case 115. The patient, aged 19, was under pressure from her parents, the putative father and her general practitioner to seek an abortion which she didn't really want herself. At follow-up she was cheerful and optimistic, glad she had completed her pregnancy, pleased with her baby and hoped to have four or five children in due course. Her marriage to the putative father was affording her happiness and sexual satisfaction.

Case 175. The patient in her early twenties never wanted an abortion but was pressed to have one by her parents. At follow-up she seemed normal in mood and was leading a normal life. Her grandmother was looking after the baby. (Comment – in this case it was possible to continue a normal life as a single girl because her grandmother was available to care for her illegitimate baby.)

Case 265. A 21-year-old clerkess whose parents were upset by the illegitimate conception and wanted it aborted, but the girl herself was not put about by the pregnancy and wanted to continue it, which she did. She looked after the baby for six weeks and it was then adopted. At follow-up she regarded the whole episode as an interesting experience and discussed it with candour and objectivity, giving no appearance of being unable to deal with any of the emotional conflicts which could be postulated. The relationship with the putative father was finished.

Case 277. A 20-year-old student, who was glad she had had the baby ('It was worth it for the week I had him') but who had been miserable at the time that it had been adopted. She was no longer interested in the putative father but was having an intense sexual relationship with a man in his forties, separated from his wife. The patient appeared cheerful at interview and reported that she was getting on well with her studies.

Case 98. A student in her early twenties who kept the baby and married the putative father. She was happy with the outcome but had abandoned her academic aspirations. (Comment – it is possible in a case such as this, that the academic aspirations were never very strong and that in some ways the pregnancy could have been a welcome or even hoped-for excuse to abandon them.)

It is notable that many of the women in category H1 were never very keen to have an abortion but were often pushed into applying by somebody else, often parents whose conventional standards were outraged. This is a group in which a psychiatric consultation can sometimes discern these doubts and help a girl to stand out for what she herself wants.

H2 ADVERSE CONTRIBUTION

Case 283. Patient aged 20. At follow-up she had broken with the putative father and was living a restricted life with her parents. She had no current boyfriend and no real plans for the future. Some days she couldn't be bothered to do anything. She was vague, fed up and not really facing her problems or her feelings. There seemed to be feelings of resentment and rejection towards the baby.

Case 294. Patient aged 23. At follow-up she had married the putative father but life was none too happy; they were living in a caravan. She was quite definite that she still wished she had had an abortion. 'Life would be very different now.'

Case 364. Patient aged 18 who at follow-up was still having a steady sexually satisfactory relationship with the putative father who would have married her when she became pregnant. She had been on tranquillisers ever since the birth of the baby and the continued pregnancy had soured the relationship with her mother. The whole affair had been concealed from her father. She was depressed, still wishing that she had had an abortion and regretting adoption, yet unable to see that things would have been any better had she kept the baby.

Case 160. A student in her early twenties who continued her pregnancy to term and had her baby adopted. She later married the putative father and, at follow-up, she reported that the marriage was going well. She was glad that she had not kept the baby, but still regretted that she had been denied an abortion which she felt would have been a better solution than adoption. (Comment – this case illustrates how the conventional belief that if the relationship with the putative father is good and the couple can marry, then the pregnancy is best continued to term, is sometimes too simplistic a view.)

H3 CONFLICTING CONTRIBUTION

H3(c) *Case 139.* A woman in her late twenties, still single at follow-up, who had gone back to live with her mother. She had stopped working and was looking after her baby. She had broken with the putative father and was having nothing to do with men. She was attending her general practitioner for nerves. In spite of the ominously retrogressive social developments and emotional disturbance she was glad that she had had the baby. (Comment – in this case, it was felt that the presence of the baby had altered the girl's life style adversely, although she professed to be glad about the way things were.)

H4 RELATIVELY UNIMPORTANT CONTRIBUTION

H4(a) *Case 250.* A passive, dependent girl of 18 unable to break away from her parents. They disapproved of the putative father but she was keen on him. At follow-up she was seeing him occasionally with no sex, refusing the financial aid which he offered for the baby, which was in his name. Patient was happy about going to term and having the baby but depressed by a situation in which she was dominated by parents. (Comment – this case differs from the previous one because it was felt that the presence of the baby was not the important factor in keeping this girl at home with her parents and depressed. Indeed it offered her an opportunity of breaking away since she and the putative father were still very interested in each other and in the baby.)

H4(c) *Case 260.* A 17-year-old girl who fell pregnant to her stepfather. At follow-up she had accepted going to term and having the baby adopted and was appropriately married.

Case 214. A stable 18-year-old girl living at home and working full-time. There was never any question of marriage to the putative father. At follow-up the patient felt that she wouldn't part with the baby now but would have been happy with an abortion.

H4(*d*) *Case 143*. The patient was 17 at the time of referral. The putative father had disappeared when the pregnancy was discovered. At follow-up the patient was living at home and had an improved understanding with her mother. She was leading a full social life (not having sexual intercourse) and was working normally. Her baby had been adopted and she had mixed feelings about going to term.

H5 SEVERELY ADVERSE BUT TRANSIENT CONTRIBUTION

Case 116. A girl in her early twenties who continued to term and had the baby adopted. She was deeply depressed, according to her own account, for about a year afterwards. At follow-up she was enjoying her work, on the pill, and sexual intercourse was now 'going OK'. (It was 'ugly' before she had the baby.) She felt more mature and glad in retrospect. 'It was a terrible experience but the best way all round.'

DISCUSSION OF CLINICAL ASSESSMENTS

The most striking finding perhaps is that only 38 (12.5 per cent) of all women who were traced were apparently severely upset by the outcome of pregnancy (Table 7:1) and by the time of the follow-up, over a third of these (14) had completely got over it (Table 7: 1, col. 5, and line C, col. 3*b*). This perhaps says more for the resilience of the human species than for the wisdom of the counselling these women obtained. If any comparison is permissible between those who had an abortion and those who had not, then a significantly smaller proportion of those aborted were severely upset (Table 7: 2), had regrets (Table 7: 3) or had been influenced adversely by what had happened (Table 7: 4). Complementarily a beneficial contribution was seen in a greater proportion of the aborted women than of those who had gone to term (Table 7: 5). Thus there was more distress occasioned by going to term with an unwanted pregnancy than by having an abortion. It should also be noted that significantly more single girls were severely upset by whatever happened to them than were married women (Table 7: 6). The stigma of pregnancy in the unmarried is so deeply rooted in our culture that a burden of guilt might colour any outcome of such an event. Thus, it is especially important to make good contraceptive facilities freely available to single women in the interests of preventive psychiatry.

The sub-group worst affected at follow-up was that composed of the 44 single women who were neither aborted nor sterilised. Fifteen were adversely affected by going to term. Seven of them were students or nurses, and some were still full of resentment towards the medical profession for not helping them. Three other girls had an illegitimate child already at the index referral. Five more were severely upset for a time although all right at follow-up. Two of these had had illegitimate pregnancies prior to referral. In contrast, there were only 2 students amongst the 10 single women who were benefited by going to term without sterilisation and none with previous pregnancies.

These results suggest that from a psychiatric standpoint single women in general, and particularly students and those who had previous pregnancies, do better if aborted than if they continue to term. There is little justification for the idea that if a girl does not 'learn her lesson' the first time, she should 'suffer the consequences' of any further 'promiscuity'. Such a policy is unlikely to convert an irresponsible girl into a competent and effective mother. The behaviour patterns in which an anti-social or quasi self-destructive element persists in spite of continual negative reinforcements, are characteristic of certain neurotic maladjustments and personality disorders. There is often a public clamour for the punishment of such people. This is understandable but unwise since it is very rarely a means of reforming the offender. In the present context, the principal sufferers from a punitive refusal of abortion in a single girl who has already had an illegitimate pregnancy are likely to be other members of society, since a child born in these circumstances may well require to be taken into 'care' and has a more than average chance of developing deviant and anti-social behaviour.

The next most unsuccessful group was the 40 ever-married women who had had no abortion and no sterilisation. Of these, 10 were adversely affected by not having had an abortion. Four of the 10 were divorced or separated and 4 had a considerable degree of marital disharmony, but the same pattern was found amongst the 12 who benefited from going to term, of whom one was divorced, one separated, one widowed, 5 had great marital difficulties at referral and 2 were married for the second time.

Sterilisation, which was not carried out in this group, might have been an advantageous procedure for 9. In 3, there was continued fear of pregnancy disrupting a normal sexual relationship and a wish for sterilisation. One had a subsequent abortion and sterilisation. In a further 4 there was gross social incompetence with the need for outside agencies to carry responsibility for the patient's offspring yet no well-integrated attempt on her part to ensure that more children were not produced. (One of these women was in the ninth month of gestation with her second illegitimate pregnancy.) One more woman made such heavy weather of the index pregnancy that it is unlikely she would welcome another.

Looking at the 47 ever-married women who had an abortion ('spontaneous' in 7 and admittedly self-induced in 2) but were not sterilised, they too were remarkable for their lack of marital success. Eight were divorced, 5 separated, 8 had marriages of miserable quality, 3 had conceived the index pregnancy adulterously although their marriages were not intolerable at the time, and 2 were widows. The frequency of marital disruption in these two groups of women reflects a selection bias against sterilisation in unstable marriages. Only 2 in this group were adversely affected by abortion. Since they had not had a sterilisation, they consoled themselves by embarking on another pregnancy. In 11, however, the lack of sterilisation was disadvantageous. One had had a further abortion, this time with sterilisation (a good marriage), one had had a ruptured ectopic pregnancy following a self-induced abortion (a good marriage), one was pregnant again and contemplating a divorce, one with financial problems, contra-indications to taking the pill and miserable sexual relations with her husband through fear of pregnancy, had had another child since the abortion, and a fifth woman had made an adulterous conception whilst her husband was in prison since the abortion. Of the other 6, 2 lived in fear of pregnancy and wanted a sterilisation, 2 were unable to make up their minds and 2 were already socially overwhelmed but lacked the drive to do anything about effective contraception.

102 women were sterilised. Only 8 had serious regrets of whom 2 were divorced and one separated. One of these divorced women was going with a man whom she hoped to marry. The other 2 had not wanted sterilisation but had felt that it was offered as a condition of abortion. Two women wanted the operation reversed – one had a stable marriage; the other, an on–off affair where the sterilisation seemed to have deprived her of the only function she knew – she already had eight children. There was one woman amongst these 8 who had to have a hysterectomy for uterine pathology and her regrets were perhaps more appropriately ascribed to this misfortune. A further 11 women had some second thoughts about sterilisation; only one of these had an unhappy marriage with a miserable sexual relationship.

As with abortion, any comparison between those sterilised and those not must be interpreted with the greatest reserve for the groups are different by selection. It may, however, be worth making the very simple observation that serious regrets and disadvantages were rare (8 per cent) following sterilisation and less rare (20 per cent) at follow-up in its absence (Table 7: 7).

Examining now the single women who were adversely affected by abortion, no feature distinguishes the group except that 8 out of 12 (two-thirds) had had a saline induction, and several of them said at follow-up how horrible they had found it. Although aborted single women who were not adversely affected had a lower proportion of saline inductions (23 out of 60 or about one-third) the difference is not significant. It is possible that the later stage of pregnancy at which this method is carried out contributes to the anguish which some recounted. At all events, this experience with saline induction and the greater prevalence of physical complications if abortion is carried out in the middle trimester, emphasise that decisions to terminate pregnancy should be made early and acted upon without delay. There were occasions when this did not happen:

Case 238. A married woman in her late twenties, who resented the way she had been 'pushed around' from one doctor to another until she was 4½ months 'gone', by which time she wasn't sure whether she still wanted an abortion since it was by then such a formidable undertaking (at least in her eyes). She decided to continue the pregnancy but by the time she had reached 7½ months she still didn't want the baby and at follow-up she was ambivalent towards him (she had wanted a girl). (See also A3(*b*), case 40.)

Perhaps if some or all of the medical people involved with making and carrying out the decision (general practitioner, gynaecologist and sometimes psychiatrist) were inherently opposed to abortion, a temptation might exist to procrastinate in case the patient changed her mind or a stage of gestation came upon them at which continued pregnancy could conscientiously be advised. Doctors should have the courage of their convictions and let their patients know where they stand with them at the earliest possible opportunity.

Although the actual number of women who suffer severe distress from either abortion or from continuing with an unwanted pregnancy is small, what can be done to alleviate this suffering or to prevent it?

Certain impressions were formed in the course of these clinical contacts with the women themselves.

Prospectively, decisions must be made expeditiously as already discussed, although pressure should not be brought to bear on the patient to change her mind: 4 out of the 10 single girls who were glad they had gone to term were uncertain themselves whether they wanted an abortion in the first place and most of the 40 who were glad about the abortion were quite clear about what they wanted – 8 were students. Nonetheless it seems unfair for a doctor to shuffle out of all responsibility for this decision and make the patient carry alone any guilt she may have. (Psychiatrists are probably more liable to adopt this stance than general practitioners or surgeons.) At a time of crisis like this women may need some support from a profession they respect and trust. It seems helpful then if, having judged the patient's real wishes, and having decided what he intends to do, the doctor then commits himself to *advising* this course. Several of the patients in the present series obviously derived much help from this approach.

After the event it was clear from several patients that they greatly appreciated the opportunity of 'a good talk' which was provided by the research interview but would otherwise never have arisen. Even the process of replying to questions in writing was found to be helpful – 'Thanks for the opportunity to get this off my chest.' Doctors, especially general practitioners, but psychiatrists if they have been involved, should perhaps be prepared to initiate an interview a few months after such a crisis. The patient may well not feel able to do so.

A more general point might be made in conclusion. For many generations in our culture large families, and a rising birth rate, have been accepted without question by the vast majority as a sign of a healthy, prosperous society with a rosy future. Small wonder that many women experience feelings of guilt and unworthiness if they contemplate abortion. Only recently have there been public stirrings of doubt over the future of mankind if his numbers continue to multiply by exponential growth. It seems inevitable, however, that a new look at what constitutes an acceptable family size to the society in the coming years cannot be long delayed, and it may well be that new attitudes towards abortion will do more than any doctor can do to remove the present psychological difficulties with which these patients have had to contend.

TABLE 7:1. *Contribution to the psychological state at follow-up, of the factor-complex abortion yes/no – sterilisation yes/no, in ever-married and single women*

	(1)	(2)	(3) Conflicting			(4) Relatively unimportant				(5)	(6)
			(a) Pregnancy outcome beneficial. Sterilisation ± adverse or regretted	(b) Sterilisation ± beneficial. Pregnancy outcome adverse or regretted	(c) Mixed picture. Ambivalent feelings	Poor state (a) Glad about outcome	Poor state (b) Regrets about outcome	Good state (c) Glad about outcome	Good state (d) Regrets about outcome	Severely adverse but transient	Data insufficient to classify in detail but not severely upset
	Beneficial	Adverse regretted									
Aborted											
Sterilised											
(A) Ever-married	30	9 (4)	6	3	4	8	2	10	3	0	1	76 (4)
(B) Single	1	0	0	1	0	0	0	0	0	0	0	2
Not sterilised											
(C) Ever-married	19	0	11	2 (2)	2	5	1	6	1	0	0	47 (2)
(D) Single	40	5 (4)	0	0	6	3	3	2	3	7 (7)	1	70 (11)
Not aborted											
Sterilised											
(E) Ever-married	4	0	2	5 (2)	4	0	0	6	1	0	1	23 (2)
(F) Single	1	0	0	0	0	0	0	0	0	0	0	1
Not sterilised											
(G) Ever-married	12	10 (7)	2	0	4	3	0	9	0	0	0	40 (7)
(H) Single	10	15 (7)	0	0	3	2	0	5	4	5 (5)	0	44 (12)
Total	117	39 (22)	21	11 (4)	23	21	6	38	12	12 (12)	3	303 (38)

NOTE. Figures in parentheses indicate number of cases severely upset.

TABLE 7:2. *Percentage distribution of those severely upset either at follow-up or for a transient period (parenthetic figures in Table 7:1) according to whether they had an abortion or not*

	All women followed up ($N = 303$)		
	Severe upset	No severe upset	Total
Aborted	8.7	91.3	100
Not aborted	19.4	80.6	100

$\chi^2 = 6.346$, d..f $= 1$, $P < 0.02$.

TABLE 7:3. *Percentage distribution of all who had felt regrets or been adversely affected by the outcome of pregnancy, according to whether aborted or not*

	All women followed up for whom detailed information was available ($N = 300$)		
	Regrets or adverse effect (Table 7:1, cols. 2, 3*b*, 4*b*, 4*d*, 5)	Benefit, satisfied or ambivalent (Table 7:1, cols. 1, 3*a*, 3*c*, 4*a*, 4*c*)	Total
Aborted	20.7	79.3	100
Not aborted	37.4	62.6	100

$\chi^2 = 8.93$, d.f. $= 1$, $P < 0.01$.

TABLE 7:4. *Percentage distribution of adverse effects of pregnancy outcome according to whether aborted or not*

	All women followed up for whom detailed information was available ($N = 300$)		
	Pregnancy outcome had an adverse effect (Table 7:1, col. 2)	Pregnancy outcome had some other effect (Table 7:1, all cols. except 2 and 6)	Total
Aborted	7.3	92.7	100
Not aborted	23.4	76.6	100

$\chi^2 = 14.4$, d.f. $= 1$, $P < 0.001$.

TABLE 7:5. *Percentage distribution of beneficial effect of pregnancy outcome according to whether aborted or not*

	All women followed up for whom detailed information was available ($N = 300$)		
	Outcome of pregnancy beneficial (Table 7:1, cols. 1, 3a)	Outcome of pregnancy adverse, conflicting or unimportant (Table 7:1, cols. 2, 3b, 3c, 4, 5)	Total
Aborted	55.4	44.6	100
Not aborted	29.0	71.0	100

$\chi^2 = 18.36$, d.f. $= 1$, $P < 0.001$.

TABLE 7:6. *Percentage distribution of severe upset at follow-up or for transient period according to marital status*

	All women followed up ($N = 303$)		
	Severe upset	Not severe upset	Total
Single	19.7	80.3	100
Ever-married	8.0	92.0	100

$\chi^2 = 7.776$, d.f. $= 1$, $P < 0.01$.

TABLE 7:7. *Percentage distribution of serious regrets or disadvantage according to whether sterilised or not†*

	All ever-married women followed up ($N = 186$)		
	Serious regrets or disadvantage	Beneficial or at worst mixed pros and cons	Total
Sterilised	8.1	91.9	100
Not sterilised	20.7	79.3	100

$\chi^2 = 5.118$, d.f. $= 1$, $P < 0.05$.

† Three *single* women who were sterilised are omitted – none had serious regrets.

8 DECISION-MAKING IN THERAPEUTIC ABORTION

Colin Farmer

DECISION-MAKING

Of the several strategies of problem-solving which appear in the literature, three will be reviewed here in the context of the therapeutic abortion programme in Aberdeen and specifically how a group of doctors there decided to terminate women of their unwanted pregnancies. These are the rational-deductive method, incrementalism and mixed scanning.

Rationalism

Naturally enough the rational-deductive strategy is built on the model of man as a rational being. Its requirements are that the decision-maker knows the full range of his options, that he can consciously and freely choose between alternatives, that he is able to assess and evaluate outcomes of them and that his choice will be made in the way which will maximise achievement of goals.[1]

However, the literature on the rational-deductive method since the 1950s has been directed mainly toward its shortcomings as a realistic explanation of the way individuals or organisations solve problems.[2] Basically these criticisms oppose the idea that all possible alternative choices can be known and that the ones which are, can be precisely weighted as to their utility. It is disputed that, even with the aid of computers, humans have the capacity to fill the requirements of the global rational model or in the case of group decisions that members can reach consensus. Humans observed in the problem-solving process respond to their values and the social structures of which they are a part as well as factual considerations. Moreover the process does not seem so much to be an outcome of balanced factual analysis as a sequence of actions based on a limited number of cues from the environment.

333

Instead of maximising utility in decisions, individuals and groups seem to accept a minimally tolerable level of improvement in outcomes consistent with their values, which Simon calls 'satisficing'.[3]

Incrementalism

Incrementalism or 'muddling through' is one strategy which answers the objections raised by the rationalistic approach to some of types of problem-solving.[4] The incrementalist approach is only concerned with choices of alternatives differing marginally from the status quo. Thus, applied to the long-run implementation of a policy or programme no single problem-solving decision takes place but instead there is a progression of minor adjustments not often in a straight line relationship to one another. In this serial adjustment process it is possible to phase current factual positions and current value positions of actors one with the other and changes in either component are consequently allowed for in decision-making over time.

In any one decision it is the best among presenting alternatives which is selected without having to consider all possible alternatives. Lindblom says that consensus among decision-making actors is not prerequisite to incrementalism but conflicts will likely arise over how different analysts assign the weights to different alternatives in choosing one over another.[5] Thus with a single evaluator, the decisions he makes will inevitably reflect his own and his social unit's normative position. Furthermore with this approach some adverse and possibly important long-run consequences arising out of the decisions made may not be considered because of the non-global, delimited nature of the strategy.

Incrementalism is therefore a relatively conservative problem-solving explanation, innovative in the slow way that judge-made law effects change. It evaluates possible outcomes of decisions in the present from activity which has taken place in the past. What incrementalism does not account for are major changes required in policies and practices when instrumental and expressive positions in society are massively out of phase with one another.

Mixed scanning

Etzioni claims the 'mixed scanning' strategy combines the advantages of rationalist and incrementalist approaches while escaping most of their imperfections.[6] It provides for two or more levels from which problems are viewed, one from which fundamental decisions about changes in policy direction are made and one from which implementing or routine decisions are made. In a sort of evolutionary cycle over time, the day-to-day incremental decisions set the stage for reviews and fundamental changes in policy while the latter, once taken, provide the base for implementing routine decisions taken on a short-run basis.

Social crises are said to set the stage for societal change where it is overdue. Crisis situations are prone to arise in democracies where decision-making at the macro-sociological level tends to be incremental in nature because of the necessity to achieve consensus from the many competing interest groups.

In this sense the democratic system inhibits orderly and progressive change which is forestalled until interest groups with particular causes are strong enough to organise and express popular opinion.

In this context decision-making elites often exhibit a double standard in making choices of alternatives: those which will promote societal goals without alienating members of the elite itself. But in the face of social change if elites are over-protective of their own position and fail for too long to consider changed societal requirements, they put themselves in jeopardy of removal from former power. As far as political elites are concerned they hold control to the extent that they can correctly gauge the power of competing societal cadres with differing goals.

Summary

If we take these strategies as a progression in the order they are described here, it is apparent that as problem-solving becomes more intensively researched the more the normative-structural components become emphasised. 'Rational' man as the model increasingly gives way to 'social' man not only in the search for more plausible explanations of the decision-making processes but also as the focal point and raison d'être for social planning.

In 1955 Simon was already casting doubts on rational strategies for problem-solving in his plea for models more consistent with man's physiological and psychological limitations in making choices.[7] More recently Cove argues that the old idea of structural-functionalism is perhaps the most useful way of looking at choice decisions since it is the decision-maker's location in the social system which influences choice. Position in the structure as he sees it is 'the locus for utilities, capabilities and uncertainties generated by the situation'.[8]

In formulating his 'active society' concept, Etzioni shows that realisation of societal values for the masses requires not only awareness of possibilities for improvement in actors but also mechanisms for control through social structures.[9] In a similar vein Ozbekhan concludes that if society is to escape the present mechanistic control by technological forces a form of social planning involving consideration of human value systems is essential.[10]

The authors of the strategies of decision-making briefly outlined here range in their arguments and examples from micro- to macro-sociological focal points depending on their interests. It is proposed here to attempt an application of these models to abortion and decisions made at the political and medical actor levels about these operations.

ORIGINS OF THE ABORTION ACT

As in other European countries reform of British abortion legislation resulted from the long-range requirement in the population for reduced fertility and the final submission of political and medical elites to that pressure.

As Davis has shown, the rates of increase in both urban and rural populations tend to decline in industrially developed countries, which occurs along with a movement of population from rural to urban locations.[11] With these demographic changes come value changes of families toward having fewer children but investing more economically and emotionally in them.

Not only do the economic costs of raising a family in the city increase but as industrially efficient countries become affluent their aspirations for an improved life style for their families increases also. Thus the value held for large families suitable in pre-industrial countries with high mortality rates becomes redundant and eventually disappears.

Goode argues that one cannot expect an immediate reliance on contraceptive practice to reduce fertility because much socialisation is required to value highly the production of children but little is required to understand death. Since it would take a generation to reinstitute values supporting high fertility if they were to be eliminated, they tend to remain as an insurance against social catastrophe. Hence the controls on high fertility tend to occur after conception through abortion or infanticide.[12]

Britain was no exception to the general pattern described above and one eventual response of parliament to the ground swell of opinion for limitation of family size was the passage of the Abortion Act in 1967. This was however vigorously opposed by some elements in the medical profession, some religious groups and citizen's groups like the Society for the Protection of the Unborn Child.

Besides the government's concern for overpopulation the support for abortion legislation largely arose from questions of national public health related to death and disablement of women from illegal abortions, obstetrical incompetence from multiparity and the minimal quality of life one expects for children in twentieth-century Britain. But the general concern with the health and welfare of the population, of which the abortion question is only a small part, had its origins in the Health Insurance Act of 1911, the Beveridge Report and the inception of the National Health Service in 1948 under the Atlee government.

The terms of the law are crucial to understanding the problems which arose in making decisions about who should be aborted of unwanted pregnancies and who should not. Many of the doctors rightly maintained that the law could be interpreted according to any meaning one wished to read into it. The three main points around which most of the contention about abortion decisions occurred were that (1) a woman's physical or mental health would likely be impaired by the continuing pregnancy, (2) the welfare of existing children would likely be affected by the addition of another child in the family, or (3) the patient's continued well-being would not be worsened by giving the abortion than if it were not done.

It was into the last category that most of the 'social' rather than purely medical decisions to terminate pregnancies fell.

THE DOCTORS

The medical mentality

The length and process of training for medicine does more than impart technical skills. The effect of five or six years' exposure to the discipline of medical school and the professional models there, is to resocialise the student to accept a special set of values enabling him gradually to think and behave like a doctor. Like members of other professions, medical practitioners become formed into a distinctly separate social group in society structured around their occupational activities. In that social position not only the formal behaviours of doctors are prescribed but informal behaviour is controlled as well.[13]

The expected normative behaviour is formally enforced through the hierarchical organisation of the profession. There is always the threat of formal sanctions for serious medical misconduct which can result in being 'struck off the list', although as Freidson indicates this is relatively rare. But ever present to the practitioner is the fear of disapproval of one's colleagues, their unwillingness to refer patients and the eventual undermining of one's reputation which can result in personal and economic hardship.[14] Plus which the long investment in training and the high income and prestige of medical practice are internal disciplining factors which make nonconformity unlikely.[15] These internalised behaviour controls and threat of sanctions together, in the nature of the case, make for a social group with a relatively conservative outlook toward value change.

Although the argument continues over what should constitute the course of training, most medical schools emphasise science subjects and the scientific method. The student is expected to recognise symptoms of disease in patients, interpret test results and arrive at diagnoses by deductive reasoning.[16] One clear training focus is to create of the student a rational problem-solver. Although as Bloom says, 'the personal attributes which the physician brings to the situation determine unconsciously much of what he will perceive and do'.[17]

Quite apart from individual differences in perception of practitioners, the variability in diagnoses through the range of ailments doctors deal with is large. This is because the symptomatology, untreated outcome and remedial action for some somatic diseases is known and for others it is not. When psychiatric disorder is considered the diagnostic variability is even greater especially when the evaluators are trained to use different diagnostic criteria.[18] But when doctors are asked to make decisions in social situations such as those presented when abortions are requested, one would expect even greater variability in judgements.

Conduct of the study

The great achievement in conducting this research was not the development of research routines but the creation of the necessary trust for a researcher who was not medically trained in respondents who were. It is true that the obstetrics and gynaecology hospital staff under the influence of Sir Dugald Baird had become accustomed to co-operate with social science research personnel but the degree to which individual consultants, registrars and nurses accepted this principle varied greatly.

The Aberdeen general practice group on the other hand had heretofor seldom entered directly into a study of their patients with anyone and never with a researcher who was not a doctor. The fundamental prerequisite to gathering the data therefore was to spend many months in contact with medical and paramedical personnel before the study began in order to be recognised as a legitimate person with whom it was proper to discuss confidential information respecting abortion applicants.

The strategy of the study was to focus on major factors contributing to termination of pregnancy decisions of Aberdeen doctors by talking to them about specific patients who requested abortions. The first to be interviewed by the researcher were the patients themselves. Through an arrangement with the hospital, interview data was obtained from a quota sample of 90 married and 85 single women over a two-year period. These were collected after the patient's referral for abortion by the family doctor but before examination by the gynaecologist. A by-product of these interviews was a short factual account of the patient's social circumstances which was sent to the consultant for his information.

Generally within a week of the patient's interview both of her doctors were questioned about her case and the final decision, if one had been taken. If the patient were subsequently referred for a psychiatric opinion the psychiatrist would ordinarily be contacted within a few days of that consultation. The data respecting the women and the psychiatric consultants will be de-emphasised in this account which will deal mainly with the referring doctors in general practice and the gynaecological consultants. The data do not exclusively refer to the specific cases in question but also include observations about the abortion issue in general which arose with both groups of doctors in the course of intensive discussions on the subject.

The general practice group

The remarkable feature of the 132 Aberdeen doctors in general practice at the time of the study is the homogeneity of their social backgrounds. Data on 90 per cent of this group of doctors were obtained regarding their social background factors.

In view of findings elsewhere[19] it is not exceptionally notable to find that 70 per cent of the group had fathers who were in social class I and II according to the Registrar General's classification of occupations. That is, their fathers were in the professional, semi-professional, executive or landowning classes. Seventeen doctors reporting had had fathers who were also doctors. A more surprising feature of the group was that nearly 50 per cent originated in Aberdeen city itself while another 20 per cent came from smaller towns in the north-east of Scotland. In all 80 per cent of the group originated in Scotland. Furthermore all except 11 in the group graduated from the University of Aberdeen Medical School.

Most of the doctors were men. Only 25 were women and some of these were members of husband and wife practices assisting their husbands part-time. Very few in the group were unmarried.

The ages of group members as of 1 January 1969 ranged from 25 to over 65 years but were over-represented in two age categories. These were the 30–34 year and 50–54 year age groups into which 30 per cent of the population fell.

As one would expect in the land of Knox, most of the practitioners were Protestant by orientation which means from a Church of Scotland background. In fact there was only one non-Protestant.

Better than 80 per cent of the group had been five years or more in practice and normally they were members of group practices. The 132 doctors on the local list comprised 50 separate practices, while 18 practised alone.

In a group with such homogeneity of background and training one could construe a great deal of consistency in decision-making among its members, but as we will see from the following such was not the case.

Decision-making patterns among general practitioners

In all except a few of the single-man practices the progress of patients through the surgeries was timed at about ten minutes per person, making the decision-making process in an abortion case or any other matter a speedy affair. There was no possibility of knowing how many women requested abortions from their doctors in the first instance since the records did not uniformly contain these data and in any case they were not made available for research purposes. However, it is known that many more referrals would have been possible than ever were sent to the hospital, as will be clarified later. Further to this there was a variation in the number of requests made not only to certain practices as against others but within one practice to one partner rather than another.

Part of this variation was due to differences in the demographic and class structure of certain practices. Some lists were made up of older populations mainly past the childbearing years and in others the preponderance of patients were at one or other end of the social class scale. The influence of social class factors on the number of requests is difficult to measure. On the one hand the women of the working classes were less sophisticated in the use of contraception and probably had more unintended pregnancies but they tended to carry them to term. On the other hand those at the upper end of the class scale were better able to prevent conception but when unwanted pregnancies occurred, tended to be more aggressive in requesting abortions. The patient's selection of one partner in a surgery over another when an abortion was to be discussed was not always possible because all patients were assigned to a specific doctor in a practice. Where it was possible and did occur, it was based on the patient's assessment of the liberality of one partner's views toward abortion over that of his colleague.

It was clear that except in a few cases the family doctors knew their patients and their families very well. The custom in Aberdeen was to stay with one doctor during one's lifetime even if the patient moved to different locations in the city. It was not uncommon for several generations of one family to have been attended by partners in the one practice even when new partners succeeded the original ones. Furthermore, it was administratively difficult for a patient to change practices very often. The National Health Service Executive Council for the city of Aberdeen listed each patient with a doctor in order that the per capita payment could be made to him. Patients could elect to change to another doctor's list but the latter had the right to refuse acceptance which he would do if a patient changed doctors too often, that is, was thought to be 'difficult'.

It was equally clear to the doctors that the childbearing population had a generally good idea about the possibilities for getting a therapeutic abortion. For one thing Sir Dugald Baird for many years as Professor of Obstetrics and Gynaecology in Aberdeen had fostered a programme of abortion with sterilisation for multiparous women. Additionally just prior to fielding this research the subject had received great publicity because of the parliamentary debates leading up to the passage of the Abortion Act. It would therefore be an exceptional case if a woman by herself or among her friends did not know that the local medical fraternity was in a position to help dispose of an unwanted pregnancy.

Abortion requests in the surgery

The doctors in this group knew that they were in a position of power relative to women requesting abortions for two reasons. In the first instance, while women knew in general that abortions were to be had under certain conditions they could not know without reference to the doctor whether they, in their circumstances, would qualify. The medical men knew the law and how the hospital system worked while the patients did not and consequently the doctors were in a position to venture opinions on the likelihood of acceptance or rejection of a referral.

Secondly, requests for abortions were characteristically made in an inarticulate way. Only an occasional patient from a middle or upper class position would verbalise her request to have her pregnancy terminated. More generally the communication was indirect, sometimes amounting to tearful pronouncements from the patient that she wouldn't be 'able to carry on' or at most putting the question as to whether 'something couldn't be done doctor?'. This great degree of delicacy in discussing abortions was variously attributed to the low level of education of many of the women, inhibitions resulting from the power incline between social positions of doctor and patient, but especially to the traditionally high value placed upon childbirth by the population. The general practitioners believed that women were often ashamed to ask for a termination of pregnancy because of guilt feelings that it aroused within them and consequently would rather have their doctor initiate the discussion and suggest the remedy. In any event the subject was or was not discussed depending on the interaction situation and the personalities of those involved in it. If the patient came by herself to the surgery, was relatively unaggressive and the doctor refused to follow up the cues beamed at him no action would likely be taken. But if the patient was aggressive, had the support of husband or mother, could articulate reasonably well and the doctor was relatively liberal, a referral to the hospital would probably be made.[20]

Two overriding factors were prerequisite to a doctor making any referral for an abortion. One was that any indication that the patient's mental or physical health was being disturbed by the pregnancy resulted in a referral. In actual fact there were few such cases outside of those in which the foetus was likely to be affected by rubella infection in early pregnancy. More typical was that a mixture of social factors such as low family income, large existing family, advanced obstetrical age, or irresponsible husband would be put forward by the patient which in addition to the pregnancy in some cases were construed to be detrimental to health.[21] There was only one clear-cut instance in the patient group under study where potential danger to physical health existed from pregnancy in a woman with a heart ailment. While the consultant did perform an abortion in that case it was clear that if she had wanted the baby she could have delivered it with special care at little risk to her health.

The other factor was that in some way the patient had to take the initiative in making the request. Any member of the group in general practice would have thought it unethical, perhaps legally dangerous and sometimes morally wrong to initiate a discussion about terminating a pregnancy when it might not be in the patient's mind to do so. The fear most often expressed was that confidence in the profession would be undermined if an abortion occurred which was advocated by the doctor on non-medical grounds but which the patient later regretted.

Referrals to hospital

This group of doctors well understood that a landmark of social planning had been reached with the passing of the Abortion Act and few members were comfortable with the repercussions resulting for them. In the days before a national abortion policy was declared in statutory form the control over referrals lay more with the family doctors who would normally refer cases to consultants they knew would be favourably disposed to accept them. After the law was passed the locus of power shifted more to the patients who tended increasingly to view abortion as a 'right' if they thought they needed one. There was a widely held belief among the doctors that they could not legally refuse a patient requesting an abortion for a second opinion from a consultant if she insisted upon it. But there was also the feeling that if doctors were too adamant in refusing these requests they would lose patients and consequently income. On the latter point it was not that the doctor would perhaps offend and lose one patient by a refusal to refer her for an abortion. It was that some feared the loss of her relatives and friends who were also consulting the same practice. This fear might not be a realistic one in a larger, more anomic setting where patients followed a market model in joining or leaving practices. However, as indicated above, doctor–patient relationships in Aberdeen were normally characterised by more enduring qualities. It is conceivable therefore that in this tightly knit city people in the same family group might be encouraged to seek alternative medical care if there were a serious disagreement between one family member and her doctor. At the same time it must be said that the population was well disciplined and if patients were aware of the amount of power they potentially retained in these circumstances, few chose to exercise it.

The increase in volume of cases coming to hospital finally led to the necessity for all the consultants to share equally these referrals. This in turn effectively reduced contact between the family doctor and a sometimes unknown consultant to formal written communications, the former requesting a consultant opinion for his patient and the latter replying as to what he was prepared to do for her. At one and the same time most general practitioners regretted the lessened control they had under the new system and were baffled by the outcomes of those they did refer because they could no longer anticipate with any assurance the decision of the consultant.

Individual doctors adjusted to the situation in different ways depending on their perspective but over time three patterns of handling abortion requests emerged. One pattern characteristic of a very small group was to routinely pass every request up to the consultant level for decision without especial involvement or comment. Explanation for this practice is made in one of three ways. Some doctors were so against abortion on moral grounds they wished not to be involved but could not bring themselves to interfere with their patient's expressed wishes. Others favoured abortion, were convinced that any woman who wanted her pregnancy terminated had a right to this care and supported every request in principle. Still others had become so demoralised because of their lack of meaningful involvement in the medical decision-making process that they felt any further attempt to try was fruitless. As one of these commented: 'Since the National Health Service was initiated we've become a group of chit signers.' To this last, perhaps atypical group, all important decisions were made in the hospital clinics anyway so in effect they saw themselves as mere conveyor mechanisms for patient requests for more expert advice.

Another small group of doctors was noted to have very low referral rates for abortion cases. These were mainly older men, close to retirement and with small, stable practices which they handled themselves. These sometimes commented that they didn't get many requests and gave two main reasons for this. Either the patient population had grown older with them and was generally past childbearing or they had long ago taken a stand against abortion and their patients knew they couldn't easily be persuaded to help procure one. When they were faced with a request they spent a lot of time trying to get the patient to accept her pregnancy, sometimes enlisting the aid of other family members in the process. Because their practices were small they could afford the time to do this and as pregnancy advanced the woman would most often become reconciled to having the baby.

By far the majority of the doctors however adopted neither of these patterns. With these doctors if a patient requested an abortion and no strong health grounds could be cited among those being put forward to support it, there was a careful examination of all other alternatives open to the patient before the referral was made which was in effect an incrementalist approach. In the case of a married woman the possibility of carrying the pregnancy to term with family help or outside assistance would be investigated. With single women the feasibility of marriage, adopting the baby, or keeping the baby with assistance from her family would be discussed. As one family doctor said, 'it's a matter of what the patient will wear'. It was clear that with this group referrals for abortion were made as a last, not a first solution to the problem of an unwanted pregnancy. While they could be persuaded to make a referral for termination of pregnancy the patient had to exert sufficient personal pressure to overcome the doctor's resistance to the principle of abortion.

Summary

The data respecting family doctors' experiences with abortion referrals show that while they remained affectively neutral[22] in their relationships with these patients it was at the expense with many of some anxiety arising from their own value considerations. The doctors reflected the traditional views of north-east Scots that unnecessary taking of life was morally wrong. Together with this was the typically Presbyterian feeling that one should be able to bear one's own responsibilities and adversities whether this be an inconvenient pregnancy or anything else. In this context the interruption of the pregnancy was too easy a solution to what should be an acceptable condition.

Coming to the effect of their medical education one realises that all procedures learned by doctors are curative or at least palliative except abortion, which is seen as destructive. Consequently termination of pregnancy was a contradiction to the training and professional orientation of many of these doctors. It is true that abortion had long been an acceptable procedure in Aberdeen medical circles in certain restricted circumstances. But the difference now was that the population who could potentially qualify for termination was enlarged and the condition of many women requesting abortions did not fit the medical criteria which their doctors had built up in their minds as a result of their experience.

Mechanic has written that much of a doctor's work throughout history has been with the social aspects of medicine.[23] Here is an example however where doctors were involved with what they realised was an extreme medical remedy for what might prove to be minor social ailments. They felt uncomfortable in making the necessary judgements because this took them outside their area of professional competence and there was little to guide them except value judgements. Consequently even though many stated that morals were outside the doctor's province, referrals for abortions were indeed made in the light of their moral perspectives whether they were for or against terminations. Those who were anti-abortion tended to argue that too free a policy would encourage a flood of applicants which would make difficulties for the hospital services, undermine a sense of responsibility in the population and besides produce guilt feelings in the patients who were terminated. Those who were pro-abortion would cite expense of unwanted children to the state, the emotional ill effects on babies who were unwanted and the lifetime consequences of forcing girls into bad marriages because of an illegitimate pregnancy.

Decision-making in the surgery was therefore not a rational process but a sort of normative incrementalism. It depended a good deal on the doctor's medical and personal value position as to what was considered the optimally effective alternative to choose: whether to have the baby or whether to have the termination. Most often weighting was against the abortion unless counterbalanced by medically persuasive factors or in marginal cases an aggressively determined patient.

In situations of this kind positions were never absolutely held and over time two changes in attitude were evident in the group. A minority adjusted to the change in law and practice regarding abortion by becoming more liberal, on the basis that no real distinction could be made between the worthiness of one case against another. The logic in that case was that all women who wanted an abortion should get one. Another small group who at first had held more liberal opinions became more restrictive in their views. They in time became convinced that many cases they reviewed were the result of irresponsible patient behaviour in allowing the pregnancy to occur in the first place. The logic of this group was that doctors who were too accepting of abortion were promoting undesirable tendencies in the population which they had a professional role to discourage. Most, however, continued relatively unchanged in their basic position on abortion during the course of the study.

The consultant group

There was a group of seven consultants to whom all women seeking abortions were referred. Their role was to carry out diagnosis and treatment of cases referred to them, to advise family doctors of the outcome of the case and when necessary to suggest post-operative community care.

They were as homogeneous in terms of background characteristics as the general practitioners. All were Scottish in origin and all were brought up in the Protestant tradition, mainly in the Church of Scotland. Their ages at the time of the study ranged from 41 to 58 years but averaged 50 years and all were married. Five of the seven came from families in which the father was in the managerial or professional occupational classes of whom two had been doctors.

All the consultants specialised in obstetrics as well as gynaecology and consequently were examining women continuing in pregnancy as well as those wishing to terminate theirs. Each consultant had responsibility for a rural gynaecological clinic as well as taking his turn at the clinics in town. Two consultants were part-time in private practice as well as public practice and the other five held full-time national health service hospital appointments.

Like the family doctors all consultants worked to a tight schedule and had little time to spend on clinic interviews. Most of the decisions made about abortion, while they were assisted by some comments from the general practitioners and the brief patient history provided by the researcher, were concluded quickly. Yet the consultants all felt these cases took the most time of all their consultations.

Since this study dealt only with national health service patients the consultants were less controlled by their patients than if they had been consulting privately. They were certainly less restricted in dealing with patients than were the general practitioners because in all cases the women were unknown to the consultants. There were consequently no effective sanctions which could be imposed by patients against consultants who made negative decisions in their cases.

Relationships with general practitioners

There was little equality in prestige between doctors in general practice and those in consultant positions. In fact there was little contact between the two groups. Only a few general practitioners held part-time hospital appointments, one of which was in obstetrics and gynaecology. If the patients under consideration had been privately referred there would have been good economic reasons for maintaining rapport and effective communications. As it was, anything other than a briefly written referral form on an abortion case was rare and the consultants did not know many of the referring doctors as personalities or by professional reputation.

Yet the more conservative consultants complained that the general practitioners were not 'holding the line' on abortion and felt they sometimes seemed to encourage referrals. In general there was a feeling among those in the hospital group that family doctors were not sufficiently involved in the decision-making process in abortion, which in most cases was true but not because they were lacking in interest. Basically their lack of involvement was a product of the operating structure of the national health service which encouraged segmentation and specialisation of medical roles which in turn inhibited communication about patients.

Conservatives and liberals

Early in the study it became apparent that the consultant group, when it came to abortion, was polarised into two sub-groups of liberals and conservatives. Not only did the members see themselves in these terms but they were able to rank their colleagues on a liberal–conservative scale. This was possible from colleagues listening to a consultant's expressed views on aspects of the abortion question and making judgements about the kinds of cases he terminated. The group was also scored on the Conservative–Radicalism continuum of the Eysenck Inventory of Social Attitudes.[24] This allowed one doctor in the group to be compared to another regarding the general tendency toward liberalism or conservatism of his outlook. The scores correlated closely with the subjective impressions of each consultant's colleagues concerning his stand on abortion.

348

Apart from the consultant's general personality pattern, his conservative or liberal attitudes toward abortion were related to two major factors: the effect of his training and his experiences with abortions. For example, two of the more liberal consultants claimed that their attitudes basically stemmed from their training under Sir Dugald Baird who had emphasised the socio-medical benefits of abortion for parous women. On the other hand two of the conservatives were strongly influenced in the opposite direction because of serious complications which arose in abortion patients under their care such that future decisions of these consultants regarding terminations of pregnancy were more cautious.

Conflict in decision-making

All consultants complained from time to time of the lack of guidelines for decision-making in abortion cases. Whereas with other conditions there was a body of research findings which helped calculate the probabilities of success in choosing one treatment alternative over another, this was not the case with abortions. In a sense this situation contradicted the thrust of their medical training and professional experience which emphasised rational choice based on predictable outcomes. One effect of having to take decisions on abortion referrals was that consultants suffered psychic abrasion because they could not escape the professional responsibility for the welfare of their patients if they made a faulty judgement and the prescribed treatment worsened the woman's condition.

Personal stress naturally mounted as the numbers of referrals increased. It was then that especially the conservative members of the consultant group began to raise objections to the way in which the abortion referral system was working. It was clear that many of these objections stemmed from personal and professional value positions.

One concern was that the pressure of referrals and the more demanding attitude of patients would change consultants into technicians and attack the basis of medical professionalism. It was said by some that the Abortion Act had opened the door to a basic change in practice. Before the Act the consultant was first asked his opinion by the family doctor on behalf of his patient and then asked if he would undertake the surgical procedure provided the opinion was satisfactory. The Abortion Act technically allowed any two doctors, who might be general practitioners, to authorise an abortion. In fact in Aberdeen by agreement between the groups one co-signer was the responsible or operating surgeon, which in practice preserved the traditional relationship. But what was likely to happen sometimes was that a first opinion advocating abortion could be obtained from a psychiatric consultant, which diluted the power of the gynaecologist in the decision-making process. He then only held a limited veto power in the event for example that gestation was too far advanced or the patient's physical health would not allow an operation to occur. Thus some of the gynaecologists contended that while formerly they were in a position of asking others to justify their requests for termination it was turning now into a situation where he had to justify why he wouldn't terminate. That is to say their former power and professional responsibility were seen to be eroding away.

It was further maintained by some that the consultants had a professional responsibility not to be too generous in carrying out abortions because of the example set to juniors in the medical team such as housemen and registrars. This obviously varied according to the consultant's definition of medical practice, its ethical boundaries, and his ideas of appropriate behaviour for a doctor. Since the Aberdeen Royal Infirmary and the Aberdeen Maternity Hospital were both teaching hospitals this was a serious consideration for some teachers.

But a very real problem with doing too many terminations was the effect on assistants in theatre, including nurses who might be unwilling participants in these decisions. It was an especial source of discontent among nurses and registrars when the consultants with liberal views on abortion authorised more abortions than they could do themselves and the registrars were left to finish the lists which contained nothing but terminations.†

At the level of personal values the anti-abortion consultants would cite the arguments of equity and responsibility. The question was often asked whether it was fair to displace to women awaiting repairs or hysterectomies from beds because of the desirability of terminating pregnancies early if they were to be done at all. The second question which went with this was how proper was it to terminate pregnancies in women who were not responsible enough to ensure effective contraceptive practices?

Principles of equity and personal responsibility run deep in Scottish traditions but they had as well a practical application regarding abortions and use of hospital facilities. The administrative questions which were

† A forthcoming article by the author analyses the attitudes of Aberdeen nurses toward therapeutic abortion.

raised were related to the appropriate choices of cases one accepts in hospital when there are limited resources in beds, theatre facilities, consulting and nursing staff. At peak periods of abortion referrals pressure would be put on the Professor by the consultants to cut back on abortion cases in order to divert beds to patients needing treatment for other ailments. However, the matter of priorities was never satisfactorily resolved and the numbers of bed days devoted to abortion cases continued to increase.

Effects of continuing abortion referrals

As time went on all the consultants perceived themselves becoming more conservative toward these operations. Those that had been liberal became less so and those that had been conservative became more so. In fact even those most favourably disposed to accepting referrals did not want to become known as abortion specialists. They found too many of these operations not only psychically wearing but technically unstimulating and lacking in variety. They further felt that if their theatre lists continued to show a high proportion of terminations it would bring them into disrepute with colleagues. The conservatives were the most conscious of the image they projected and feared that if they became too liberal word would filter back to the general practitioners who would then flood them with unwanted referrals.

There were short-run control mechanisms which also influenced the numbers of cases accepted for abortion. If a consultant on his ward rounds or in his clinics saw too many beds occupied by these cases or was asked to give too many opinions in a day or in one week this tended to bring about more refusals of marginal cases. The same thing was true of the types of cases being referred. If more single girls presented in a certain time period and the consultant was strongly opposed to pre-marital intercourse fewer were likely to be terminated.

Besides these short- and long-run controls on the acceptance rate there were a number of other adjustments which consultants made to cope with the flow of referrals for abortion. One was that even the liberals started to insist that each consultant take his share of these cases. Otherwise all the referrals would have gone to half the consultants who feared they eventually would have been doing little else but terminating pregnancies.

Secondly, more of those patients presenting at a later stage of gestation tended to be refused as time went on. This was associated with not only the consultants' requirements for psychic preservation but also the necessity to preserve the morale of the theatre and ward staffs. It became evident that the nursing staff and patients were more upset by hysterotomies and saline terminations and accordingly these methods were less favoured than dilatation and curettage and suction methods which could only be used where gestation was not far advanced.

A third pattern which became established with certain consultants, although not necessarily routinely, was to refer more cases for second opinions to a psychiatrist. If the patient showed signs of emotional disturbance it was the cautious habit of some to find out through the second opinion whether a termination was likely to make her even more disturbed. However, psychiatrists were also used in the hope that their opinion would confirm a tentative refusal on the part of the gynaecologist. In these cases the gynaecologist was using psychiatrists in the same way as some general practitioners used the gynaecologists: as a means of opting out of the decision-making process. Ironically there was only one gynaecologist who was prepared to accept the psychiatric opinion unequivocally. Others wanted the second opinion either to confirm that there was no indication for abortion or to indicate that there was a clear need in precise terms which they could comprehend. A few of the gynaecologists consequently accused their psychiatric colleagues of being overly permissive and unclinical in their judgements. These kinds of criticisms arose from several sources. For one thing the two disciplines viewed the patients from very different perspectives, the psychiatrists using the more 'gestalt' approach of seeing the patient in her total social environment. Secondly, having had different kinds of training the two groups spoke a different medical language. The nuances of psychiatric diagnosis were not completely understood by some gynaecologists. Thirdly, the gynaecologist was the one who finally had to perform the operation which was not made more palatable by knowing that the psychiatrist would escape major responsibility if anything went wrong as a result of the surgery.

Summary

Like those for the group of general practitioners, the data concerning consultants showed a variation of position on the abortion issue. This depended on basic personality patterns overlaid on which were value orientations congruent with the social background and the view of medical practice held by the consultant.

The difference in situation between the two groups was that the consultant's role required him to make the final decision for a termination and be responsible for the outcome. It was also clear as with the family doctors that there was little guidance available to consultants in accomplishing this other than their moral stance. It was not only the patient's welfare they felt they had to consider in the decision. Responsibilities to preserve their own psychic stability, to society and the profession in keeping the abortion situation within reasonable bounds and to hospital staff and administration were all balancing factors in decision-making. The crucial variable was the fluctuation in the flow of referrals through the consultants' clinics, which in the ways indicated above, affected the acceptance–refusal rate: that is to say, made the consultant give greater or less weight to alternatives other than abortion.

DISCUSSION

In the Aberdeen abortion situation doctors can be seen as a conservative elite in a changing society where the population is demanding additional options for limiting family size. The Abortion Act requires the medical profession to implement its provisions, giving doctors a legal monopoly in addition to their monopoly on skills to terminate pregnancies. However, this study shows that members of the profession are often unwilling repositories of these responsibilities.

The work of a doctor involves taking responsibility for health of people in his care and that means making decisions about medical interventions which will probably work to the patient's advantage. While their medical training prepares them to accept this responsibility doctors are indoctrinated in the rational tradition of problem-solving where outcomes are ideally predictable with some certainty. But with abortion requests, the research information which could have assisted in making the process of decision more rational was basically lacking. Where a clearly medical factor qualified the patient under the Act there was some security for a doctor to think the decision to terminate was professionally correct. But where judgements were required to assess the weights of social factors provided for in the legislation the situation produced doubt and conflict in the minds of family doctors and consultants alike. Medical practice in such circumstances became more art than science and inevitably doctors relied on their individual value positions in making their judgements. The outcome was an apparent lack of uniformity or consistency in decision-making even with respect to the same medical actor from case to case.

Two concomitant factors made decisions in therapeutic abortion even more atypical from the doctor's point of view. One clear ethical responsibility incumbent upon medical professionals is to preserve life and all their training is directed to that end. In abortion however the doctor is often required to decide on the quality of life of the pregnant woman and her existing children as against the continued existence of the unborn foetus.

Another difference between diagnosing in abortion and in other conditions is that the Act provides for remedies of a specific condition, pregnancy, which has traditionally not been thought of as an illness. Medical men are not only being asked to accept that in one woman's case the pregnancy will be considered a normal healthy condition and in another abnormal, unhealthy and requiring medical intervention. But in a rather exceptional way the law on abortion was seen by some to restrict the normal options of doctors not to take action if they felt it inadvisable. There was some reduction in the normal freedom of action which prevailed in other medical situations. A certain amount of power therefore passed over to the patient in a way not typical of the patient role in any other sense.

In such a decision-making situation the family doctor typically adopted an incremental strategy wherein his values as a person and as a professional were weighed against the severity of the patient's circumstances and the strength of her wishes to terminate her pregnancy. Similarly the consultants operated incrementally, wherein their value positions plus the psychic drain of doing these operations and their responsibility to other patients and to the hospital were balanced against their judgement of the patient's ability to accept the pregnancy and manage with another child.

This meant that there were two filtering mechanisms for abortion applicants, one at the general practitioner and one at the consultant level. Both of these consultations presented barriers to the woman trying to have her pregnancy terminated and in effect reduced the number of abortions. There was no guarantee that the perception of the situation by the first medical viewer would be consistent with that of the second. So that even when the family doctor did willingly refer for abortion the chance of the assigned consultant accepting the case was less than certain.

Before and during the study the number of referrals was shown to be increasing but this appears to be a function of the increasing number of requests. As far as the individual applicant was concerned the outcome was never predictable unless medical factors predominated in the application, but such cases were rare. Most of the time the successful outcome of an abortion application depended on the woman's luck: that is to say, in having a family doctor–consultant set both of whom were liberal toward accepting social factors in abortion and being referred at a time of low volume for cases of her type. The probable long-range consequences to the patient of terminating or not terminating her pregnancy resulted from individual, that is variable, judgements of the professionals which once taken were normally irreversible. The perception of the situation and the goals of patient and doctor interacting in the decision-making process might be quite opposed but the difference of their position in the social structure at this time makes the force of the medical opinion more powerful.

Looked at from the political policy-making level the approach to the abortion question was clearly one of mixed scanning. There was the inexorable build up of social pressure to limit family size resulting in political action sufficient to produce a private member's bill on abortion. Pressure was sustained over considerable opposition such that the Abortion Act became law in 1968. Following Etzioni's argument a need for change had been correctly perceived to exist by the government of the day which bent to the popular wish. This was only done at the expense of some reduction in power of the medical elite which as a conservative political force had resisted a more permissive policy in terminating pregnancies.

The abortion programme has been proceeding in the interim in incremental fashion but against continued opposition which led to the establishment, in 1971, of the Committee of Inquiry into the Working of the Abortion Act. The political function of the Committee is to allow the government the option of retaining its policy on abortion, revising it or abolishing it depending on its reading of the power of opposing wishes of segments in the society.

British abortion applicants in the mass do not have the awareness, position or control over the social structure which allows women in other European countries to be the major determiners of whether a termination is in their best interests. This would only happen if further legislative change allowed abortion on demand within a certain number of weeks of conception. In that event greater uniformity of the decisions made and abortion rates would ensue and the absolute numbers of abortions would increase. However, such legislation would likely be resisted by the profession.

. Operating under the present statute the abortion programme will always result in variability of rates of abortion throughout the country. This is because the Act lends itself to incrementalism since it can be interpreted in any way a pair of doctors decide it is to be construed. As long as there are spheres of influence of medical schools which are liberal or conservative toward abortion, and within these areas there are liberal and conservative practitioners, there can be no other result.

REFERENCES

1 See for example discussions of variants of rational decision-making by: M. Shubik, 'Studies and theories of decision-making', *Admin. Sci. Quart.*, 3, 1958, 289–306, esp. 297; Amitai Etzioni, *The Active Society*, Free Press, New York, 1968, p. 264; H. A. Simon, 'A behavioral model of rational choice', *Q. J. Econ.*, **69**, 1955, 99–118, esp. 100–3; D. Braybrooke and Charles E. Lindblom, *A Strategy of Decision*, Free Press, New York, 1963, ch. 3, esp. pp. 37–41.

2 Among which are Simon, 'A behavioral model of rational choice', pp. 104–13; Etzioni, *The Active Society*, pp. 264–8; Braybrooke and Lindblom, *A Strategy of Decision*, pp. 48–56.

3 H. A. Simon, *Administrative Behaviour*, Macmillan, New York, 1959, p. 83.

4 See Braybrooke and Lindblom, *A Strategy of Decision*, pp. 83–110, and Etzioni, *The Active Society*, pp. 268–73.

5 Braybrooke and Lindblom, *A Strategy of Decision*, pp. 87 and 90.

6 Etzioni, *The Active Society*, pp. 282–300.

7 Simon, 'A behavioral model of rational choice', pp. 99–100.

8 John J. Cove, 'Back to structural functionalism: an old approach for new models of decision making', unpublished paper presented at the 70th Annual Meeting of the American Anthropological Association, November 1971.

9 Etzioni, *The Active Society*, pp. 12–15. Briefly, the 'active' orientation involves human collectivities which are informed of natural laws so as to be able to control their destinies optimally through social units in response to perceived needs for change.

10 H. Ozbekhan, 'Toward a general theory of planning', in E. Jantsch, *Perspectives of Planning*, OECD, Paris, 1969, pp. 47–104.

11 Kingsley Davis, 'Recent population trends in the New World', in S. N. Eisenstadt (ed.), *Comparative Perspectives on Social Change*, Little Brown, Boston, 1968. See also Kingsley Davis, 'Population', *Scientific American*, **209**, 3, 1963, 62–71.

12 W. J. Goode, 'Changes in family patterns', in John N. Edwards (ed.), *The Family and Change*, Knopf, New York, 1969, pp. 23–4.

13 Samuel W. Bloom, *The Doctor and his Patient*, Free Press, New York, 1965, p. 88.

14 Eliot Freidson, *Profession of Medicine*, Dodd, Mead, New York, 1970, pp. 180–3.

15 W. J. Goode, 'Encroachment, charlatanism and the emerging profession: psychology, sociology and medicine', *Am. soc. R.*, **25**, December 1960, 902–14. His point 10 in the list of characteristics of a profession embodies this idea.

16 H. S. Becker and B. Geer, 'Medical education', in H. E. Freeman, S. Levine and L. G. Reeder (eds.), *Handbook of Medical Sociology*, Prentice Hall, Englewood Cliffs, 1963, p. 171.

17 Bloom, *The Doctor and his Patient*, p. 61.

18 D. Mechanic, *Medical Sociology, a Selective View*, Free Press, New York, 1968, ch. 3. See also T. Szasz, 'The myth of mental illness', *American Psychologist*, **15**, 113–18.

19 See for example, C. F. Shumacher, 'The 1960 medical school graduate; his biographical history', *J. med. Educ.*, xxxvi, 1961, 401; D. Fish, C. Farmer and R. Nelson-Jones, 'Some social characteristics of students in Canadian medical schools 1965–1966', *Can. Med. Ass. J.*, **99**, 1968, 950–4; O. Hall, 'The stages of a medical career', *Am. J. Soc.*, liii, 1948, 328.

20 On one author's explanation as to why doctors tend to have definite opinions when giving advice to patients see M. Balint, *The Doctor, his Patient and the Illness*, Pitman Medical Publishing Co. Ltd., London, 1964, esp. chs. 16 and 17. Also see T. J. Scheff, 'Typification in rehabilitation agencies', in E. Rubington and H. S. Weinberg (eds.), *Deviance – the Interactionist Perspective*, Collier-Macmillan Canada Ltd., Toronto, 1968, pp. 120–4.

21 For a fuller discussion of presenting problems in this group of patients see C. Farmer, 'Mechanisms of selection and decision-making in therapeutic abortion', in G. Horobin (ed.), 'Therapeutic abortion in North-East Scotland', *J. biosoc. Sci.*, **3**, 1971, 121–7.

22 Affectively neutral as used by T. Parsons, along with universalism and functional specificity as characteristics of modern medical practice, in T. Parsons, *The Social System*, Collier-Macmillan, Toronto, 1951, p. 438.

23 Mechanic, *Medical Sociology*, p. 111.

24 This test is described in H. J. Eysenck, *The Psychology of Politics*, Routledge and Kegan Paul, London, 1954, ch. 4.

9 CONCLUSIONS

Gordon Horobin

It is customary to end with a concluding chapter drawing together the threads of the foregoing argument, summarising the main findings and finally expressing the need for further research. In a sense this task is superfluous in that each individual author has summarised his own conclusions. Each chapter furthermore represents a different style of work, asks different types of question and uses different models of explanation. Any attempt on my part to summarise further necessarily involves a selectivity which may not coincide with that used by my colleagues. It has to be, in other words, a personal view of what is important and worthy of emphasis, and must reflect a sociological bias. Although this might be thought to do less than justice to the clinical and psychological perspectives employed in the rest of the book, I can only acknowledge this bias or selectivity and absolve my colleagues from any responsibility for what is written here.

The study set out to document abortion policy and practice in one city over a period of eight or nine years. Data on the years 1963–8 were collected retrospectively from case records and for the years 1968–9 prospectively from interviews, tests, etc. Finally it has been possible to include epidemiological data for 1970 and 1971, again from routinely compiled case records.

TRENDS

Looking at the complete period certain trends are apparent. Using the ratio of abortions to live births there was a doubling between 1963 and 1966, a further doubling in the next two years and again in the three-year period 1969–71. The ratio per 1000 live births increased sevenfold during the period 1963–71, but this is in some degree inflated because of the falling birth rate and the latter is in any case partly a function of the increase in abortions. The rate of abortions per 1000 women at risk

358

is therefore a more meaningful statistic and this increased over the eight-year period by 550 per cent (Tables 1:1 and 1:2).

The greatest increase occurred in the young single woman category, the rate among ever-married women rising only threefold (Tables 1:4 and 1:5). An increase in abortions was however apparent before the Act came into effect and reflects less a change in abortion policy than the consequences of increasing illegitimate conceptions. Of course more women were requesting abortions and were being referred by GPs in greater numbers, but the proportion of women referred who were aborted did not change dramatically following the Abortion Act (Tables 1:6 to 1:12).

One of the most interesting findings of the epidemiological study is the social class differential in referrals of single women. While over three-quarters of professional workers, students and schoolgirls who were illegitimately pregnant and over a half of clerical, distributive and skilled manual workers, only a quarter of pregnant, single fish-workers were referred to the gynaecologists (Table 1:10). Jean Aitken-Swan comments on this phenomenon and speculates about some of the reasons for it (see Chapter 1, pp. 22–4). Unfortunately we cannot know how many women are 'refused' referral for abortion by their GPs but it would seem unlikely that family doctors are consciously adopting a class-biassed referral policy. It may be that the answer lies more in the social interaction of doctor and patient with the request for abortion as an emergent outcome of the interaction, a point made by Colin Farmer in Chapter 8 (p. 342). A vast array of 'factors', some internal, some external to the interaction are potentially relevant to the outcome but at least two are worthy of special note. Firstly there is no doubt that doctors employ typifications of patients just as they typify illnesses.[1] As Scheff argues: 'The more the status of the client is inferior to and different from that of the staff, whether because of economic position, ethnicity, race, education, etc., the more inaccurate and final the "normal case" will be.'[2] It seems likely that, on the basis of 'common knowledge', doctors will attribute feelings and motives to their clients which will be less accurate the greater the social distance between the interactants. Specifically, if in the past women in unskilled manual occupations, particularly in the fish trade, were (or were reputed to be) more tolerant of illegitimacy, then the typification may persist when direct evidence to refute it is not available to the doctor. Secondly, the interaction strategies or 'techniques of impression management' employed by patients undoubtedly vary with social class.[3] This is not to say that the techniques employed by working class women are necessarily more crude than those of the middle or professional class but that they are less effective because they are missed or misunderstood by the doctor.[4]

There is some slight evidence from the figures of abortion for 1971 that the trend is levelling off at around 400 per year or 10 per 1000 women at risk (Table 1:1 and Fig. 1:1). Referrals of ever-married women in fact showed a very slight reduction in 1971, evidence perhaps of the long-term effects on the married population of sterilisation and readier availability of adequate contraception. A further slight increase in referrals of single women occurred during the year, but the rate of increase was considerably less than in the previous five years, but it is too early to judge whether this relative stability is likely to continue. A greater willingness on the part of general practitioners to prescribe the 'pill' for unmarried patients and a more 'open door' policy operated by the Aberdeen Family Planning Clinic may partly account for the change in the trend.

THE CLIENT'S PERSPECTIVE

At the same time we should not expect readier access to contraception to replace abortion for not only will 'mistakes' occur but some women are unwilling to use oral contraceptives from what some family planning 'experts' might consider to be irrational motives. But the meanings which women attribute to contraception are socially constructed and acquire a sort of objectivity having the force of external constraint.[5] Thus for example some single women appear to define taking the pill as indicative of moral laxity in making the woman as it were 'available'. In planning ahead against the contingency of a sexual encounter the woman comes to see herself as 'that kind of woman' who allows casual encounters to occur, and this is evidently different in meaning from being seduced. Some of the single women see this in more instrumental terms, preferring the risk of pregnancy to the possible reputation of being 'available'. The meaning of immunisation through oral contraception to the unmarried woman who is 'going steady' may be quite different, although there is no direct evidence of this in the present study since abortion applicants have not used a reliable contraceptive technique with complete regularity. The technique which appeared to provide the most efficient means of prevention and which is within the control of the woman is by the same token the technique which, because of its effect on the single woman's self-concept, she may prefer not to use (see Chapter 4, pp. 134-7).

The process by which the pregnant woman becomes an abortion applicant is, as was noted above, rather obscure. We know too little about the meaning of pregnancy, the ways in which pregnancy in some cases acquires the status of a problem and how in turn solutions to that problem are sought. A variety of significant others enter into the process of meaning construction and decision-making including family members, friends and the helping professions. Enough has been said or implied throughout this work about the relevant career contingencies of clients to underline the fact that the decision to apply for abortion is neither straightforward nor necessarily complete by the time the woman reaches the gynaecologist or psychiatrist.[6] I would suggest that the extent to which the client 'knows what she wants' is often exaggerated by the protagonists of 'abortion on demand' as much as it is minimised by those who resist any liberalisation of the law. Certainly a sizeable minority of the women referred to Aberdeen consultants during the period of this study changed their minds at some point between referral and operation. 137 women changed their minds, representing 5 per cent of all women referred during 1963-71 and 14 per cent of those referred but who were not aborted. The circumstances of a few of these cases are reported in Chapters 3, 4 and 6 from which it is clear that pressure from other interested parties – e.g. husbands, boyfriends and parents – is one important factor. It is also clear that the consultants are aware of the possibility of ambivalence, and establishing the degree of certainty in the request is an important part of the decision-making process.

Partly because of what may be seen by some clients as unnecessary probing of their commitment to the request, the results of the follow-up interviews show a remarkably high proportion of satisfaction with the decision. Thus 10 out of 18 married women and 7 of the 17 single women who were refused later said they were glad they had continued with the pregnancy. Higher proportions (over 90 per cent) of those aborted reported satisfaction with the decision but very few single or married women expressed strong resentment at having been refused. It could be argued that this finding is evidence of good selection procedures on the part of consultants but it is equally consistent with an attitude on the part of clients that 'the doctor knows best'.

Expressed satisfaction or lack of regret following abortion are in themselves evidence of the value of the operation to the successful applicants, but there are other indicators for those who require 'harder' data to convince them. Such data come independently from the social, gynaecological and psychiatric follow-up studies. There were apparently a large number of marital problems mentioned in the requests of the married women, especially in the lower social class groups. Thirty of the 85 interviewed by JA-S reported such problems, ranging from alleged cruelty or inadequate support by the husband to overt break-down of the marriage. Significantly, however, some of these women reported a marked improvement in their relationships afterwards with deserting husbands returning home or dropping plans for legal separa-tion. It should be mentioned however that the effects of sterilisation cannot be distinguished from those of abortion in such instances. The evidence from the clinical psychiatric interviews at follow-up tend to support these findings, with a majority of the married women who were both sterilised and aborted and of the single women who were aborted having a relatively beneficial outcome (see Chapter 7). Further, although it is rather more difficult for a sociologist to interpret data derived from psychological tests, I would regard as extremely important Dr Olley's finding that 'highly disturbed and depressed groups at referral had been transformed into groups with essentially normal scores eighteen months later. The aborted groups . . . showed the greatest improve-ment' (Chapter 6, p. 255). Finally, as a negative rather than a positive finding, gynaecological morbidity was no more evident at follow-up in the aborted than in the non-aborted women.

From the point of view of the client therefore there is a good deal of evidence from this study to strengthen the view of those who believe that abortion is justifiable and in most instances beneficial in cases where (a) alternatives to unwanted pregnancy have been carefully considered and found inadequate, and (b) careful assessment by both client and practitioner has been possible. This is not to say that 'abor-tion on demand' would necessarily lead to bad choices and hence to unfortunate sequelae. It is rather that under the present law and in present conditions of practice, the client places some reliance on the doctor's professional judgement. If she had the burden of responsibility herself her actions and choices might or might not be the same as now.

THE PROFESSIONAL PERSPECTIVE

Two cardinal features of the organisation of medical work in Britain seem crucial to an understanding of abortion policy and practice. We may term these the principles of 'professional autonomy' and 'clinical judgement'. In the first place, the medical profession claims autonomy over the content of its work on the basis of expertise only available to those properly selected and adequately trained. Further the profession claims the knowledge and hence the right to define the area of its work, i.e. what is within the province of medicine, and in the main this claim is socially legitimated. Each member of the profession in turn is granted similar licence to determine for each client the nature and degree of the medical component of the presenting problem, to act accordingly and to control the extent of the involvement of others in the treatment process.

Whilst in general the claim of modern medicine to a monopoly of the right to diagnose and treat illness rests on its 'rational', scientific base, it is also held that successful practice is an art rather than an exact science and that the practitioner therefore needs experience and judgement as well as training. Thus it is that variations between doctors in diagnosis, in therapy and in management can be accounted for and accepted both within the profession and by the public. This is the concept of clinical judgement which, provided there is no evidence of either incompetence or 'bad faith', is held to justify any action on the part of the practitioner.

Both of these principles are clearly relevant to abortion in this country. In the first place, abortion, involving as it has in the past surgical intervention, is defined as within the professional and technical sphere of medicine. Whilst the surgical techniques of abortion are relatively straightforward, however, the grounds upon which gynaecologists are legally empowered to terminate a pregnancy and which they, as doctors, feel adequate to justify termination are inevitably vague and indeterminate. Put in another way, having been licensed to practice abortion, the medical profession has insisted upon retaining the power of decision (professional autonomy), basing such decisions upon doctors' (in practice, gynaecologists') criteria (clinical judgement). Unlike many, but not all, doctors' decisions, however, abortion decisions almost always involve moral judgements and assessments of social deprivation, and such 'non-medical' elements are clearly not within the province of their professional expertise.

363

It seems inevitable that doctors who have tried conscientiously to work within the terms of the Act have faced this dilemma and it is not surprising that there exist wide variations in acceptance rates as between hospital regions, hospitals and between doctors within hospitals. Excluding at one extreme those who have virtually opted out on conscientious grounds and at the other those who have chosen to provide abortion 'on demand' in the private sector, there are still extreme conservatives and extreme liberals. By and large, the conservatives have been amongst the leaders of that group who have pressed for repeal, reform or at least clarification of the 1967 Act. Clearly they have found it increasingly difficult to cope with the rising demand for abortion and would prefer a more restrictive legal framework to the often painful process of decision and rejection.

More moderate gynaecologists – most of the Aberdeen consultants would enter that loose category – have had relatively little difficulty in operating with the law and have indeed rather welcomed the freedom it allows the individual practitioner to exercise his clinical judgement. Effective medical practice has always and necessarily involved 'taking social factors into account'. This is so because all illness and all therapy have some implications for the social relationships of the patient and his family. The patient's age, sex, family and occupational roles are, for example, almost always relevant to clinical decisions, never more so than in the geriatric field. Even so, the more 'purely medical' the problem, the more secure does the practitioner feel in carrying out his professional tasks, for his training and his more general philosophy insist on the centrality of the bio-physical, with the psychological and the social elements in the total situation providing no more than the context within which his technical skills are to be employed.

There is, I would argue, a strain toward the 'medicalisation' of problems presented to members of the medical profession so that 'one small symptom is worth a cart-load of social factors' might be a common decision rule. This is exemplified in the tendency to couch discussion of abortion in the language of disease: there are 'indications' for which abortion is a possible 'treatment'. Whilst this terminology seems appropriate for the rather restricted range of circumstances in which abortion was erstwhile permitted (if the continued pregnancy threatened the life of the mother or, in Judge Macnaghten's words, would 'make the woman a physical or mental wreck'), it appears, at least from the sociologist's perspective, increasingly artificial to continue such usage. Some of the difficulties inherent in any attempt to categorise abortion applications in terms of indications were mentioned in Chapter 2, but this does not mean that the exercise is of no consequence. If distinctions are drawn between, for example, 'social indications' and 'medical indications', and the latter are thought to be more important, or at least more tangible, these distinctions will be apparent in variations in acceptance rates. Thus, as was shown in Table 2:3, only 37.5 per cent of women referred with what were (retrospectively) classified as social indications were terminated, while all other labelled categories showed at least a two-thirds success rate. The point is not whether medical or psychiatric indications are more urgent or serious or carry greater risk than social indications – the comparison is probably meaningless in any case – but that consultants feel more secure in recommending abortions when the presenting problem is within their own or contiguous professional expertise. While the power to decide continues to lie with the medical profession it is likely that this imbalance in acceptance rates will remain, at least in the public sector, although there is reason to suppose that the reverse situation may obtain in the private sector.

Talcott Parsons, in his now famous analysis of modern medical practice, declared:

The physician is not by virtue of his modern role, a generalised 'wise man' or sage – though there is considerable folklore to that effect – but a specialist whose superiority to his fellows is confined to the specific sphere of his technical training and experience . . . Affective neutrality is also involved in the physician's role as an applied scientist. The physician is expected to treat an objective problem in objective, scientifically justifiable terms. For example, whether he likes or dislikes the particular patient as a person is supposed to be irrelevant, as indeed it is to most purely objective problems of how to handle a particular disease.[7]

Whilst Parsons' concern was essentially with the formal functional requirements of the medical system and his formulation of the role of the physician did not therefore preclude individual variations – it is obvious that not all doctors can be ethically neutral all the time – the basic presuppositions of this formulation have only recently been challenged. Freidson, for example, takes a different view:

However, while the label of illness does seem to function to discourage punitive reactions, it does not discourage condemnatory reactions. The 'illness' is condemned rather than the person, but it is condemned nonetheless . . .

365

Moral neutrality exists only when a person is *allowed* to be or do what he will, without remark or question . . . Clearly, the physician neither approves of disease nor is neutral to it. When he claims alcoholism is a disease, he is as much a moral entrepreneur as a fundamentalist who claims it is a sin. His mission is to impute social and therefore moral meaning to physical and other signs that are, but for such meaning, fit only for the licking and biting by which animals treat themselves.[8]

The doctor's position in regard to abortion is clearly more complicated than is the case with what one may call 'normal' disease. In the first place abortion is a treatment rather than a disease, and moreover, that which is 'treated' – pregnancy – is generally regarded as a non-pathological, indeed a desirable condition. When he is asked to intervene in pregnancy, therefore, he is obliged to consider the possibly undesirable consequences of an essentially 'normal' condition rather than the pathological consequences of a pathological condition which is the more usual concern of medicine. When the pregnancy can be defined as in some senses pathological, as, for example, when a 'medical' condition associated with the pregnancy arises, the gynaecologist can rely on his clinical judgement and, as we have argued earlier, a decision to abort occasions relatively less heart-searching. In all other cases, however, it would seem that the gynaecologist is forced to make what are partly clinical and partly moral judgements.

Such mixed judgements are not, of course, confined to the field of abortion. A geriatrician's decision whether or not to admit a patient to hospital may, for example, depend as much on his assessment of whether the patient's relatives 'deserve' a rest, as on the physical condition of the patient. What is perhaps unique about abortion is its apparent violation of the taboo on killing in combination with the array of moral attitudes surrounding sexual behaviour. This is a potent mixture indeed, for no other issues in contemporary society arouse quite such intensity of emotional response as these, and it is not surprising that some in the medical profession feel that the role of guardian of the public morality has been offered to, if not thrust upon them. To quote Professor Jeffcoate as an extreme example of this stance: 'Is it right that the promiscuous girl, who has not troubled to practise contraception, should have priority over the decent married woman who has been waiting perhaps twelve months for admission for investigation of sterility?'[9]

Implicit in this statement is the idea that whether or not according to some more or less objective criteria a woman 'needs' an abortion, the question 'does she *deserve* it?' is also a relevant one. Such moral arguments were commonly expressed during the debate surrounding the 1967 Abortion Act, as were issues – some might say non-issues – like 'abortion is the thin end of the wedge that leads to Belsen, euthanasia of the old . . .' or the concern for what abortion might do 'to youth, to marriage and the family'.[10]

It is not suggested that members of the medical profession *should not* make such value judgements, nor that moral sentiments *should not* play any part in medical practice, for, despite the claims of many both within and outwith the profession that the role of the doctor is ethically neutral, it is extremely difficult to see how such judgements could be eschewed. Putting the point more colloquially, neither the clients nor the doctors can have their cake and eat it. If patients wish to be treated 'as human beings' and not simply as bodies to be mended or diseases to be cured, then they cannot object to the social nature of their humanity being scrutinised and its relevance to therapy assessed. By the same token, since modern medicine aims to promote health rather than simply treat disease, doctors cannot claim to be good practitioners of medicine and at the same time declare that their concern is with the 'purely medical', whatever that may mean. It may be remarked in passing that the hospital consultant is perhaps less often concerned with the patient 'in his social setting' than is the general practitioner who may refer for abortion a wider selection of cases, particularly those where the social component is considerable, than the consultant is prepared to accept. This occurs in other conditions than unwanted pregnancy, of course, and results partly from diagnostic uncertainty on the part of the non-specialist and partly through the GP's greater vulnerability to suggestion and pressure from the patient and his or her family.

If there is any force in the foregoing argument it would seem that 'clinical judgement' frequently involves some element of moral judgement and that this element is likely to be largest in those areas of medicine which have to do with issues of social and even religious concern. But this does not mean that such judgements must remain unchallenged, for they are not part of that corpus of knowledge and expertise which is the basis of the doctor's claim to professional autonomy. This tension between professional autonomy and the enlarged clinical judgement appropriate to abortion decision-making is central to the issue of abortion policy and practice in this country and gives rise to what often seem to be conflicting statements from members of the profession. Thus, for example, the Royal College of Obstetricians and Gynaecologists in its evidence to the Committee of Inquiry into the working of the Abortion Act says, 'So long as termination of pregnancy necessitates an operation and possibly anaesthesia surgeons cannot be expected to be told when to undertake it', and later in the same document, 'It seems to us . . . that the time has come for the public and the legislators to decide if they want abortion on demand or request, with or without limitation on the latest time in pregnancy at which the operation is permitted.'[11] Given this uncertainty and ambivalence many practitioners as well as clients will welcome the proving and perfecting of the newer techniques of abortion which may soon make surgery unnecessary.

METHODOLOGICAL CONSIDERATIONS

How credible are the conclusions derived from data gathered by field work? If we enter to some degree into the lives of the people we study, take part in their daily round of activity and observe the scenes and sites where it occurs; if we talk with them both informally and in relatively organised interviews; if we inspect organisation records, official documents, public media, letters, diaries, and any other records and artifacts we can find; if we record systematically all the information we acquire in these ways; and if, finally, we assess that information systematically to see what evidence it provides for what conclusions – if we do all that, should people take our conclusions to be highly credible? Or should they find it risky to give much evidentiary value to conclusions so arrived at?[12]

The question must occur to all but the most smug or insensitive worker in the human sciences. Sometimes it is phrased in technical terms and is answered by tests of validity (does the research instrument measures what it claims to measure?) and reliability (does the instrument consistently produce the same results when applied to the same sample?) The more general formulation adopted by Becker is however more appropriate in the present instance, with the possible exception of the research conducted by Peter Olley, using standard psychological tests. The problem arises explicitly in Jean Aitken-Swan's and Colin Farmer's interview studies where the accounts given by the actors, women applying for abortions, general practitioners and consultants, constitute the data. In effect the researcher asks two separate but related questions: how do I know that what my respondents tell me is true? and, given this uncertainty, how do I know that my interpretation of their stories is valid?

Clearly a concluding chapter to a long and detailed monograph, consisting of the work of several authors, is not the place to engage in an extended discussion of research methodology, still less of the problem of 'truth'. A brief comment however is in order. A concern with 'facts' is, of course, very proper in any research enterprise, but that concern must not blind either the researcher or his audience to the essentially interactional nature of the interview situation. It is interactional in two senses. The first and most obvious is the face-to-face social interaction of the interviewer and respondent, involving a social relationship, however impermanent. Each engages in role-taking which, in Turner's words, consists in 'devising a performance on the basis of an imputed other-role'.[13] Each has expectations, more or less explicit, of the other, but the rules of the game are not necessarily shared knowledge. The rules are 'written' by the interviewer but she has no way of knowing if the respondent understands or accepts the rules. Intentions are imputed as well as meanings other than those assumed by the questioner. What the respondent answers therefore, leaving aside deliberate distortion, is contingent on her interpretation of what the question meant, the intention behind the question, the implications of her reply for the continuation of the respondent role, its possible consequences for her own intentions and so on. Her replies, in short, constitute a 'situated account'.[14]

The second sense in which interview (or indeed any) research is interactional refers to the relationships between theory and observation. As Denzin says,

Theory dictates a sampling model which in turn demands certain empirical observations. Those observations must be reliable and valid and they must flow from the theory. At every point in the cycle the world is seen through the eyes of the scientist for his definitions dictate his activities. A test's reliability rests on the interactions directed towards it. Validity, as I have conceptualised it arises out of the interactions between a researcher's definition of a theory and his attempts to translate that theory into concrete empirical activity.[15]

Concretely, the researcher's 'theory' about, for example, the reasons why women apply for abortion determine the questions which are put and further, what count as answers to those questions. The relevance of an item of information – be it an opinion, a reason or a 'fact' – is determined, in what is often called positivistic research, by the researcher and not by the respondent.

From both points of view, then, the interactional nature of empirical research renders truth relative: relative to the theories of the researcher and to the respondent's definition of the situation. What emerges as data from an interview, therefore, is a combination of what the interviewer regards as relevant and what the respondent regards as relevant and acceptable. In many instances the outcome can be treated as relatively unproblematic; presumably there is less scope for misunderstanding and reinterpretation of the question 'How old are you?' than 'What happened when you first went to see your doctor about the pregnancy?'

It should be stressed that the intention in raising this methodological issue is not to cast doubt on the appropriateness of the interviewing technique nor the value of the information derived. It is rather to underline the point made by Jean Aitken-Swan (see Chapter 3, p. 97) about the respondent's perception of the interviewer's role in relation to her, the respondent's, inter-personal task of trying to obtain an abortion. The story that emerges from the interview then represents the respondent's attempt to specify, on the basis of cues received from the questions and the context in which they are put, what she considers relevant to the attainment of her objective. In this sense the story is 'true', although a different 'truth' might be revealed in a different situation with different cues.

External measures of consistency are difficult to apply in such circumstances, but it is worth noting that follow-up interviews allowed some opportunity to check back on the information provided at first interview. Of course, part of the purpose of the follow-up was to ascertain what changes may have occurred in the woman's situation following the abortion or continued pregnancy. Nevertheless some feedback on the original interview was possible and it is interesting to note that questions from the original interviews which were asked in appropriate form at follow-up produced very few changed stories. Thus, in general, there is reason to believe that there was relatively little deliberate distortion although it should be emphasised again that, in this instance, it was the *woman's* story and not that of the husband, doctor or any other interested party.

Clearly much the same might be said of the section by Colin Farmer, where data derived from interviews with general practitioners and consultant gynaecologists are reported and analysed. He notes that it was 'clear to the doctors that the childbearing population had a generally good idea about the possibilities for getting a therapeutic abortion' (Chapter 8, p. 341). It is beside the point whether the women *did* know about the possibilities in any detail; a request from a woman for referral is likely to be construed by the practitioner as evidence of knowledgeability, even though she may only have heard of the legal possibility and known nothing of the content of the Act. Further, the GP's impression of the public's state of awareness is gained from those who do know something about the possibilities and make a request, however tentative, but he is unlikely to know how many other women might have requested a referral if they had known it was possible. The practitioners' perceptions of the state of knowledge of their patients, derived mainly from the more knowledgeable patients, help explain their concern that the Abortion Act had placed more power in the hands of the applicants.

To generalise these points still further, then, we can conclude that the attitudes, ideologies, interpretations and explanations offered by the participants in interactions concerning abortion constitute data which can then be used in second-order interpretations of their behaviour. In this sense the subjective becomes objective and is at least as salient as externally validated data about 'what was *"really"* the case'. It would also be possible to treat the researchers' own behaviour and explanations as further data to be used in third-order analyses of the interactions between theory and empirical activity, although that is an exercise which might better be left to the more phenomenologically oriented reader than attempted here.

For present purposes it is enough to note that the kinds of data deemed relevant by the researcher and the types of explanation he attempts are the products of theory whether explicitly or implicitly held. Such theories are likely to differ as between workers within a discipline and are of course even more radically different between disciplines. We do not expect, for example, the theories of psychologists and sociologists to coincide and we take for granted that the explanations of behaviour which they offer will be different. It is for this reason above all that no wider synthesis has been attempted in this concluding chapter, and that perhaps undue emphasis has been placed on the methods used by the sociologists and their conclusions. My perspective in other words is that of a sociologist and I have no competence beyond that of an interested layman to comment upon the psychologists' use of their particular techniques and of concepts such as 'character disorder'. No doubt each reader will select, interpret and synthesise on the basis of his own theories; we can at least claim that we have jointly and severally provided material upon which the reader can exercise his critical judgement.

I should like to conclude by returning to a point made in the introductory chapter. Answers to the questions: what are the characteristics of women referred for abortion?; how are the decisions made?; what are the consequences of the decision? depend as much on the context in which they are asked as on the methods by which answers are sought. Abortion in Aberdeen 'means' something different from abortion in for example Birmingham or Glasgow, and a full account of that meaning to the clients, the professionals and to the policy-makers would entail far more than has been attempted in this book. Amongst other things it would be necessary to examine all the alternatives to abortion including contraception services, family support services, adoption, etc. It would further be necessary to place the meanings of abortion within a context of the meanings of childbirth, sexuality, marriage and family living. All that we have been able to undertake and to some degree accomplish is to sketch in the narrower context – some of the characteristics of the population, medical practice and specialist services. These are necessary but not in themselves sufficient to answer the three broad questions we set out to answer.

REFERENCES

1 See for example, T. Scheff, 'Typification in the diagnostic practices of rehabilitation agencies', in *Sociology and Rehabilitation*, ed. Marvin B. Sussman, American Sociological Association, Cleveland, 1966, pp. 139–44.
2 Ibid. p. 143. The term 'normal case' is adapted from the term 'normal crime' coined by Sudnow to refer to stereotypes of what is commonly found by an agency.
3 Techniques of impression management are discussed by Erving Goffman in *The Presentation of Self in Everyday Life*, Allen Lane, The Penguin Press, London, 1969.
4 Some further discussion of doctor–patient interaction is also contained in M. J. Bloor and G. W. Horobin, 'Conflict and conflict resolution in doctor–patient interactions', in A. Mead and C. Cox (eds.), *The Sociology of Medical Practice*, Collier-Macmillan, forthcoming.
5 There is now a large literature on the social construction of knowledge and meaning. See for example P. L. Berger and T. Luckmann, *The Social Construction of Reality*, Penguin Books, London, 1966.

6 'Career' is used here in the same sense as that used by Erving Goffman in 'The moral career of the mental patient', in *Asylums*, Penguin Books, London, 1968.

7 Talcott Parsons, *The Social System*, Routledge and Kegan Paul, London, 1951, p. 435.

8 Eliot Freidson, *The Profession of Medicine*, Dodd, Mead and Co., New York, 1970, p. 253.

9 T. N. A. Jeffcoate, 'Abortion', in *Morals and Medicine*, BBC, London, 1970, p. 34.

10 These statements by Professors I. Donald and H. MacLaren are discussed, together with many others, by Sally Macintyre in 'The medical profession and the 1967 Abortion Act in Britain', *Social Science and Medicine*, 1973, **7**, 2, 121–34.

11 Royal College of Obstetricians and Gynaecologists, Evidence to the Committee of Inquiry into the Working of the Abortion Act (1967), paras. 59 and 68.

12. Howard Becker, *Sociological Work*, Allen Lane, The Penguin Press, London, 1971, ch. 3.

13 Ralph H. Turner, 'Role taking: process versus conformity', in A. M. Rose (ed.), *Human Behaviour and Social Processes*, Routledge and Kegan Paul, London, 1962, p. 23.

14 Marvin B. Scott and Stanford M. Lyman, 'Accounts', *Am. soc. R.*, **33**, 1968, 46–62. For a more extended discussion of these and related problems of interviewing see Aaron B. Cicourel, *Methods and Measurement in Sociology*, Free Press, New York, 1964, esp. ch. 3, as well as Becker, *Sociological Work*.

15 Norman K. Denzin, *The Research Act in Sociology*, Butterworth & Co., London, 1970, p. 105.

NAME INDEX

375

SUBJECT INDEX

Note: Psychological symptoms and personality factors as measured by the psychological tests and interview are dealt with extensively in the text and tables of Chapters 5, 6 and 7, and are not, for the most part, separately indexed. Abortion applicants who continued with their pregnancies are compared throughout with women who were aborted, and are not separately indexed.